Baillière's
CLINICAL
OBSTETRICS
AND
GYNAECOLOGY
INTERNATIONAL PRACTICE AND RESEARCH

Baillière's

CLINICAL OBSTETRICS AND GYNAECOLOGY

INTERNATIONAL PRACTICE AND RESEARCH

Volume 6/Number 3
September 1992

The Immune System in Disease

G. M. STIRRAT MA, MD, FRCOG
J. R. SCOTT MD
Guest Editors

Baillière Tindall
London Philadelphia Sydney Tokyo Toronto

This book is printed on acid-free paper.

Baillière Tindall   24–28 Oval Road,
W.B. Saunders   London NW1 7DX

The Curtis Center, Independence Square West,
Philadelphia, PA 19106–3399, USA

55 Horner Avenue
Toronto, Ontario M8Z 4X6, Canada

Harcourt Brace Jovanovich Group (Australia) Pty Ltd,
30–52 Smidmore Street, Marrickville, NSW 2204, Australia

Harcourt Brace Jovanovich Japan, Inc,
Ichibancho Central Building,
22-1 Ichibancho, Chiyoda-ku, Tokyo 102, Japan

ISSN 0950–3552

ISBN 0–7020–1634–9 (single copy)

Baillière's Clinical Obstetrics and Gynaecology is published four times each year by
Baillière Tindall. Annual subscription prices are: £65.00 (annual subscription); £27.50 (single
issue); all other countries, please consult your local Harcourt Brace Jovanovich office for dollar
price.

The editor of this publication is Catriona Byres, Baillière Tindall,
24–28 Oval Road, London NW1 7DX.

Baillière's Clinical Obstetrics and Gynaecology was published from 1983 to 1986 as
Clinics in Obstetrics and Gynaecology.

Typeset by Phoenix Photosetting, Chatham.
Printed and bound in Great Britain by Mackays of Chatham PLC, Chatham, Kent.

Contributors to this issue

W. D. BILLINGTON MA, BSc, PhD, Reader and Head of Honours School, Department of Pathology and Microbiology, School of Medical Sciences, University of Bristol, University Walk, Bristol BS8 1TD, UK.

D. WARE BRANCH MD, Department of Obstetrics and Gynecology, University of Utah Medical Center, 50 North Medical Drive, 28200, Salt Lake City, UT 84132, USA.

JUDITH N. BULMER MB, ChB, PhD, MRCPath, Senior Lecturer and Honorary Consultant in Pathology, School of Pathological Sciences, University of Newcastle upon Tyne, Royal Victoria Infirmary, Newcastle upon Tyne NE1 4LP, UK.

DONALD J. DUDLEY MD, Assistant Professor, Department of Obstetrics and Gynecology, University of Utah School of Medicine, 50 North Medical Drive, Salt Lake City, UT 84132, USA.

AGAMEMNON A. EPENETOS MB, ChB, MRCP, PhD, Consultant in Clinical Oncology and Reader in Developmental Cancer Therapeutics, Imperial Cancer Research Fund Oncology Group, Hammersmith Hospital, Du Cane Road, London W12 0HS, UK.

ROSEMARY A. FISHER BA, MPhil, PhD, Research Fellow, Department of Medical Oncology, Charing Cross Hospital, Fulham Palace Road, London W6 8RF, UK.

JOSEPH A. HILL MD, Associate Professor, Department of Obstetrics, Gynecology and Reproductive Biology, Brigham and Women's Hospital, Harvard Medical School; Fearing Research Laboratory, 250 Longwood Avenue, Room 204, Boston, MA 02115, USA.

CHRISTOPHER H. HOLMES BSc, PhD, Research Fellow, University of Bristol Department of Obstetrics and Gynaecology, St Michael's Hospital, Southwell Street, Bristol BS2 8EG, UK.

G. MARC JACKSON MD, Assistant Professor, Department of Obstetrics and Gynecology, University of Utah Medical School, 50 North Medical Drive, Salt Lake City, UT 84132, USA.

WARREN R. JONES MD, BS, PhD, DGO, FRACOG, FRCOG, Professor, Department of Obstetrics and Gynaecology, Flinders Medical Centre, Bedford Park, SA 5042, Australia.

SALEEM T. A. MALIK MA, MB, ChB, PhD, MRCP, Medical Oncologist, Ontario Cancer Research and Treatment Foundation, Thunder Bay Regional Cancer Center, 290 Munro Street, Thunder Bay, Ontario P7B 7T1, Canada.

HOWARD L. MINKOFF MD, Dir. MFM, Professor of Obstetrics and Gynecology, Department of Obstetrics and Gynecology, SUNY Health Science Center at Brooklyn, Box 24-450 Clarkson Avenue, Brooklyn, New York 11203-2098, USA.

EDWARD S. NEWLANDS PhD, FRCP, Professor of Cancer Medicine, Department of Medical Oncology, Charing Cross Hospital, Fulham Palace Road, London W6 8RT, UK.

LOUISE PRIOLO MD, Department of Obstetrics and Gynecology, SUNY Health Science Center at Brooklyn, Box 24-450 Clarkson Avenue, Brooklyn, New York 11203-2098, USA.

C. W. G. REDMAN MA, MB, BChir, FRCP, Clinical Reader, Nuffield Department of Obstetrics and Gynaecology, John Radcliffe Hospital, Oxford OX3 9DU, UK.

FRANCES SEARLE BSc, MSc, PhD, Principal Biochemist, Department of Medical Oncology, Charing Cross Hospital, Fulham Palace Road, London W6 8RF, UK.

JAMES R. SCOTT MD, Professor and Chairman, Department of Obstetrics and Gynecology, University of Utah Medical School, 50 North Medical Drive, Salt Lake City, UT 84132, USA.

ROBERT M. SILVER MD, Department of Obstetrics and Gynecology, University of Utah Medical Center, 50 North Medical Drive, 28200, Salt Lake City, UT 84132, USA.

KAREN L. SIMPSON BSc, Research Assistant, University of Bristol Department of Obstetrics and Gynaecology, St Michael's Hospital, Southwell Street, Bristol BS2 8EG, UK.

GORDON M. STIRRAT MA, MD, FRCOG, Dean of Faculty of Medicine and Professor, University of Bristol, Department of Obstetrics and Gynaecology, St Michael's Hospital, Southwell Street, Bristol BS2 8EG, UK.

DOUGLAS A. TRIPLETT MD, FACP, Professor of Pathology, Assistant Dean, Indiana University School of Medicine; Director of Hematology, Ball Memorial Hospital, 2401 University Avenue, Muncie, Indiana 47303, USA.

Table of contents

Foreword/G. M. STIRRAT & J. R. SCOTT ix

1 The immune system in health and disease 393
D. J. DUDLEY

2 The normal fetomaternal immune relationship 417
W. D. BILLINGTON

3 Complement and pregnancy: new insights into the
immunobiology of the fetomaternal relationship 439
C. H. HOLMES & K. L. SIMPSON

4 Immune aspects of pathology of the placental bed
contributing to pregnancy pathology 461
J. N. BULMER

5 Immunological contributions to recurrent pregnancy loss 489
J. A. HILL

6 Obstetrical implications of antiphospholipid antibodies 507
D. A. TRIPLETT

7 The immune system in disease: gestational trophoblastic
tumours 519
E. S. NEWLANDS, R. A. FISHER & F. SEARLE

8 Alloimmune conditions and pregnancy 541
G. M. JACKSON & J. R. SCOTT

9 Autoimmune disease in pregnancy 565
R. M. SILVER & D. WARE BRANCH

10 Immunological aspects of pre-eclampsia 601
C. W. G. REDMAN

11 HIV infection in women 617
L. PRIOLO & H. L. MINKOFF

12 Contraception 629
W. R. JONES

13 The immune system and gynaecological cancer 641
S. T. A. MALIK & A. A. EPENETOS

14 Overview and future perspectives 657
G. M. STIRRAT & J. R. SCOTT

Index 669

PREVIOUS ISSUES

December 1989
Psychological Aspects of Obstetrics and Gynaecology
M. R. OATES

March 1990
Antenatal Care
M. HALL

June 1990
Medical Induction of Abortion
M. BYGDEMAN

September 1990
Induction of Ovulation
P. G. CROSIGNANI

December 1990
Computing and Decision Support in Obstetrics and Gynaecology
R. J. LILFORD

March 1991
Factors of Importance for Implantation
M. SEPPÄLÄ

September 1991
Human Reproduction: Current and Future Ethical Issues
W. A. W. WALTERS

December 1991
Hormone Replacement and its Impact on Osteoporosis
C. CHRISTIANSEN

March 1992
HIV Infection in Obstetrics and Gynaecology
F. D. JOHNSTONE

June 1992
Assisted Reproduction
L. HAMBERGER & M. WIKLAND

FORTHCOMING ISSUE

December 1992
Prostaglandins
M. G. ELDER

Foreword

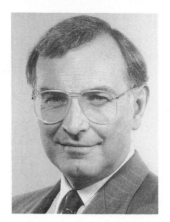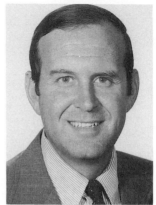

The medical profession can be divided into two distinct groups: those who find the subject of immunology difficult because it had not been 'invented' when they were at medical school and those who have the same problem because it *was* taught at medical school. Why should this almost universal apprehension about immunology exist?

The first reason is that the teachers themselves did not really understand it clearly and could not, therefore, describe it satisfactorily. The second is that too much was made of postulated mechanisms rather than principles and, thirdly, too many firm conclusions were drawn from inconclusive data. The reader must always keep in mind the underlying principle of immunology first enunciated by a founding father of the discipline—Sir Macfarlane Burnet. Immunology is basically about self and its protection and non-self and its elimination. Self discrimination is so fundamental to our integrity as individuals that the graft/host relationship of viviparous pregnancy immediately poses conceptual difficulties (in more senses than one).

The purpose of this volume is to provide a succinct, critical and authoritative update on the role of the immune system in obstetric and gynaecological conditions. One of its most important functions is to elucidate the enigmatic relationship between mother and fetus in health and disease. Conditions such as auto-immune disease and HIV infection in which the immune system is pathologically involved are considered. 'State of the art' reviews of conditions in which the immune system may be causally involved such as pre-eclampsia and recurrent pregnancy loss are included. Deviations of immune processes for therapy are discussed in chapters on trophoblastic and other gynaecological tumours and on contraception.

The immune system is not a discrete entity within the body. The manner in which it is integrated with other cellular recognition processes and the implications that may have for our future understanding are outlined in the final chapter. If the reader is better informed and less afraid of 'immunology' after reading this volume its aim will have been achieved. If not, then we will have to try harder in future.

G. M. STIRRAT
J. R. SCOTT

1

The immune system in health and disease

DONALD J. DUDLEY

The immune response to each foreign antigen is a highly regulated and non-random process. For a specific immune response to a non-self-antigen, a precise series of basic events occurs. These events include: (1) antigen processing and presentation, (2) recognition of the processed foreign antigen by a specific T cell, (3) clonal expansion of T cells and elaboration of lymphokines, and (4) the final immune response (e.g. antibody versus cytotoxicity). Regulatory influences upon each step determine the ultimate immune response to specific antigen. Recent investigations have highlighted the complexity of immune regulation and demonstrated that disturbances in the regulation of the immune response result in aberrant and abnormal immune function. This chapter will describe these basic immune concepts, focusing on new insights into the regulation of the immune response.

INNATE VERSUS ADAPTIVE IMMUNITY

An important, often overlooked, distinction is that between the innate and adaptive immune system (Figure 1). These systems represent two different, but interactive, hierarchies of immune responsiveness (Roitt et al, 1989). The innate immune system is populated by phagocytic cells (such as macrophages, monocytes, and neutrophils) or natural killer (NK) cells which recognize foreign antigen indiscriminately. After ingestion, phagocytes and NK cells enzymatically destroy these foreign antigens. A feature of innate immunity is that activation of these cells depends only upon the foreign nature of the eliciting antigen. This lack of specificity for antigen is a hallmark for 'immune surveillance' in which the scavenger phagocytic cells continuously seek foreign antigens. Another key feature of innate immunity is that host resistance to a particular antigen is not enhanced by repeated exposure (i.e. lack of memory).

Recognition of foreignness by the innate immune system is critical to the function of adaptive immunity. Phagocytic cells, or antigen-presenting cells (APC), ingest antigen, process the antigen, migrate to secondary lymphoid tissues, and then present processed fragments of the antigen to cells of the adaptive immune system, including T and B cells. The hallmark of adaptive immunity is the precise specificity of antigen recognition and memory, such that repeated exposures to a specific antigen elicit exaggerated immune

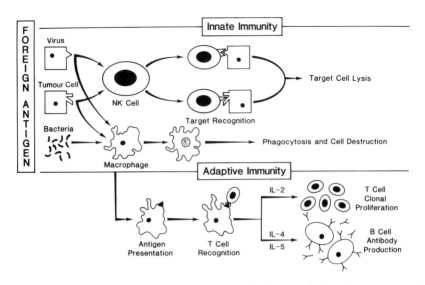

Figure 1. Innate versus adaptive immunity. Foreign antigen is recognized by phagocytic cells of the innate immune system (e.g. macrophages or NK cells). This foreign antigen can be microbial pathogens, viral antigens, or tumour antigen. Innate immune responses result in direct cytotoxicity or destruction of the pathogen. Activation of the adaptive immune system is dependent upon interaction with processed antigen provided by cells of the innate immune system. T cell and B cell activation results in T cell clonal proliferation and B cell antibody production, respectively.

responsiveness. Antigen recognition is genetically predetermined for each particular T cell. Each T cell possesses on its cell surface a specific T cell receptor which recognizes only one specific antigen presented by APCs. Similarly, each B cell recognizes specific antigen via surface immunoglobulins, often without prior antigen processing (Male et al, 1987). The T cell receptor (TCR) and surface immunoglobulin of T and B cells are members of a class of membrane proteins referred to as the 'immunoglobulin gene superfamily' (Williams and Barclay, 1988). Both of these cell receptors are characterized by their specificity for foreign antigen. Complex and highly regulated genetic rearrangements of the TCR and immunoglobulin genes result in the seemingly never-ending array of specific receptors for almost any possible antigen, including novel artificial antigens (Kronenberg et al, 1986).

ANTIGEN PROCESSING AND PRESENTATION

APC and major histocompatibility complex molecules

Cells of the innate immune system which function as antigen-presenting cells (or accessory cells) include macrophages, dendritic cells, fibroblasts,

Kupffer cells of the liver, Langerhans' cells of the skin, and endothelial cells (Roitt et al, 1989). Also, B cells of the adaptive immune system may present processed antigen. APC exist in almost every tissue and circulate in the blood. In general, these cells account for the ability of the innate immune system to recognize almost any foreign invader in almost any tissue. However, while antigen processing and presentation may occur at the site of inflammation or in secondary lymphoid tissues (including lymph nodes and spleen), antigen recognition by T cells usually occurs in the spleen or lymph tissues. Adaptive immune responses usually do not occur at sites of local inflammation where the antigen is initially recognized. After random recognition of foreignness by APC, the non-random process whereby T cells orchestrate the immune response is initiated.

Processed antigen is presented in physical association with a cell surface protein known as the major histocompatibility complex (MHC). MHC molecules are grouped into two general classes, class I MHC and class II MHC. Class I MHC (subclassified in the human into HLA-A, B, or C) molecules are expressed on almost every cell in the body and are crucial to the immune system by defining self. APC may present endogenous antigen from virally infected cells in association with class I MHC directly to cytotoxic T cells and NK cells.

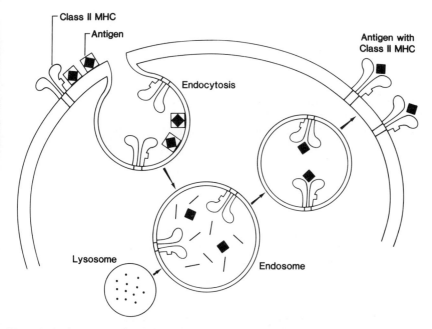

Figure 2. Antigen processing and presentation. Antigen recognized by the antigen-presenting cell (APC) is endocytosed with MHC class II molecules. After digestion of the antigen in the endosome with the assistance of lysosomal contents, the processed antigen associates with the class II MHC molecules and this combined molecule is then expressed on the surface of the APC. This proposed model is a simplification of the model described by Brodsky and Guagliardi (1991).

Table 1. Inflammatory cytokines.

Cytokine	Molecular weight	Cellular sources	Target cells	Principal activities
IL-1α IL-1β	15 kDa	Macrophages, monocytes, LGL, B cells, fibroblasts, endothelial cells	T and B cells, macrophages, endothelial cells, fibroblasts	Lymphocyte activation, prostaglandin production, macrophage stimulation, pyrexia, enhanced leukocyte–endothelial interactions, tissue regeneration, enhanced MHC expression
TNF	17 kDa	Macrophages, CTL, NK cells	Macrophages, neutrophils, fibroblasts	Cachexia, enhanced leukocyte–endothelial interactions, macrophage activation, enhanced cytotoxicity
IL-6	26 kDa	Macrophages, fibroblasts	Macrophages, endothelial cells, hepatocytes	Acute phase response, T cell activation, B cell antibody production, prostaglandin production
IL-8	6–10 kDa	Macrophages, monocytes, endothelial cells, keratinocytes, fibroblasts	Neutrophils, T cells, basophils	Neutrophil activation and degranulation, chemotactic for neutrophils and T cells

Almost all other exogenous antigens, e.g. proteins and bacteria, are expressed in association with class II MHC. Expression of class II MHC by the APC is the key to antigen presentation. When foreign antigen is recognized by APC a specific sequence of energy-dependent biochemical events takes place within the cell (Figure 2). After stable membrane-bound exogenous protein is endocytosed and proteolytically fragmented into peptide fragments, fragments of preferably 10–20 amino acids in length fit into an antigen-binding groove on internalized MHC molecules (Lanzavecchia, 1990; Brodsky and Guagliardi, 1991). The class II MHC molecule-processed antigen complex is then exported to the cell surface membrane. Antigen processing and presentation with class II MHC molecules is almost always required for T cell recognition of antigen, although there are a few T cell-independent antigens which stimulate B cells directly (e.g. lipopolysaccharide). The requirement for direct interaction between APC and T cells is but one example of the integrated defence mechanism provided by innate and adaptive immune responses.

Cytokines and cytokine networks

In conjunction with antigen processing and presentation, APC elaborate proteins known as cytokines (Table 1). Almost any cell can secrete cytokines when injured, thus establishing a site of local inflammation where other inflammatory cells are recruited and activated. Inflammatory cytokines produced by injured cells and inflammatory cells of the innate immune system amplify and perpetuate the inflammatory response, ensuring involvement of the adaptive immune response when appropriate. Predominant among these cytokines included interleukin 1α and β (IL-1α and IL-1β), tumour necrosis factor (TNF), interleukin 6 (IL-6), and interleukin 8 (IL-8).

IL-1 and TNF are secreted by activated macrophages and other cells after cellular injury. IL-1 comes in two separate and distinct forms, α and β, corresponding to a membrane-bound and soluble protein, respectively (Dinarello, 1989). Macrophages appear to be the most important source of IL-1, and macrophages can be stimulated to produce IL-1 after phagocytosis of bacteria, viruses, and yeasts. Immune activation by T cells, immune complexes, and activated complement also stimulates IL-1 production. IL-1 has both autocrine and endocrine activities. Local actions include augmentation of T and B cell activation, neutrophil activation and degranulation, and stimulation of prostaglandin E_2 (PGE$_2$) production by macrophages, fibroblasts, and endothelial cells. Endocrine function of IL-1 includes the induction of fever, demargination of neutrophils from the bone marrow, and the potentiation of the hepatic acute phase response (in association with IL-6). TNF and IL-1 share many of these activities and often act synergistically (Beutler and Cerami, 1989). TNF (cachectin) also comes in an α and β form, and the T cell-derived β form is also known as lymphotoxin (see below). TNF, like IL-1, stimulates procoagulant properties of vascular endothelium, enhancing fibrin deposition and perhaps contributing to the pathogenesis of diffuse intravascular coagulation. TNF also mediates tumour cell killing and may be crucial to innate immunity against microbial pathogens.

IL-6 is a pleiotropic cytokine produced by almost any cell in response to injury (Le and Vilcek, 1989). IL-6 stimulates macrophage production of PGE_2, acts with other cytokines to potentiate the activation of T and B cells, and is essential to the hepatic acute phase response (Heinrich et al, 1990). Conversely, IL-8 has no modulatory effects on macrophage PGE_2 production but is a potent chemoattractant and activating molecule for neutrophils (Baggiolini et al, 1989).

Based upon observations in several tissues, activation of the inflammatory response results in a complex interplay of these cytokines known as a 'cytokine network'. Such networks have been hypothesized to contribute to the pathophysiology of psoriasis (Luger and Schwarz, 1990), adult respiratory distress syndrome (Kunkel et al, 1991), rheumatoid arthritis (Seitz et al, 1991), and infection-induced preterm labour (Dudley et al, submitted). Interleukin 1 is initially elaborated in response to tissue injury and foreign antigen invasion and drives the elaboration of other inflammatory cytokines, including IL-6 and IL-8, from macrophages, fibroblasts, endothelial cells, and human gestational tissues (Le and Vilcek, 1989; Dudley, in press and submitted). IL-6 is responsible for the acute phase response characteristic of inflammation. Finally, IL-8 is produced in inflammatory cells and attracts neutrophils to the inflammatory site. While IL-8 has not been shown to induce the production of other cytokines or prostaglandins, this cytokine may act to perpetuate inflammatory responses via secondary mediators derived from neutrophils and other inflammatory cells.

Along with the inflammatory cellular infiltrate, cytokine production, and prostaglandin production, APC-derived cytokines are important co-stimulators of T and B cell activation and differentiation (Roitt et al, 1989). IL-1 is an obligatory co-factor involved in specific T cell activation and lymphokine production, and IL-6 also acts to potentiate the activation of T cells and the differentiation of B cells into plasma cells. These autocrine and paracrine factors thus are one link between the activation of the innate immune system (i.e. inflammation) and the activation of adaptive immune cells.

LYMPHOCYTE MIGRATION AND HOMING

Before T cells can recognize antigen, they undergo a complex and specific series of differentiation events in the thymus (Dudley and Weidmeier, 1991). After completing thymic maturation, immunologically competent T cells migrate into the circulation and then 'traffic' into specific secondary lymph organs including the spleen, peripheral lymph nodes, and mucosal-associated lymphoid tissue (Ford, 1975). Lymphocyte homing into these secondary lymph organs is dependent upon the association of specific vascular 'addressins' and T cell-membrane associated ligands (Figure 3). Addressins and attachment sites for T cells and are found in specialized areas of vascular endothelium in the postcapillary venules of lymph nodes known as 'high endothelial venules (HEV)'. HEV are lined by cuboidal endothelial cells which possess surface addressins that associate with specific

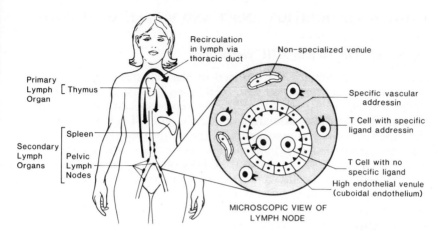

Figure 3. Lymphocyte migration and homing. After maturation in the thymus, differentiated T cells are released into the circulation and migrate to specific secondary lymphoid organs. Migrating T cells with specific ligands interact with addressins on the cuboidal high endothelial venules (HEV) in the lymph node. These T cells enter the parenchyma of the lymph node and are available to interact with processed antigen on the surface of an APC. The T cells then re-enter the circulation via efferent lymphatic drainage. (Reprinted with permission from Dudley DJ & Weidmeier S (1991) The ontogeny of the immune response: perinatal perspectives. *Seminars in Perinatology* **15:** 184–195, W.B. Saunders, Orlando, FA.)

ligands on the surface of circulating T cells (Stamper and Woodruff, 1976). After attachment of lymphocytes via a specific addressin–ligand interaction, the lymphocyte passes through the HEV, enters the parenchyma of the secondary lymph tissue and becomes available for interaction with specific antigen presented by APC. Lymphocytes then leave the lymph node via the efferent lymphatics, empty into the thoracic duct, and recirculate into the circulation via the subclavian vein. When antigen enters a lymph node of an animal previously sensitized to that specific antigen, then lymphocyte traffic is shut down for approximately 24 h, ensuring that antigen-specific T cells remain in the affected lymph node.

The process of lymphocyte migration and homing to secondary lymph tissue is a specific and complicated process which does not occur randomly (Butcher, 1986). In this manner, T cells continually recirculate among lymphoid tissues via the blood stream and lymphatics. The recirculation of mature T cells among secondary lymphoid tissues ensures that the full immunological repertoire of antigen specificities is available throughout the organism, facilitating the interactions between antigen-specific T cell and processed antigen (Berg et al, 1989). Since only 1–2% of the available lymphocyte pool recirculates each hour, lymphocytes isolated from peripheral blood represent only the pool of recirculating and relatively inactive lymphocytes. Data obtained from functional studies on peripheral lymphocytes must therefore be carefully interpreted since the biological activities of peripheral lymphocytes may not reflect the biological activities of lymphocytes from specific tissue sites (Dudley et al, 1990).

ANTIGEN RECOGNITION AND T AND B CELL ACTIVATION

Antigen recognition and MHC restriction

After processed antigen is expressed on the cell surface of the antigen-presenting cell in association with MHC class II molecules, the antigen is recognized by T cells possessing a T cell-receptor specific for that particular antigen. The close approximation of an APC with a T cell is dependent not only upon the physical association of the antigen with the TCR and the macrophage MHC class II molecule but also with an adhesion molecule of the surface of the T cell known as the CD4 molecule. The term 'CD' stands for 'cluster designation' and refers to a wide variety of cell surface molecules and markers on immune effector cells (Table 2). Activation of T cells via different CD markers result in the utilization of different signal transduction pathways and confer different properties to these activated T cells (Altman et al, 1990).

Table 2. Summary of important CD molecules.

Cell source	CD antigen	Common name	Molecular weight	Function
Macrophage	CD11b	MAC-1	160 kDa	Complement receptor
	CD25	IL-2R	55 kDa	IL-2 receptor
Leukocytes	CD11a	LFA-1 (α)	180 kDa	Adhesion molecule
	CD18	LFA-1 (β)	95 kDa	Adhesion molecule
	CD45	LCA	180 kDa	Leukocyte common antigen
T cells	CD2	T11	50 kDa	T cell activation via interaction with CD3
	CD3		20–26 kDa	T cell activation
	CD4		60 kDa	Class II MHC restriction
	CD5	Lyt-1		Accessory molecule for T cell activation
	CD8		32 kDa	Class I MHC restriction
	CD28		80–90 kDa	T cell activation distinct from CD3 pathway
B cells	CD20	Bp 35		B cell activation
	CD22	Bp 130		Enhances B cell activation
	CD23		45 kDa	IgE receptor
	CD35	CR1	220 kDa	Complement receptor 1

In general, APC with class II MHC stimulate T cells with the CD4 surface adhesion molecule while APC or cells possessing class I MHC molecules associate with and stimulate T cells possessing the CD8 adhesion molecule in its surface membrane (Figure 4) (Schwartz, 1985). The stringent association of a specific MHC molecule with a T cell-derived adhesion molecule is known as 'MHC (or genetic) restriction'. Traditionally, CD4+ T cells have been termed helper T cells and CD8+ T cells have been termed 'suppressor' T cells. However, the terms helper and suppressor are too vague to describe adequately the functions and properties of these two T cell subclasses. Therefore, the terms 'CD4+ T cells' and 'CD8+ T cells' will be used to

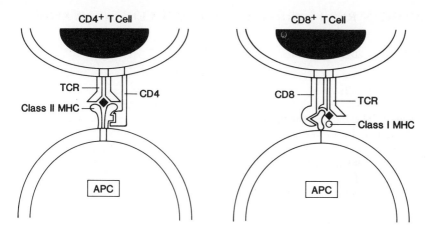

Figure 4. MHC restriction. In general, specific processed antigen is recognized by T cells via a T cell receptor (TCR) specific for the antigen. T cells also express accessory adhesion molecules termed CD4 or CD8. As noted on the left of this figure, T cells which bear the CD4 adhesion molecule recognize processed antigen on the surface of an APC which expresses MHC class II molecules. As depicted on the right, T cells with CD8 adhesion molecules recognize antigen in association with class I MHC molecules.

describe these T cell populations. Because macrophages and most APC utilize class II MHC molecules to present processed antigen, CD4+ T cells most likely orchestrate adaptive immune responses (Janeway et al, 1988).

T cell activation

After the processed antigen is recognized by specific TCR, the T cell is activated via the CD3 molecule (Figure 5). The CD3 molecule is a group of five membrane-bound proteins in intimate association with the TCR which, when the TCR recognizes antigen, mediates T cell activation (Clevers et al, 1988). Activation of the CD3 molecules results in an increase of intracellular calcium via inositol phospholipid hydrolysis and activation of protein kinase C (Altman et al, 1990). Recognition of processed antigen by the TCR-CD3 complex is the principal means by which T cells are activated, although some T cells can be activated via other surface molecules (Altman et al, 1990). Upon activation of T cells, the cell surface expresses new receptors for IL-1 and interleukin 2 (IL-2), the primary T cell growth factor. Activated T cells also produce IL-2, which then acts in an autocrine and paracrine fashion to stimulate T cell clonal proliferation (Farrar et al, 1982). Additionally, activated T cells induce expression of class II MHC molecules, facilitating interactions between APC and antigen-specific CD4+ T cells.

The TCR consists of a heterodimer with polymorphic chains which insert into the cell membrane, with the CD3 proteins interspersed among these two chains. Greater than 90% of T cells which have completed thymic maturation possess a type of TCR known as alpha/beta (α/β). In the α/β T cells, there are two chains, one α- and one β-chain, in which there are

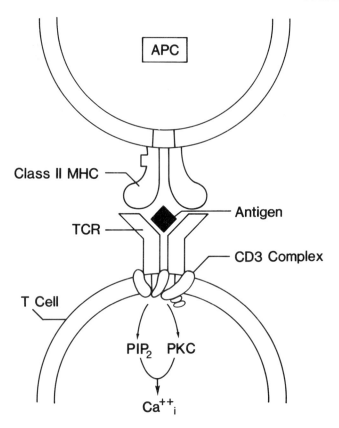

Figure 5. The TCR–CD3 complex. This figure depicts a simplified model of the biochemical events during T cell activation. After recognition of processed antigen by the T cell receptor (TCR), the five proteins of the CD3 complex transmit an activation signal across the T cell membrane. This activation signal then stimulates protein kinase C (PKC) and inositol phospholipid metabolism, resulting in an increase in the intracellular calcium concentration. The T cell will undergo cell division and produce lymphokines. (The CD4 molecule was not included in this figure for clarity.)

variable regions at the N terminus which confers antigenic specificity (Kronenberg et al, 1986). T cells with the α/β TCR–CD3 complex and CD4 adhesion molecule direct the immune response.

Another T cell population bear γ- and δ-chains for their heterodimer TCR. The function of γ/δ T cells is unclear, but these cells are either CD4−CD8− or CD4−CD8+ and often reside in the epithelium of skin, uterus, lung, and gut (Allison and Havran, 1991). Gamma/delta T cells may be activated by heat shock proteins during stress responses and some γ/δ T cells do not appear to be MHC-restricted (Raulet, 1989). These findings suggest that γ/δ T cells may be involved in the pathogenesis of autoimmunity (Born et al, 1990).

B cell activation

Recognition of specific antigen by surface immunoglobulin by sensitized B cells stimulates antibody production and cell division in a T cell-independent manner. However, optimal B cell activation, proliferation, and differentiation occurs in the presence of processed antigen with activated T cells. These T cells provide a wide array of growth factors which stimulate antibody production by B cells (see below).

LYMPHOKINES AND CYTOTOXICITY

Lymphokines and growth factors

After T cells have been activated by interaction between processed antigen and their specific TCR, clonal proliferation of the activated T cell occurs. Clonal proliferation results in a rapid expansion of T cells responsive to the eliciting antigen and is dependent upon the elaboration of immune effector proteins known as lymphokines. Lymphocytes residing in secondary lymph tissues generally do not produce significant levels of lymphokines until specific T cell activation. While cytokines may be produced by several different cell types, lymphokines are produced by activated T cells. The predominant lymphokines produced by T cells include interleukins 2 through 6 (IL-2, IL-3, IL-4, IL-5, IL-6) and interferon-γ (IFN-γ) (Table 3).

The production of these lymphokines by activated T cells in turn helps to direct the function and properties of other adjacent immune effector cells. IL-2 is secreted primarily by CD4+ T cells after specific antigenic stimulation, although NK and CD8+ T cells can produce detectable IL-2 after appropriate stimulation (Roitt et al, 1989). Thus, IL-2 is the primary T cell growth factor and its elaboration is crucial to the process of T cell clonal proliferation, the proliferation and generation of cytotoxic T lymphocytes (CTL), and the proliferation and antitumour activity of NK cells (Farrar et al, 1982; Robertson and Ritz, 1990). IL-2 regulates the progression of immune responses via the autocrine and paracrine stimulation of T cell proliferation and the induction of other lymphokines, including IFN-γ. IFN-γ is a pleiotropic lymphokine with multiple effects throughout the immune system. Most important among these immunological activities, IFN-γ stimulates the differentiation of immune effector cells, upregulates the expression of class II MHC molecules on APC, and stimulates NK and CTL antiviral and antitumour activity while inhibiting haematopoiesis (Male et al, 1987).

B cell activation, proliferation, and differentiation is mediated by IL-4, IL-5, and IL-6. Formerly known as BSF-1 and BCGF-I, IL-4 is a pleiotropic lymphokine which exerts effects on several different facets of the immune response. With regard to B cell function, IL-4 activates resting B cells, acts as a growth factor for previously activated B cells, and enhances expression of class II MHC on the surface of B cells and monocytes (Paul, 1991). IL-4 induces antibody isotype switching and is important for the production of

Table 3. T cell-derived lymphokines.

Lymphokine	Molecular weight	Cellular sources	Target cells	Principal activities
IL-2	15 kDa	Activated Th1 CD4+ T cells, NK cells	CD4+ and CD8+ T cells	T cell growth and proliferation
IL-3	15 kDa	Activated Th1 and Th2 CD4+ T cells	Haematopoietic precursors, stem cells, mast cells	Promotes growth and differentiation of myeloid progenitor cells
IL-4	18 kDa	Activated Th2 CD4+ T cells	B cells, eosinophils	B cell growth and differentiation, IgE production, eosinophilia
IL-5	≈ 15 kDa	Activated Th2 CD4+ T cells	B cells	B cell differentiation, antibody isotype switching
IL-6	26 kDa	Activated Th2 CD4+ T cells	B cells	B cell differentiation into plasma cells with high-rate antibody production
IFN-γ	40–50 kDa	Activated Th1 CD4+ T cells, NK cells	CD4+ and CD8+ T cells, macrophages	Enhance MHC class II expression, macrophage activation, enhance endothelial–leukocyte interaction

Table 4. Growth factors.

Growth factor	Molecular weight	Cellular sources	Target cells	Principal activities
IL-3	15 kDa	T cells	Stem cells, haematopoietic progenitors, mast cells	Promotes growth and differentiation of myeloid progenitor cells
IL-6	26 kDa	Macrophages, T cells, fibroblasts	T and B cells	Enhances T cell growth and proliferation, promotes B cell differentiation
GM-CSF	23 kDa	Macrophages, T cells	Myeloid stem cells, T cells	Promotes granulocyte and macrophage differentiation from myeloid precursors
G-CSF	19 kDa	Macrophages, fibroblasts	Myeloid stem cells	Promotes differentiation of granulocyte precursors
M-CSF (CSF-1)	21 kDa	Macrophages, monocytes	Myeloid stem cells	Promotes differentiation of macrophage precursors

IgG$_1$ and IgE (Lebman and Coffman, 1988). IL-4 is also a growth factor for T cells, stimulates haematopoiesis of granulocytes, and enhances proliferation of mast cells (Paul, 1991). IL-5 plays an essential role in B cell growth at every stage of the cell cycle and augments primary B cell responses to T cell-independent antigens (Takatsu, 1988). Additionally, IL-5 enhances antibody isotype switching to produce IgM, IgG, and IgA. IL-5 also stimulates eosinophil differentiation and induces IL-2 receptor expression of T cells. Lastly, IL-6 stimulates the differentiation of B cells into high-rate antibody-producing plasma cells (Heinrich et al, 1990). Other lymphokines have been isolated and characterized, including IL-7, IL-9, IL-10, and IL-11. These lymphokines are currently being intensively investigated.

Another class of proteins elaborated by T cells and other cells are termed growth factors (Table 4). Four primary growth factors have been identified, including interleukin 3 (IL-3), granulocyte-macrophage colony-stimulating factor (GM-CSF), granulocyte colony-stimulating factor (G-CSF), and macrophage colony-stimulating factor (M-CSF), also known as colony-stimulating factor-1 (CSF-1). These colony-stimulating factors may constitute a related family of proteins since they have a common glycoprotein structure, their genes are adjacent and probably functionally linked, and three CSF receptors have sequence similarity (Metcalf, 1991). IL-3 and GM-CSF have overlapping and synergistic effects, including the stimulation of monocytes and macrophages to produce M-CSF, GM-CSF, G-CSF (Groopman et al, 1989). IL-3 stimulates the activation and proliferation of mast cells and basophils, and GM-CSF enhances viability and activities of neutrophils, eosinophils, and macrophages (Groopman et al, 1989). G-CSF and M-CSF/CSF-1 induce and support the differentiation and proliferation of neutrophil and macrophage lineages, respectively. M-CSF/CSF-1 is produced primarily by monocytes, and is also found in relatively large concentrations in the murine uterus and placenta (Pollard, 1990). In general, IL-3 and GM-CSF act on early multipotential haematopoietic progenitors, while G-CSF and M-CSF stimulate more differentiated myeloid progenitor cells.

The primary role of these haematopoietic growth factors is to regulate the proliferation and differentiation of haematopoietic progenitor cells. However, growth factors also enhance the function of mature myeloid cell lineages and IL-3 and GM-CSF are products of activated T cells, suggesting that these growth factors may play a pivotal role in the host response to infection and antigenic challenge (Groopman et al, 1989). Since T cells can produce lymphokines which effect cell destruction and growth factors which stimulate differentiation, determining how lymphokine and growth factor production is regulated is crucial to understanding the resulting predominant immune response.

T cells, NK cells and cytotoxicity

Cell killing, or cytotoxicity, is the final result of cell-mediated immunity. Cytotoxicity may be mediated by the adaptive immune system (T cell-dependent cytotoxicity) or the innate immune system (T cell-independent cytotoxicity). There are three general circumstances in which cytotoxic mechanisms will be activated, depending primarily upon target recognition (Roitt et al, 1989). In adaptive immune cytotoxicity, target recognition is via antigen presented in association with an MHC molecule. The macrophage and cytotoxic CD8+ T cell (or CTL) play central roles. As described previously, the macrophage presents processed antigen to CD4+ T cells which elaborate lymphokines, such as IL-2, which activate CTL to effect their cytotoxic role. CD8+ CTL also will eliminate virally infected host cells via association of antigen with class I MHC. CTL may also directly recognize allograft class I MHC without previous antigen presentation or the assistance of CD4+ T cells since these foreign-class I MHC mimic self-class I MHC with associated antigen (Roitt et al, 1989).

The innate immune system mediates the other two circumstances of cytotoxicity via NK cells. These cells may either recognize foreign antigen directly or via antibody-dependent mechanisms by 'killer' cells. Killer cells are in fact NK cells which recognize the attachment of antibody to its specific target. NK cells undergo maturation in the bone marrow and seem to be of their own unique lineage (Robertson and Ritz, 1990). Also referred to as large granular lymphocytes (LGL), NK cells constitute 5–15% of circulating peripheral blood lymphocytes and can be found in the spleen, bone marrow, and lymph nodes. NK cells do not express either the TCR or the CD3 activation molecule, and target recognition and cell activation pathways have yet to be completely elucidated. Therefore, NK cells are not restricted by MHC or prior sensitization to eliciting antigen, suggesting that these cells evolved prior to the development of adaptive immunity. The primary function of NK cells appear to be: (1) resistance to microbial pathogens, particularly viruses; (2) elimination of neoplastic cells, although the experiment proof for this activity is unclear; and (3) regulation of haematopoiesis (Robertson and Ritz, 1990).

Regardless of target recognition and the cells mediating the cytotoxic response, the mechanism of cell killing is similar (Tschopp and Nabholz, 1990; Podack et al, 1991). After target recognition and effector cell activation, a calcium-dependent phase occurs in which cytoplasmic granules are secreted into the effector–target cell junction. These granules contain monomeric precursor proteins known as perforins. After insertion into the target cell membrane, perforins polymerize and form channels through the cell membrane. Attachment of perforins to the cell membrane and polymerization is calcium-dependent. Polyperforins function similarly to the serine proteases of the final step of complement-mediated cytotoxicity (the so-called 'lethal hit'). Pore formation in the target cell membranes is not sufficient for cell death and NK cell cytotoxic factors, including the elaboration of TNF, are essential components in effecting cell death. Other additional proteases contribute to target cell destruction.

The final phase of cytotoxicity is a programmed sequence of intracellular events termed 'apoptosis'. TNF inserted into the target cell activates an endonuclease which fragments target cell DNA resulting in 'blebbing' with subsequent chromatin disintegration. The effector cell, either the CTL or NK cell, is resistant to these mechanisms of cell death, allowing the effector cell to move on to another target cell. Thus, immune effector cells of the adaptive and innate immune systems effect target cell death via a final common pathway.

THE REGULATION OF IMMUNE RESPONSES

Th1 and Th2 CD4+ T cells

If activated T cells produced lymphokines maximally and indiscriminately, the resulting immune response would undoubtedly be disorganized and inappropriate. It is becoming evident from recent studies that lymphokine production is tightly regulated and is a critical determinant of a concerted immune response. Utilizing murine T cell clones, Mossman and Coffman (1989) described two functional subsets of CD4+ T cells, known as Th1 and Th2 (Figure 6). Th1 CD4+ T cells produce IL-2, IFN-γ, and lymphotoxin after activation, and are required for delayed-type hypersensitivity and cytotoxic T cell responses (Janeway et al, 1988; Mossman and Coffman, 1988). Th2 CD4+ T cell clones produce IL-4, IL-5, and IL-6 after stimulation and are essential for antibody responses. While these initial studies described T cell clones, such functional phenotypes of CD4+ T cells appear to function in vivo in mice (Hayakawa and Hardy, 1988) and humans (Rotteveel et al, 1988). These findings highlight the exquisite regulation of

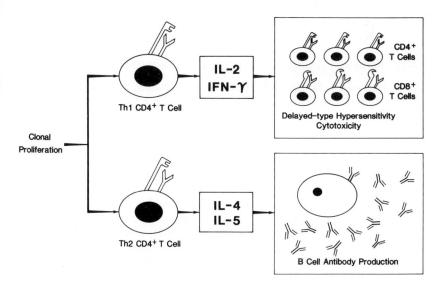

Figure 6. Th1 versus Th2 CD4+ T cell responses. With T cell activation and clonal proliferation, T cells elaborate a wide variety of lymphokines. If the CD4+ T cell produces primarily IL-2 and IFN-γ, a Th1 response predominates including T cell-mediated cytotoxicity and delayed-type hypersensitivity. If a CD4+ T cell produces IL-4 and IL-5, then antibody production by B cells is the primary response. During the immune response to a specific antigen, both of these responses probably occur to varying degrees depending upon the external regulatory influences acting on the activated CD4+ T cell.

lymphokine production that must occur in order for a specific immune response to occur. T cell-mediated lymphokine production appears to be regulated by a variety of mediators, including steroid hormones, prostaglandins, and other cytokines (Table 5).

Table 5. Factors which regulate lymphokine production.

Regulatory factor	Lymphokines			
	IL-2	IFN-γ	IL-4	Other
Steroid hormones				
DHEA	Enhances	Enhances	No effect	
Glucocorticoids	Inhibits	Inhibits	Enhances	
1,25-(OH)$_2$D$_3$	Inhibits	Inhibits	??	
Oestrogen	No effect	No effect	No effect	Stimulates CSF-1
Progesterone	No effect	No effect	No effect	Stimulates secondary inhibitor and CSF-1
Arachidonic acid metabolites				
PGE$_2$	Inhibitory	Inhibitory	No effect	May stimulate IL-5
LTB$_4$	Enhances	Enhances	??	
Cytokines				
IL-1	Enhances indirectly	Enhances indirectly	??	Stimulates IL-6 and IL-8 production
IL-6	Enhances indirectly	Enhances indirectly	??	Co-factor for T cell activation
GM-CSF	??	??	??	Co-factor for T cell activation

Steroid hormonal regulation of lymphokine production

Glucocorticosteroids have long been known to have 'immunosuppressant' activity (Cupps and Fauci, 1982). However, the exact mechanism of this immunosuppression has only recently been elucidated. In mice, corticosteroids at physiological concentrations inhibit IL-2 production and stimulate IL-4 production (Daynes and Araneo, 1989). At pharmacological concentrations, glucocorticoids inhibit the production of both IL-2 and IL-4. These actions occur at the level of the glucocorticoid hormone response element (Daynes and Araneo, 1989). Therefore, glucocorticosteroids exert their influence directly at the gene level upon lymphokine production by T cells. Similar to the glucocorticoids, 1,25-dihydroxyvitamin D$_3$ inhibits IL-2 (Tsoukas et al, 1984), IFN-γ (Reichel et al, 1987), and GM-CSF (Tobler et al, 1988) production by T cells in a concentration-dependent fashion. Thus, lymphocytes activated in the presence of physiological concentrations of glucocorticoids or 1,25-dihydroxyvitamin D$_3$ appear to favour a Th2 CD4+ phenotype.

Conversely, dehydroepiandrosterone (DHEA) stimulates T cell production of IL-2 in vitro and in vivo (Daynes et al, 1990a). At physiological concentrations of DHEA (10^{-10} M to 10^{-8} M), DHEA enhances IL-2 production significantly. The IL-2 enhancing effects of DHEA overcomes the IL-2 inhibitory influences of glucocorticoids, suggesting a direct genetic influence of DHEA. Of note, the sulphated form of DHEA has no effect upon IL-2 or IL-4 production. DHEA is produced by adrenal gland in larger quantities than any other steroid, and DHEA is the only adrenal steroid produced in its sulphated form (Baulieu et al, 1965). Further, DHEA has been found to have significant antiviral (Loria et al, 1988) and anticarcinogenic properties (Schwartz et al, 1988). Additionally, circulating DHEA-S levels in human serum decreases with age, peaking in the 20s and then decreasing until levels at the age of 70 are about one-third of peak levels (Orentreich et al, 1984). These findings suggest that DHEA may play an important role in promoting adaptive immune responses in vivo.

Further supporting the role of DHEA, the amount of IL-2 produced by lymphocytes isolated from secondary lymphoid tissue, including spleen, peripheral lymph nodes, mesenteric lymph nodes, and gut lymphoid tissue (Peyer's patches) correlates with the degree of steroid sulphatase activity (Daynes et al, 1990b). Secondary lymphoid tissues in which T cells produce large amounts of IL-2 (spleen and peripheral lymph nodes) have greater degrees of steroid sulphatase activity and thus more bioavailable DHEA, while tissues in which T cells produce minimal IL-2 after stimulation (e.g. gut lymphoid tissue) have low steroid sulphatase activity. These findings suggest that the steroid hormonal content of each lymphoid tissue exerts regulatory control over the relative amount of lymphokines produced by T cells derived from each distinct lymphoid tissue. Thus, the lymphoid microenvironment for each tissue is different depending upon the steroid hormonal milieu present in each lymphoid tissue. These findings also reveal that T cell lymphokine production is not preprogrammed, and that lymphokine production is readily altered by exogenous regulatory influences.

Sex steroids clearly affect immune function, but the precise mechanisms involved have not been elucidated. Both progesterone and oestrogen modulate DTH and suppress T cell proliferation (Ahmed et al, 1985). Progesterone induces other proteins which have 'immunosuppressive' activity (Szekeres-Bartho et al, 1985), while oestrogen depletes the functional activity of CD8+ T cells. Neither oestrogen nor progesterone appears to act via direct alterations of lymphokine production (Daynes et al, 1990a), but both of these hormones can stimulate CSF-1 expression in the murine uterus and placenta (Pollard, 1990).

Prostaglandins modulate T cell function and lymphokine production

Among the products of cyclo-oxygenase and lipoxygenase activity, prostaglandin E_2 (PGE_2) and leukotriene B_4 (LTB_4), respectively, have important immunomodulatory effects. Perhaps the best characterized is PGE_2, which has been previously described as an immunosuppressant. PGE_2 inhibits the proliferation and differentiation of macrophage precursors, T cells, and B cells (Hwang, 1989). Additionally, PGE_2 inhibits macrophage production of IL-1 and TNF and expression of class II MHC molecules (Hwang, 1989). PGE_2 inhibits T cell activation by cross-linking the TCR–CD3 complex at early stages of T cell activation (Vercammen and Ceuppens, 1987), preventing the initiating stimulus for signal transduction. PGE_2 does not affect

IL-2-mediated T cell proliferation after initial T cell activation has occurred. Long known to inhibit the production of IL-2 (Rappaport and Dodge, 1982), Betz and Fox (1991) recently reported that PGE$_2$ altered lymphokine production by stimulated T cells so that their lymphokine profiles resembled those of Th2 CD4+ T cells. IL-2 and IFN-γ production was markedly inhibited, IL-4 production was not inhibited, and IL-5 production was slightly enhanced. Moreover, PGE$_2$ will act synergistically with IL-2 to induce production of GM-CSF by CD4+ T cells, indicating that PGE$_2$ can be a positive signal for lymphokine production in certain T cells (Quill et al, 1989). Hence PGE$_2$ acts not as an immunosuppressant, but rather as an immunomodulator.

LTB$_4$ is a lipoxygenase product secreted by activated macrophages and neutrophils which effects neutrophil attraction and degradation (Ford-Hutchinson et al, 1980). Previously described as an 'immunostimulant', LTB$_4$ also enhances NK cell and CTL cytotoxicity by increased effector to target binding and improved lytic efficiency (Rola-Pleszczynski et al, 1983). While LTB$_4$ is a stimulatory co-factor of IFN-γ and IL-2 production, the net effect of T cell activation in the presence of LTB$_4$ appears to be suppression of CD4+ T cell proliferation with enhancement of the CTL, or CD8+ T cell population (Payan et al, 1984). The effect of LTB$_4$ on T cells, like PGE$_2$, depends upon the external conditions in which T cell activation occurs and is thus immunomodulatory rather than uniformly immunostimulatory.

Cytokine regulation of lymphokine production

Other cytokines have important effects upon T cell activation and lymphokine production. IL-1, IL-6 and GM-CSF all potentiate T cell activation and proliferation in response to specific antigen. IL-1 appears to be a critical co-factor for optimal T cell stimulation, while IL-6 and GM-CSF enhance T cell proliferation. Synergism of cytokine activities appears to be a common mechanism to further stimulate T cell activation. However, it is not clear how these cytokines affect lymphokine profiles by CD4+ T cells (Th1 versus Th2).

The predominant immune response

Given the great variety of immunoregulatory influences that alter the lymphokine production of activated T cells, how then do these cells decide which immune response predominates? Experimental evidence supports three possible immune responses: Th1 only, Th2 only, and a mixed Th1 and Th2 response (Mossman and Coffman, 1989). If a Th1 response predominates, then DTH with cytotoxicity will be evident with little antibody production. In Th2 responses, high titre antibody production will result. Most immune responses are probably of the mixed variety, with some cytotoxicity (but little DTH) and moderate antibody production. Such mixed responses account for local cytotoxicity, antibody responses, and memory (or sensitization) against an invading pathogen. The nature of antigen presentation may determine the relative propensity of the Th1 versus Th2 response. Both macrophages and B cells may present antigen and stimulate both Th1 and Th2 cell responses. Macrophage production of inflammatory cytokines, prostaglandins, and leukotrienes may determine which lymphokine profile is produced by the activated T cell. Thus, macrophages may dictate to antigen-specific T cells the nature of their immune response (Th1 versus Th2) while other exogenous immunoregulatory factors (e.g. steroid hormones) in the lymphoid microenvironment determines the degree of the immune response by modulating the amount of lymphokines produced.

THE IMMUNE RESPONSE AND DISEASE

Based upon these new insights into how immune responses are regulated, recent investigations have elucidated the basic immune response to several diseases. Three well-studied examples will be discussed to highlight these principles.

Nippostrongylus brasiliensis

Most helminth infections are characterized by extremely high serum IgE levels with a marked eosinophilia. *N. brasiliensis* is a helminth parasite in which the murine immune response has been thoroughly investigated. Not only is IL-4 and IL-5 production from splenocytes markedly elevated in mice infected with *N. brasiliensis*, but IL-2 and IFN-γ production by these splenocytes is substantially decreased (Mossman and Coffman, 1989). These findings suggest a preferential Th2 type response in response to infection with helminths.

Leishmaniasis

After infection of mice with the obligate intracellular parasitic protozoon *Leishmania major*, two different responses are noted depending upon the murine strain infected. In Balb/c mice, a susceptible strain, *L. major* infection results in a severe unremitting disease resulting in animal death (Locksley et al, 1987). The immune response to *L. major* in Balb/c mice is characterized by high antibody serum levels (predominately IgE), no DTH, and splenocytes which produce high levels of IL-4 and low levels of IFN-γ, i.e. a Th2 response. Conversely, infection of a resistant strain of mice, e.g. C57Bl/6, with *L. major* results in local infection with ultimate complete resolution. The immune response in these animals is typically Th1, characterized by a strong DTH response, low antibody, and splenocytes which produce large amounts of IFN-γ and small amounts of IL-4 (Mossman and Coffman, 1989). An interesting clinical parallel in the human is *L. donovani* infection. Some individual response to *L. donovani* with a strong DTH response and have a mild self-limiting disease, while other individuals produce large amounts of antibody, low DTH, and contract a severe disseminated visceral disease known as kala-azar (Sacks et al, 1987). Although there are as yet no firm experimental data, it seems likely that a similar pattern of immune responses as that seen in mice infected with *L. major* exists in the human immune response to *L. donovani*.

Bacterial sepsis

In several experimental models, including the mouse and baboon, injection of lethal doses of *Escherichia coli* results in a characteristic pattern of cytokine release (see cytokine networks above). Initially, TNF and IL-1 are elaborated, probably from a wide variety of cells that could potentially be damaged by lipopolysaccharide including macrophages and endothelial cells (van Deventer et al, 1990). IL-1 and TNF release occurs within minutes, peaks quickly, and then disappears from the circulation relatively rapidly (Creasy et al, 1991). Overexuberant production and release of IL-1 and TNF into the circulation, rather than LPS, may account for the hypotension characteristic of severe sepsis (Tracey et al, 1987). Following IL-1 and TNF, IL-6 levels gradually rise and then sustain a relatively high serum concentration for several hours (Creasy et al, 1991). Lastly, IL-8 is elaborated and sustained for up to 24 h and may function to perpetuate the inflammatory response via the prolonged recruitment of neutrophils (DeForge and Remick, 1991). Similar findings have been found in human whole peripheral blood and volunteers administered LPS or *E. coli* intravenously (van Deventer et al, 1990). Systemic administration of antibody against endotoxin improves outcome in patients experiencing septic shock (Ziegler et al, 1991), and anti-TNF antibody has been shown to prevent septic shock in primates given lethal doses of bacteria (Tracey et al, 1987).

The future

These examples exemplify the rapid progress that has been made into the understanding of the immune response. Because of these insights, more rational immunotherapy can be developed for a wide variety of human diseases. Moreover, better understanding of the host–parasite relationship and the host immune response will result in the development of more effective vaccines.

SUMMARY

For an immune response against an eliciting antigen, innate and adaptive immune mechanisms interact to provide a specific and appropriate response characterized by self–non-self discrimination and memory. This non-random process involves antigen presentation followed by T cell recognition and activation with the elaboration of T cell-derived lymphokines. The nature and amount of lymphokine production from antigen-activated T cells then determines the predominant immune response (e.g. cytotoxicity versus antibody). Exogenous regulatory factors, including steroid hormones, prostaglandins, and cytokines, modulate immune responsiveness. How these regulatory factors influence the immune response during specific host–parasite interactions determines the predominant immune response to specific antigen. As the regulation of the immune response is unravelled, new and powerful immunomodulatory therapies will be developed and utilized to improve the immune response and host survival.

Acknowledgements

This work was supported by a Kennedy-Dannreuther Fellowship from the American Gynecologic and Obstetrical Society. The author gratefully acknowledges the expert artistic contributions of Nancy Shaskey.

REFERENCES

Ahmed SA, Penhale WJ & Talal N (1985) Sex hormones, immune responses, and autoimmune diseases: mechanisms of sex hormone action. *American Journal of Pathology* **121**: 531–551.
Allison JP & Havran WL (1991) The immunobiology of T cells with invariant gamma/delta antigen receptors. *Annual Review of Immunology* **9**: 679–705.
Altman A, Mustelin T & Coggeshall KM (1990) T lymphocyte activation: a biological model of signal transduction. *Critical Reviews in Immunology* **10**: 347–391.
Baggiolini M, Walz A & Kunkel SL (1989) Neutrophil-activating peptide-1/interleukin-8, a novel cytokine that activates neutrophils. *Journal of Clinical Investigation* **84**: 1045–1049.
Baulieu EE, Corpechot C, Dray F et al (1965) An adrenal secreted androgen: dehydroepiandrosterone sulfate. Its metabolism and a tentative generalization on the metabolism of other steroid conjugates in man. *Recent Progress in Hormone Research* **21**: 411–500.
Berg EL, Goldstein LA, Jutila MA et al (1989) Homing receptor and vascular addressins: cell adhesion molecules that direct lymphocyte traffic. *Immunology Reviews* **108**: 5–61.
Betz M & Fox BS (1991) Prostaglandin E_2 inhibits production of Th1 lymphokines but not of Th2 lymphokines. *Journal of Immunology* **146**: 108–113.
Beutler B & Cerami A (1989) The biology of cachectin/TNF—a primary mediator of the host response. *Annual Review of Immunology* **7**: 625–655.
Born W, Hall L, Dallas A et al (1990) Recognition of a peptide antigen by heat shock—reactive gamma/delta T lymphocytes. *Science* **249**: 67–69.
Brodsky FM & Guagliardi LE (1991) The cell biology of antigen processing and presentation. *Annual Review of Immunology* **9**: 707–744.
Butcher EC (1986) The regulation of lymphocyte traffic. *Current Topics in Microbiology and Immunology* **128**: 85–122.
Clevers H, Alarcon B, Wileman T & Terhost C (1988) The T cell receptor/CD3 complex: a dynamic protein ensemble. *Annual Review of Immunology* **7**: 629–662.
Creasy AA, Stevens P, Kenney J et al (1991) Endotoxin and cytokine profile in plasma of baboons challenged with lethal and sublethal *Escherichia coli. Circulatory Shock* **33**: 84–91.
Cupps TR & Fauci AS (1982) Corticosteroid-mediated immunoregulation in man. *Immunological Reviews* **65**: 133–155.
Daynes RA & Araneo BA (1989) Contrasting effects of glucocorticoids on the capacity of T cells to produce the growth factors interleukin 2 and interleukin 4. *European Journal of Immunology* **19**: 2319–2325.
Daynes RA, Araneo BA, Dowell TA, Huang K & Dudley DJ (1990a) Regulation of murine lymphokine production in vivo: III. The lymphoid tissue microenvironment exerts regulatory influences over T helper cell function. *Journal of Experimental Medicine* **168**: 1825–1838.
Daynes RA, Dudley DJ & Araneo BA (1990b) Regulation of murine lymphokine production in vivo: II. Dehydroepianodrosterone is a natural enhancer of IL-2 synthesis by helper T cells. *European Journal of Immunology* **20**: 793–802.

DeForge LE & Remick DG (1991) Kinetics of TNF, IL-6, and IL-8 gene expression in LPS-stimulated human whole blood. *Biochemical and Biophysical Research Communications* **174:** 18–24.

Dinarello CA (1989) Interleukin-1 and its biologically related cytokines. *Advances in Immunology* **44:** 153–205.

Dudley DJ & Wiedmeier S (1991) The ontogeny of the immune response: perinatal perspectives. *Seminars in Perinatology* **15:** 184–195.

Dudley DJ, Mitchell MD, Creighton K & Branch DW (1990) Lymphokine production during term human pregnancy: differences between peripheral leukocytes and decidual cells. *American Journal of Obstetrics and Gynecology* **163:** 1890–1893.

Dudley DJ, Trautman MS, Araneo BA, Edwin SS & Mitchell MD. Decidual cell biosynthesis of interleukin-6: regulation by inflammatory cytokines. *Journal of Clinical Endocrinology and Metabolism* **74:** 884–889.

Farrar JJ, Benjamin WR, Hilfiker ML et al (1982) The biochemistry, biology, and role of interleukin 2 in the induction of cytotoxic T cell and antibody-forming B cell responses. *Immunological Reviews* **63:** 29–66.

Ford WL (1975) Lymphocyte migration and immune responses. *Progress in Allergy* **19:** 38–59.

Ford-Hutchinson AW, Bray MA, Doig MV, Shipley ME & Smith MJ (1980) Leukotriene B$_4$, a potent chemokinetic and aggregating substance released from polymorphonuclear leukocytes. *Nature* **286:** 264–265.

Groopman JE, Molina JM & Scadden DT (1989) Hematopoietic growth factors: biology and clinical applications. *New England Journal of Medicine* **321:** 1449–1459.

Hayakawa K & Hardy RR (1988) Murine CD4+ T cell subsets defined. *Journal of Experimental Medicine* **168:** 1825–1838.

Heinrich PC, Castell JV & Andus T (1990) Interleukin-6 and the acute phase response. *Biochemical Journal* **265:** 621–636.

Hwang D (1989) Essential fatty acids and immune response. *FASEB Journal* **3:** 2052–2061.

Janeway CA, Carding S, Jones B et al (1988) CD4+ T cells: specificity and function. *Immunological Reviews* **101:** 39–79.

Kronenberg M, Siu G, Hood LE & Shastri N (1986) The molecular genetics of the T-cell antigen receptor and T-cell antigen recognition. *Annual Review of Immunology* **4:** 529–591.

Kunkel SL, Standiford T, Kasahara K & Strieter RM (1991) Interleukin-8 (IL-8): the major neutrophil chemotactic factor in the lung. *Experimental Lung Research* **17:** 17–23.

Lanzavecchia A (1990) Receptor-mediated antigen uptake and its effect on antigen presentation to class II-restricted T lymphocytes. *Annual Review of Immunology* **8:** 773–793.

Le J & Vilcek J (1989) Interleukin-6: a multifunctional cytokine regulating immune reactions and the acute phase protein response. *Laboratory Investigation* **61:** 588–602.

Lebman DA & Coffman RL (1988) Interleukin 4 causes isotype switching to IgE in T cell-stimulated clonal B cell cultures. *Journal of Experimental Medicine* **168:** 853–862.

Locksley RM, Heinzel FP, Sadick MD, Holaday BJ & Gardner KD (1987) Murine cutaneous leishmaniasis: susceptibility correlates with differential expansion of helper T-cell subsets. *Annals Institute Pasteur/Immunology* **138:** 744–749.

Loria RM, Inge TH, Cook SS, Szakal AK & Regelson W (1988) Protection against acute lethal viral infections with the native steroid dehydroepiandrosterone (DHEA). *Journal of Medical Virology* **26:** 301–314.

Luger TA & Schwarz T (1990) Evidence for an epidermal cytokine network. *Journal of Investigative Dermatology* **95:** 100S–104S.

Male D, Champion B & Cooke A (1987) *Advanced Immunology*. Philadelphia: J.B. Lippincott Co.

Metcalf D (1991) Control of granulocytes and macrophages: molecular, cellular, and clinical aspects. *Science* **254:** 529–533.

Mossman TR & Coffman RL (1989) TH1 and TH2 cells: different patterns of lymphokine secretion lead to different functional properties. *Annual Review of Immunology* **7:** 145–173.

Orentreich N, Brind JL, Rizer RL & Vogelman JH (1984) Age changes and sex differences in serum dehydroepiandrosterone sulfate concentrations throughout adulthood. *Journal of Clinical Endocrinology and Metabolism* **59:** 551–555.

Paul WE (1991) Interleukin-4: a prototypic immunoregulatory lymphokine. *Blood* **77:** 1859–1870.

Payan DG, Missirian-Bastian A & Goetzl EJ (1984) Human T-lymphocyte subset specificity of the regulatory effects of leukotriene B_4. *Proceedings of the National Academy of Sciences (USA)* **81:** 3501–3505.

Podack ER, Hengartner H & Lichtenheld MG (1991) A central role of perforin in cytolysis? *Annual Review of Immunology* **9:** 129–157.

Pollard JW (1990) Regulation of polypeptide growth factor synthesis and growth factor-related gene expression in the rat and mouse uterus before and after implantation. *Journal of Reproduction and Fertility* **88:** 721–731.

Quill H, Gaur A & Phipps RP (1989) Prostaglandin E_2-dependent induction of granulocyte-macrophage colony-stimulating factor secretion by cloned murine helper T cells. *Journal of Immunology* **142:** 813–818.

Rappaport RS & Dodge GR (1982) Prostaglandin E_2 inhibits the production human interleukin 2. *Journal of Experimental Medicine* **155:** 943–948.

Raulet DH (1989) The structure, function, and molecular genetics of the gamma/delta T cell receptor. *Annual Review of Immunology* **7:** 175–207.

Reichel H, Koeffler HP, Tobler A & Norman AW (1987) 1alpha,25-dihydroxyvitamin D3 inhibits gamma-interferon synthesis by normal human peripheral blood lymphocytes. *Proceedings of the National Academy of Sciences (USA)* **84:** 3385–3389.

Robertson MJ & Ritz J (1990) Biology and clinical relevance of human natural killer cells. *Blood* **12:** 2421–2438.

Roitt I, Brostaff J & Male D (1989) *Immunology*, 2nd edn. Philadelphia: J.B. Lippincott Co.

Rola-Pleszczynski M, Gagnon L & Sirois P (1983) Leukotriene B_4 augments human natural cytotoxic cell activity. *Biochemical and Biophysical Research Communications* **113:** 531–537.

Rotteveel FTM, Kokkelink I, Van Lier RAW et al (1988) Clonal analysis of functionally distinct human CD4+ T cell subsets. *Journal of Experimental Medicine* **168:** 1659–1673.

Sacks DL, Lal SL, Shrivastava SN, Blackwell J & Neva FA (1987) An analysis of T cell responsiveness in Indian Kalaazar. *Journal of Immunology* **138:** 908–913.

Schwartz AG, Whitcomb JM, Nyce JW, Lewbart ML & Pashko LL (1988) Dehydroepiandrosterone and structural analogs: a new class of cancer chemopreventive agents. *Advances in Cancer Research* **51:** 391–424.

Schwartz RH (1985) T-lymphocyte recognition of antigen in association with gene products of the major histocompatibility complex. *Annual Review of Immunology* **3:** 237–261.

Seitz M, Dewald B, Gerber N & Baggiolini M (1991) Enhanced production of neutrophil-activating peptide-1/interleukin-8 in rheumatoid arthritis. *Journal of Clinical Investigation* **87:** 463–469.

Stamper HB & Woodruff JJ (1976) Lymphocyte homing into lymph nodes: in vitro demonstration of the selective affinity of recirculation lymphocytes for high endothelial venules. *Journal of Experimental Medicine* **144:** 828–833.

Szekeres-Bartho J, Kilar F, Falkay G et al (1985) Progesterone-treated lymphocytes release a substance inhibiting cytotoxicity and prostaglandin synthesis. *American Journal of Reproductive Immunology* **9:** 15–24.

Takatsu K (1988) B-cell growth and differentiation factors. *Proceedings of the Society for Experimental Biology and Medicine* **188:** 243–258.

Tobler A, Miller CW, Norman AW & Koeffler HP (1988) 1,25-Dihydroxyvitamin D_3 modulates the expression of a lymphokine (granulocyte-macrophage colony-stimulating factor) posttranscriptionally. *Journal of Clinical Investigation* **81:** 1819–1823.

Tracey KJ, Fong Y, Hesse D et al (1987) Anti-cachectin/TNF monoclonal antibodies prevent septic shock during lethal bacteremia. *Nature* **330:** 662–664.

Tschopp J & Nabholz M (1990) Perforin-mediated target cell lysis by cytolytic T lymphocytes. *Annual Review of Immunology* **8:** 279–302.

Tsoukas CD, Provvedini DM & Manolagas SC (1984) 1,25-Dihydroxyvitamin D_3: a novel immunoregulatory hormone. *Science* **224:** 1438–1440.

van Deventer S, Buller HR, ten Cate JW et al (1990) Experimental endotoxemia in humans: analysis of cytokine release and coagulation, fibrinolytic, and complement pathways. *Blood* **12:** 2520–2526.

Vercammen C & Ceuppens JL (1987) Prostaglandin E_2 inhibits human T-cell proliferation after crosslinking of the CD3-Ti complex by directly affecting T cells at an early stage of the activation process. *Cellular Immunology* **104:** 24–36.

Willams AF & Barclay AN (1988) The immunoglobulin superfamily—domains for cell surface recognition. *Annual Review of Immunology* **7:** 381–405.

Zeigler EL, Fisher CJ, Sprung CL et al (1991) Treatment of Gram-negative bacteremia and septic shock with HA-1A human monoclonal antibody against endotoxin. *New England Journal of Medicine* **324:** 429–436.

2

The normal fetomaternal immune relationship

W. D. BILLINGTON

INTRODUCTION

The immune system has evolved to provide a complex yet highly efficient mechanism for the recognition and elimination of foreign material entering into the body. It is therefore paradoxical that the survival of our species should depend upon a method of reproduction that involves the introduction into the female of genetically alien spermatozoal cells (and seminal plasma proteins) that must not be allowed to activate immunological effector processes leading to their destruction. Additionally, the successfully fertilized oocyte that develops to the blastocyst stage and implants into the uterine endometrium initiates an intimate anatomical relationship between one organism, the conceptus, with both paternally derived and developmentally regulated (differentiation) cell surface molecules (antigens), and another, the pregnant female, who herself lacks many of these molecules and yet possesses an immune system that should be fully competent to recognize and react against them. The conceptus is therefore a highly successful allogeneic graft that appears to contradict the basic law of transplantation immunology that states that genetic disparities between graft and host will inevitably lead to immunologically mediated rejection reactions. The purpose of this review is to identify the antigens that have the potential to stimulate maternal immune responses, to examine the timing of their expression during development, and to assess the nature and extent of any maternal antibody and cell-mediated immunity directed against them during normal pregnancy. Germane to this is a consideration of the transmission of maternally produced antibodies across the placenta and the ontogeny of the immune response in the developing fetus.

INSEMINATION

Most women do not develop detectable levels of antibody or evidence of cell-mediated immunity following exposure to the components of the semen, even when this amounts to multiple inseminations over a prolonged period of time. In those women where such an immune response does occur it is often, but not inevitably, associated with some degree of infertility, with local synthesis of IgA and IgG antibodies within the reproductive tract that

Baillière's Clinical Obstetrics and Gynaecology—
Vol. 6, No. 3, September 1992
ISBN 0–7020–1634–9

are able to bind to the spermatozoal cell surface and affect either their viability or motility within the cervix or uterus, or their ability to attach to the zona pellucida of the oocyte at the site of fertilization. On very rare occasions, there can be acute hypersensitivity and local allergic reactions to the seminal plasma proteins with unexpected and upsetting effects for the individual, including cardiovascular distress, swollen joints, and even diarrhoea.

The reason for the failure of most women to mount an immune response to inseminated spermatozoa has yet to be established. Although the numbers of spermatozoa in the normal ejaculate are significant in terms of their potential to stimulate an immune response ($50-150 \times 10^6$/ml in an average volume of 3.5 ml) a substantial proportion of them are almost certainly lost by vaginal leakage. Those that remain in the reproductive tract and pass through the cervical canal are believed to be rendered non-immunogenic by the presence of one or more components of the seminal plasma, particularly spermine or prostaglandins of the E series, that are suggested, on the basis of in vitro experiments, to act as local immuno-suppressive factors (Quayle et al, 1989). It is difficult to determine the extent to which this immunosuppressive activity is operative in vivo.

Molecular biological and biochemical studies are now being employed to identify the precise molecular structures on the spermatozoal cell surface that are responsible for the elicitation of antibodies in infertile women. When this is achieved it will be possible to correlate more effectively the specific nature of the immune response in the individual patient and her fertility status. Antispermatozoal antibodies are not directed against the classical HLA antigens that are involved in transplantation rejection reactions. Despite some contradictory reports in the literature it is now widely accepted that HLA antigens are not expressed on spermatozoa. This has the clinical implication that any antisperm antibody-associated female infertility cannot be overcome simply by donor insemination, as it will be related to sperm-specific and not individual HLA-specific antigens.

EARLY EMBRYONIC DEVELOPMENT

Although many studies have been carried out to determine the nature of the antigens expressed on the surface of the pre-implantation embryo in numerous laboratory and farm animal species, relatively little is known about the human embryo. From the limited data available at present, it would appear that neither the oocyte nor the early cleavage and blastocyst stages of development express HLA antigens (Desoye et al, 1988; Roberts et al, 1992). Whether or not there are other, non-HLA, antigens present, there is as yet no evidence for maternal recognition of any embryonic antigens at this stage of pregnancy nor that any form of maternal immunity can have deleterious effects on pre-implantation embryonic development. Although immunoglobulins, and possibly sensitized lymphocytes, may potentially be able to gain access to the lumen of the fallopian tube and the uterus, they will have no damaging effect unless they have specific reactivity against an appropriate (and exposed) target antigen on the embryo. The evidence is that this is not the case.

The pre-implantation embryo, encapsulated in its zona pellucida, and developing in an environment normally devoid of antigen-presenting cells (APC) and helper T lymphocytes that could trigger immune recognition, or potentially damaging immune effector agents and effective components of complement, is unlikely to be involved in maternal immunological interactions, whatever embryo-associated antigens may eventually prove to be expressed.

IMPLANTATION

Loss of the zona pellucida and attachment of the blastocyst to the uterine epithelium marks the end of the free-living stage of embryonic development. The single-celled outer layer of the blastocyst, the trophectoderm, and its cellular descendants, the cytotrophoblast and syncytiotrophoblast, come into direct and increasingly intimate contact with maternal host tissues. From implantation onwards, the fetomaternal immune relationship assumes an increasing importance. It is, however, necessary to bear in mind two significant points. First, there is never any vascular continuity between mother and fetus: the circulatory systems of the two individuals remain entirely separate throughout the whole of gestation. Secondly, trophoblast is the *only* fetal tissue to have direct and continuous contact with the maternal environment. This trophoblastic interface with the mother develops at three major anatomical sites as the pregnancy becomes established.

THE FETOMATERNAL INTERFACE

The early cytotrophoblast undergoes rapid proliferation and differentiation, possibly under the control of a regulatory cytokine network, and gives rise continuously to an overlying syncytial layer, the syncytiotrophoblast. Further differentiation of these two forms of trophoblast ultimately leads to the variety of subpopulations that constitute the fetal interface throughout the remainder of pregnancy. Following the formation of the definitive placenta, this interface is composed of:

(1) the placental chorionic villi, where the covering layer of villous syncytiotrophoblast is bathed by the maternal blood in the intervillous spaces. An underlying layer of villous cytotrophoblast is present until the latter stages of gestation.

(2) a diverse cytotrophoblastic cell population within the placental bed, where there is direct contact with maternal uterine (decidual) cells and with maternal blood. Some of the cytotrophoblast cells invade further and into the myometrium whilst others enter into the uterine spiral arteries and come to line, and even replace, the endothelial surface.

(3) the cytotrophoblast population, 2–10 cells thick, that forms part of the

amniochorionic membrane at the non-placental region of the implantation site. The cytotrophoblast cells are in direct apposition to the maternal decidual cells.

It is apparent that the developing foreign fetus has no physical association with its maternal host and is protected by an unbroken anatomical barrier of trophoblastic tissue. The trophoblast constituting this barrier is, of course, of embryonic origin and in order to survive and fulfil its functions it must avoid recognition and rejection by the maternal immune system with which it has direct and continuous contact. The manner in which this is achieved is considered below.

DUAL FUNCTION: THE PLACENTA AS A BARRIER AND A PATHWAY

It should be remembered that the trophoblast has not only to perform a barrier role but also that of a transmission pathway for the exchange of a variety of substances from mother to fetus and vice versa (Figure 1). Such exchanges take place largely across the placental syncytiotrophoblastic surface of the chorionic villi. This is not a simple semipermeable membrane but rather a sophisticated selective transfer system, permitting the passage

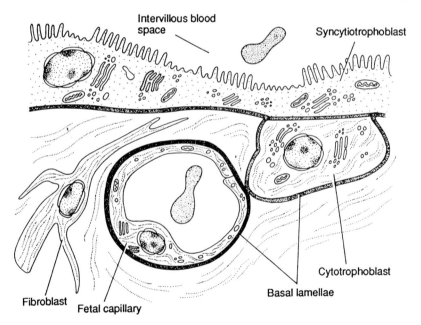

Figure 1. Ultrastructure of the human placental barrier. The only continuous cellular layers between the two circulations are the syncytiotrophoblast and the fetal endothelium, each attached to its own basal lamella. The intervening connective tissue is thin and is unlikely to form an important barrier. From Begley et al (1980).

of certain materials whilst preventing that of many others. This selectivity is exercised in a number of different ways and with varying degrees of specificity depending upon the nature of the materials transferred. The immunological aspects of maternofetal transmission are critically important in both normal and pathological pregnancies and are discussed later in this review as well as elsewhere in this volume.

Non-rejection of the fetal trophoblast

The central issue is whether fetal trophoblast expresses HLA, or other, cell surface antigens capable of being recognized and reacted against by the immunocompetent pregnant female. If such antigens are entirely absent, then the trophoblastic tissue will be a 'passive' graft as far as the mother is concerned and will not elicit immune rejection reactions. No other explanation would be required for the so-called 'immunological paradox of pregnancy', the successful implantation and development of a genetically disparate embryo. On the other hand, if trophoblast were to express any paternally encoded HLA antigens not represented in the maternal genome then it would be necessary to identify the mechanism(s) responsible for its non-recognition or its failure to induce an effective rejection response. Trophoblast would then take the form of an 'active' graft requiring immunoregulatory control processes to allow its survival.

Antigenic status of the trophoblast

The question of the HLA antigen status of the trophoblast has not been an easy one to answer. This is largely because trophoblast exists as a variety of subpopulations and in complex anatomical relationships with both other fetal cells and maternal cells. Trophoblast cannot therefore readily be separated into purified single-cell suspensions and subjected to cell-surface phenotype analysis or employed in culture for functional assay purposes. This has to some extent been overcome by examination of trophoblast in situ using immunohistological techniques with monoclonal antibodies, although this can still present some technical difficulties and depends also on the ability to identify with certainty the specific trophoblast populations within the tissue.

Advances have been made recently in techniques for the isolation, separation and culture of some, but not all, of the relevant trophoblast populations (Loke, 1990). Totally homogeneous cell preparations remain elusive. The syncytiotrophoblast is, by definition, lacking in cellularity and, as it is also a mitotic end-stage, cannot therefore be maintained as a cell culture. Cytotrophoblastic cells of the amniochorionic membrane and from the chorionic plate and placental bed have been more commonly employed as sources for trophoblast cultures.

Immunohistological studies on first trimester and term placentae, supported by molecular biological analyses, have provided definitive evidence for the absence of HLA antigens from the syncytiotrophoblast of the chorionic villi (Bulmer and Johnson, 1985; Hunt and Hsi, 1990). This most important of trophoblastic tissues has therefore developed a genetic mechanism, probably by hypermethylation of the DNA of the genes for HLA, by which it is able to avoid recognition as a foreign tissue. It is not yet certain that the same is true for all the other trophoblastic populations. Villous and non-villous cytotrophoblast cells of the placenta and cyto-trophoblast cells of the amniochorion, although also apparently failing to express paternally encoded classical HLA antigens, have been shown to exhibit a newly discovered HLA molecule, designated HLA-G (Ellis et al, 1990; Kovats et al, 1990, 1991). Current evidence indicates that this is a non-polymorphic form of HLA. If this is confirmed, and it is incapable of being recognized by the T lymphocytes of the maternal immune system, then these trophoblastic cells also will be regarded as a 'passive' graft. The significance and biological role of the HLA-G expression on cytotrophoblast remains to be established.

Implications of an HLA antigen-deficient trophoblast

The lack of HLA antigens on the syncytiotrophoblast and the presence only of the non-classical HLA-G antigen on the cytotrophoblast cells would appear to preclude the involvement of the fetal trophoblast in currently recognized types of allogeneic immune reactions, which involve major histocompatibility complex (MHC) class I and II associated cellular recogni-tion processes (see Chapter 1). This would apply both to the recognition (generative) and effector phases of the immune response. The maternal immune system would therefore not be stimulated by allogeneic trophoblast nor would trophoblast provide a recognizable target for any maternal cytotoxic T cells that might be generated by any other HLA-positive fetal cells. Furthermore, assuming that the phenomenon of MHC restriction applies equally to trophoblast, the absence of classical MHC class I antigens would prevent the co-recognition of any other form of cell surface antigen that trophoblast might express. The relevance of the reported trophoblast-specific (Davies and Browne, 1985a) and trophoblast-associated (trophoblast-lymphocyte cross-reactive, TLX) (McIntyre et al, 1984) anti-gens would then be called into question, at least in this context.

Insusceptibility of trophoblast to immune attack

Trophoblast is remarkably resistant to immune lysis. Attempts to kill tro-phoblast in vitro by cell-mediated or antibody-mediated mechanisms have generally proved unsuccessful, unless extreme measures, such as interferon-γ boosting, are taken to enhance the cytotoxic activity of the effector cells (Pross et al, 1985). Such conditions are unlikely to prevail in the pregnant female. Lysis by non-MHC related mechanisms, such as natural killer (NK) cell activity, is also unlikely, given the failure of trophoblast cells to exhibit NK target molecules (King et al, 1990). Antibody-mediated lysis, even in vitro, demands appropriate levels of specific antibody and effective components of complement. There is little evidence for either as far as in vivo placental trophoblast is concerned.

IMMUNOREGULATION IN PREGNANCY

Despite the accumulating evidence that trophoblast survival as an intrauterine graft is afforded solely by the unique feature of non-expression of classical HLA antigens, there remains a school of thought that there are important immunoregulatory mechanisms that prevent either the generation or effector activity of a maternal allogeneic immune response. Largely on the basis of in vitro studies on experimental animals, but supported by some data from in vivo investigations and from human pregnancies, there is evidence for the downregulation of maternal immune responses against histocompatibility antigens. Factors of placental (trophoblastic) origin (Menu et al, 1989) and molecules secreted by novel forms of maternal lymphocytes within the decidua (Michel et al, 1989), both as yet poorly characterized, appear able to inhibit the generation of cytotoxic T cells (Tc), and in some cases to induce the formation of suppressor cells, as well as to prevent the effector activity of experimentally generated Tc cells, in the pregnant female. The need for any such mechanisms remains to be proven.

There are other forms of immunoregulation deemed by some investigators to be relevant for the establishment and maintenance of normal pregnancy but these are still in the realms of hypothesis and are based on few, if any, widely accepted data.

ANTI-FETAL ANTIBODY IN PREGNANCY

The pregnant female is undoubtedly able to recognize the paternally inherited histocompatibility antigens of her fetus and to response by the production of antibodies. This was first recorded almost 40 years ago and pregnancy sera have proved valuable as the source of anti-HLA antibodies used as reagents for tissue typing in clinical transplantation. They are not, however, detectable in all pregnancies. Using standard complement-dependent lymphocytotoxicity tests, anti-HLA antibodies are commonly reported to be present in only 10–15% of primiparous women and fewer than 60% of multiparous individuals (Doughty and Gelsthorpe, 1976). Not all centres in fact are able to detect even this level of response; one careful study identified antibody in only 38% of all pregnant women (Regan and Braude, 1987; Figure 2). Antibodies may develop against HLA-A, B, C (class I) or HLA-DR (class II) antigens, and may develop together or independently (Vives et al, 1976; Borelli et al, 1982).

The kinetics of anti-HLA production are not known in detail. Although they might occasionally arise earlier, they are more likely to be detectable by 12 weeks' gestation, are present in those women who are going to respond by 28 weeks, and reach peak levels before undergoing a decline in the third trimester, followed by a postpartum increase. This is, however, a very imperfect view of the antibody response of pregnancy. More recent studies using assays that are capable of detecting antibodies other than those that fix complement have demonstrated a greater frequency of antibody response

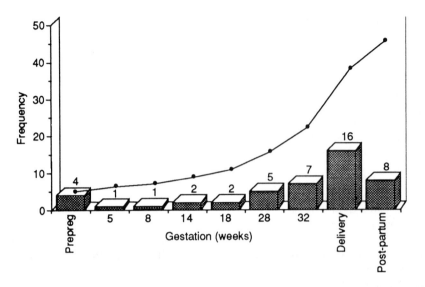

Figure 2. Histogram showing the time of first detection of antipaternal cytotoxic antibody in 120 women having a livebirth. The number of women with positive tests at each gestational time interval is denoted above each histogram bar. The cumulative frequency of antipaternal cytotoxic antibody is shown by the solid line (———). From Regan & Braude (1987) with permission.

(Antczak, 1989; Gilman-Sachs et al, 1989). Additionally, the levels of antibody detected reflect only those that are present as free molecules in the serum. It is clear, however, from recent studies that the presence of anti-HLA antibodies can be masked by the ability of these antibodies both to complex with soluble HLA antigens and to induce the development of maternal antibodies to them (anti-anti-HLA, or anti-idiotypic, antibodies) (Reed et al, 1991).

To obtain a fuller picture of the antibodies in normal pregnancy it would be necessary to consider at least the following factors: degree of materno-fetal incompatibility; parity status; stage of gestation; antibody isotype; rate of synthesis and catabolism of the antibody; degree of antigen–antibody complexing; formation of anti-idiotype antibodies; binding of antibody to placental cells; rate of transport to fetus.

The stimulus for anti-HLA antibody production

It has for long been assumed that fetal leukocytes are able to leak into the maternal circulation and provide the stimulus for maternal antibody formation. Attempts to demonstrate this were, however, unsuccessful until the availability of the fluorescence-activated cell sorter (FACS), which is capable of identifying very small numbers of cells following fluorescent antibody labelling. Cells reacting with specific antipaternal HLA antibody and containing Y chromatin have been detected in maternal blood samples taken from as early as the 15th week of gestation in women carrying a male fetus, as established either by amniocentesis or delivery (Iverson et al, 1981). The normal variation in the frequency, timing and extent of ante-partum leukocyte leakage is not known. It possibly occurs at a rather low level and not in all pregnancies. Haemorrhage at delivery almost certainly augments any earlier stimulus and is hence responsible for the typical postpartum increase in detectable anti-HLA antibody. Earlier suggestions that the stimulus may arise from trophoblast, either in normal or molar pregnancies, should now be discounted with the present evidence of lack of classical HLA antigens on this fetal tissue.

Relevance of anti-HLA antibodies

A major question is whether the antifetal HLA antibodies have a biological function or are merely a trivial consequence of fetal leukocyte leakage. This is a controversial issue currently unresolved. It could be argued that unless these antibodies are produced by all women then they cannot subserve an essential function. Fetomaternal HLA incompatibilities almost certainly exist in every pregnancy; these occur in 98% of all cases even on the basis of typing only for HLA-A, B and DR antigens. At present, antibodies are unable to be detected in all pregnancy sera. Whether more extensive screening, using newer assays, will alter this picture remains to be seen.

An alternative view is that maternal alloantibody production is necessary for the maintenance of normal pregnancy. This is based upon experiments showing that lymphocyte activities in vitro can be inhibited or 'blocked' by pregnancy serum (Takeuchi, 1990). Antifetal antibody can be demonstrated to be one of the components capable of effecting this blocking action. Various hypotheses have been constructed to suggest how this blocking activity could operate in vivo in order either to prevent the generation of a deleterious cell-mediated immune reaction or to inhibit any already sensitized lymphocyte population (Davies, 1986). The former would be the more likely as there appear to be no cytotoxic T cells against fetal HLA antigens in other than a few isolated cases (Sargent et al, 1987).

Although there is no definitive evidence for the existence of any such blocking system, this notion has been further extended to explain the failure of pregnancies in recurrent spontaneous miscarriage (RSM) in terms of an immune rejection through lack of blocking antibodies in these women. Additionally, this has then provided the rationale for immunotherapeutic approaches to RSM by infusion of paternal or third party pooled leukocytes in order to stimulate the production of the absent blocking antibodies (Taylor and Faulk, 1981; Beer at al, 1981; Mowbray et al, 1985). This controversial area is discussed in detail in a current review (Billington, 1992b) and in Chapter 5.

Maternal antibodies can be detected against fetal antigens other than those encoded by the major histocompatibility complex. Apart from those against fetal red blood cells, there are non-HLA antibodies directed against such structures as Fc receptors (Power et al, 1983), fetal IgG molecules (Grubb, 1970) and trophoblast cell surface molecules (Davies and Browne,

1985b). These have not, however, been fully characterized, nor are they a consistent feature of pregnancy. Whether they have any biological function remains a matter of speculation.

TRANSMISSION OF PASSIVE IMMUNITY

The immune system of the neonate, although structurally fully developed, does not reach adult levels of functional immunocompetence until several months after birth (see below). Protection of the neonate against a variety of environmental pathogens is assisted by the acquisition of maternal pre-formed antibodies. These are provided in two ways; by transfer across the placenta during the antenatal period and by uptake from colostrum and milk during breast-feeding. In the latter case, the immunoglobulins are of the IgA class and have a valuable role in the protection of the neonatal gut against enteric infections, acting as an 'antiseptic paste' and preventing bacterial uptake (Hanson et al, 1984). The prenatal transmission is a more complex phenomenon and restricted to the IgG class. All four subclasses of IgG are transferred across the placenta, although apparently at differing relative rates and stages of gestation.

Placental transfer of IgG

The selective transfer of IgG is determined by the Fc portion of the immuno-globulin. This binds to specific receptors (Fcγ) on the syncytiotrophoblast surface and the immunoglobulin is subsequently transferred into the fetal circulation. The Fcγ receptor shows greater affinity for IgG$_1$ and IgG$_3$, with considerably less for IgG$_2$. The degree of affinity for IgG$_4$ is presently unknown.

The details of the mechanism of IgG transfer following Fc receptor engagement are not fully established. It is necessary for the IgG to be protected from proteolytic degradation during its intracellular passage across the syncytiotrophoblast. There is good evidence to support the view that this is achieved by uptake of the IgG into clathrin-coated micropinocytic vesicles which protect and transport the antibody across the trophoblast and discharge it by exocytosis (Wild, 1983). Other proteins are taken up non-selectively into macropinocytic vesicles which then fuse with lysosomes and undergo degradation.

Active transport of IgG to the fetus may possibly begin as early as 6 weeks of gestation. It is well documented to occur by 12 weeks and appears to continue at a relatively low and steady rate until 16–22 weeks. There is then a rapid increase and by 26–34 weeks the concentrations in the fetus reach and then soon exceed those of the maternal circulation (Figure 3). Data on transmission of IgG subclasses indicate that IgG$_1$, IgG$_2$ and IgG$_3$ can be detected in the fetus at 11 weeks, whereas IgG$_4$ is seen occasionally at 14 weeks but normally only after 19 weeks. IgG$_2$ is transferred less readily than the others, which is in accord with the evidence of its lower affinity binding with the Fc receptor (see Wild, 1983). Paired sera analyses show that the

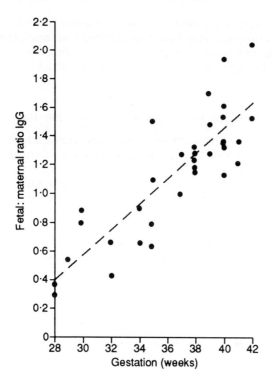

Figure 3. Fetal:maternal ratio of IgG related to gestational age. From Pitcher-Wilmott et al (1980).

total IgG levels, and those of all four subclasses, are greater in the cord blood than the maternal circulation at term (Pitcher-Wilmott et al, 1980) (Table 1).

It is possible to identify the maternal origin of immunoglobulins in the fetal or neonatal circulation and to distinguish them from those that may be being produced by fetal or neonatal synthesis. IgG molecules have allotypic antigenic sites which act as genetic markers (Gm groups). Gm allotype

Table 1. IgG subclass levels in fetal cord blood and maternal sera at term*.

	IgG_1 (%)	IgG_2 (%)	IgG_3 (%)	IgG_4 (%)	Total IgG (u/ml)
Fetus†	127(38)	95(43)	165(89)	90(62)	148(36)
Mother†	85(31)	72(40)	132(72)	58(39)	106(23)
Mean difference‡	42	23	33	32	42

* Data from 19 paired sera, expressed as percentages with regard to the concentrations in a reference serum standard.
† Means, with standard deviation in parenthesis.
‡ Paired t-tests all show highly significant differences.
(Adapted from Pitcher-Wilmott et al, 1980)

analysis can therefore be used to demonstrate the relative proportions of maternal and fetal immunoglobulins and to follow the rate of replacement of the maternal IgG molecules during the early months after birth. By about 1 year of age all the IgG molecules express only the child's own Gm markers (Grubb, 1970).

Implications of placental transmission of immunoglobulins

The acquisition of passive immunity by transplacental transfer of maternal antibodies against a variety of pathogens is clearly of benefit for the newborn. Unfortunately the Fc receptor-mediated mechanism of the syncytiotrophoblast is unable to distinguish between IgG antibodies that are beneficial and those that are potentially harmful. The antifetal HLA antibodies are partly absorbed out by binding to macrophage and endothelial cell Fc receptors in the core of the chorionic villi of the placenta (Johnson et al, 1976) and are partly transferred to the fetus (Tongio et al, 1975; Jones and Need, 1988). They probably bind harmlessly to fetal tissue and are eventually cleared. Although antifetal HLA antibody has cytotoxic potential in vitro, this is manifest only in artificial assay conditions and employing heterologous complement, i.e. obtained from a different species. In the fetal environment, at least at the earlier stages of gestation, there will only be small quantities of fetal complement which, being homologous, is likely to be ineffective in mediating antibody cytotoxicity.

Isoantibodies

Deleterious effects on the fetus and neonate can occur with the transmission of maternal IgG elicited by isoimmunization with fetal erythrocytes, leukocytes and platelets (Jones and Need, 1988). These blood elements commonly gain access to the maternal circulation during parturitional haemorrhage and to a lesser extent by breaching the placental barrier earlier in gestation. Therapeutic termination of pregnancy in the first trimester is also known to allow maternal isoimmunization. The most severe effects are seen in Rhesus haemolytic disease where the maternal antibodies (mainly IgG_1 and IgG_3) against the Rh(D) antigen of fetal erythrocytes effect their lysis by binding to the red cells and acting as opsonins, leading to intracellular destruction within phagocytes. Neonatal leukopenia and neonatal thrombocytopenia are occasional consequences of isoimmunization against fetal leukocytes and platelets, respectively. The clinical aspects of these immune diseases are considered in Chapter 8.

Autoantibodies

Autoimmune diseases in the pregnant female can also have consequences for the fetus and neonate (Taylor, 1988). Maternal IgG autoantibodies are able to cross the placenta and produce pathological effects by binding to fetal cellular receptors (thyrotoxicosis and myasthenia gravis), by forming circulating immune complexes (systemic lupus erythematosus) or by activating complement and effector cells (autoimmune haemolytic anaemia). The effects are normally seen only in the neonate and are almost always transient, disappearing within 3 months, reflecting the catabolism of the maternal immunoglobulins (see Chapter 9). Neonatal diseases of this kind can sometimes be identified in mothers who are asymptomatic and thus provides the opportunity to initiate treatment of the individual at an earlier stage in the development of the autoimmunity.

PASSAGE OF MATERNAL CELLS TO THE FETUS

Contrary to an apparently common belief, there is little, if any, evidence of passage of immunocompetent maternal cells across the placenta into the fetal circulation and tissues in normal pregnancy (Hunziker and Wegmann, 1986; Billington, 1992a). As there is no vascular continuity between mother and fetus such passage would require transmission from the intervillous spaces of the placenta across the syncytiotrophoblast of the chorionic villi, a cellular cytotrophoblast layer (unbroken in the earlier stages of gestation), trophoblastic basement membrane and walls of the fetal blood vessels within the mesenchyme of the villi. This is an unlikely process unless the physical barriers were to be damaged in some way.

Graft-versus-host disease

The extremely rare occurrence of fetal/neonatal graft-versus-host disease (GVHD), where there may or may not be evidence of maternal cells in the newborn (Pollack et al, 1982), is a clear indication of the impermeability of the placental barrier in normal pregnancy. The situation in neonatal GVHD is in fact more complicated. GVHD outside pregnancy is always associated with primary or secondary immunodeficiency. It is not yet clear whether the maternal–fetal GVHD is triggered by fetal immunodeficiency, nor the extent to which maternal T cell activity is actually involved in the pathogenesis of the disease (Ammann, 1986).

Limitations of most technical approaches make it difficult to establish the maternal origin of any cells in the fetal tissues. Karyotype analysis, seeking to detect XX cells in male neonates, has been the main method employed. Newer immunological and molecular genetic techniques may, however, prove much more sensitive as probes for maternal cell markers.

Cord blood sampling

Examination of cord blood samples at delivery represents a more straightforward approach to the detection of maternal cell transfer to the fetus. It is, of course, limited to one very brief phase in the maternofetal relationship, which may not be representative of the situation occurring throughout most of pregnancy. Nevertheless, there are no convincing reports of maternal lymphoid cells in cord blood samples (Adinolfi, 1988).

There have been suggestions that small numbers of maternal cells passing into the fetal circulation would be undetectable owing to their elimination by the developing immune defences of the fetus, perhaps by cytotoxic antibody, cytotoxic cells, or suppressor cells. Of these potential effector mechanisms there is good evidence for the presence and functional activity of fetal suppressor T cells in the cord blood (Papadogiannakis et al, 1990). Although their precise surface phenotype and mode of suppression remain to be established, it is clear that these fetal cells, at least in vitro, are able to exert a strong, non-specific suppressor influence on both the proliferation and effector function of both T and B lymphocytes of maternal origin.

It is clearly a difficult, it not impossible, task to determine the true extent of any maternal cell passage into the fetus throughout the different phases of gestation. On present evidence, it would appear either that this does not occur at all or does so in such small numbers that it is of no biological or clinical relevance. Only when pathological events prevail might maternal cell passage be significant and deleterious, although even here it must be convincingly demonstrated that maternal T cells are present in the fetus or neonate and that they are causally related to the disease process concerned. This issue is discussed further in Chapter 8.

DEPORTATION OF TROPHOBLAST

Trophoblast embolism of the lungs, originally believed to occur only in eclamptic patients, is now known to be a normal physiological process in many, possibly all, normal pregnancies (Douglas et al, 1959; Billington, 1992a). From as early as the 26th day post-fertilization portions of the syncytiotrophoblast break away from the chorionic villi into the intervillous spaces. This trophoblast is usually in the form of small multinucleate syncytial clumps ('sprouts') which become pinched off from the villous surface during development. On rare occasions, larger villous fragments may be shed. The trophoblast is deported from this site into the uterine veins and subsequently into the inferior vena cava. It is estimated that 100 000 sprouts (1 g) may enter the maternal circulation each day (Iklé, 1964). Lytic enzymes destroy a large proportion of these sprouts but significant numbers survive and are eventually filtered out by becoming lodged in the capillaries of the maternal lungs. Recent claims that small numbers can pass from the pulmonary capillary bed and reach the peripheral circulation have now been discredited (Covone et al, 1988). This therefore precludes the possibility of isolating fetal trophoblast from maternal blood for the prenatal diagnosis of genetic defects.

The biological significance of trophoblast deportation is unknown. One recurring suggestion has been that it may provide an additional signal for the induction of some form of immune response that may act as a regulatory (protective) mechanism, such as blocking antibodies, against transplantation rejection reactions. As this trophoblast does not express HLA antigens, either class I or class II, any immune response would have to be against the ill-defined trophoblast membrane antigens. The nature, and even the existence, of antitrophoblast antibodies is controversial and their function is therefore a matter only of speculation (Billington and Davies, 1987; Hole et al, 1987). There is no evidence of any local response to the pulmonary trophoblast, which slowly degenerates and disappears.

It is quite possible that sprout formation and venous deportation merely represents the physiological desquamation of an ageing syncytial tissue that has reached its terminal postmitotic stage. This would follow from the fact that it is a non-replicating form of trophoblast that is derived and sustained by the proliferation and differentiation of the underlying cytotrophoblast layer.

ONTOGENY OF IMMUNITY IN THE FETUS AND NEONATE

The fetus develops in an intrauterine milieu that is largely, but not entirely, protected from invasion by pathogens that have entered the maternal host. The placenta and fetal membranes act as a barrier to all but a few potentially deleterious viruses, bacteria and protozoa. From birth onwards, however, the neonate is exposed to all the considerable array of pathogenic organisms in its new external environment. The immune system must therefore be competent to deal with infections during both fetal and neonatal life. This is achieved partially through the acquisition of preformed maternal IgG antibodies, as described earlier in this review, and partially by the maturation of the fetal immune cell repertoire necessary for the recognition of foreign antigens and the elicitation of specific humoral and cellular immune responses against them, aided also by the synthesis of non-antigen-specific protective substances, such as complement, lysozyme and interferon (Adinolfi, 1988).

IgA antibodies in breast milk

The normal neonate is immunologically well protected, especially if it is also in receipt of secretory IgA antibodies from breast milk (Hanson et al, 1984). Up to 1 g/day of IgA is provided by colostrum/milk. A large proportion of this passes quickly through the gut but up to 30% binds to the intestinal epithelial surfaces and provides a more prolonged protective effect. A small quantity of IgA is also taken up across the gut epithelium, but this transfer is restricted to only the first 24 h of life, owing to closure of the transepithelial transport mechanism, probably by steroid hormone control processes.

IgA, principally the IgA_2 subclass, which is the predominant form in breast milk, provides protection against a wide range of pathogens in the gut and, surprisingly, against respiratory tract infection by respiratory syncytial virus (RSV) (Downham et al, 1976). The way in which the IgA reaches the respiratory mucosa and the precise mode of its protective action are not yet established.

Breast milk also contains a variety of non-immunoglobulin substances that have a wide spectrum of protective effects on the neonate against bacterial, viral and protozoal infection (Goldman et al, 1985). The extent to which the cellular components of breast milk (which includes T and B lymphocytes, macrophages and polymorphs) (Head, 1977; Goldman et al, 1985) participate in the immune defence system of the neonate is an interesting question which has not yet been satisfactorily answered. It is in fact unclear whether they are able to cross the intestinal epithelium and assume functional activity within the lymphoid tissues or circulation of the genetically alien neonate. Such allogeneic immune cell chimaerism would appear to be an unlikely phenomenon but cannot be dismissed.

Development and maturation of fetal immunocompetence

It is frequently stated that the neonate has not reached full immune competence. However, analysis of the surface phenotypes and investigation of the in vitro functional capabilities of the cellular components of the cord blood at delivery indicates that neonatal immune responses can be comparable to those generated by adults (Adinolfi, 1988). The differences normally observed are due to the fact that the adult immune system has had the opportunity to be primed and activated by prior exposure to the antigens involved, whereas the fetal immune system has, with few exceptions, been isolated from such stimulatory influences. This is the main reason why the young infant requires protection by its maternally acquired IgG antibodies, as it would be vulnerable to infection with only its own slowly maturing primary immune responses on first exposure to the antigen. Once specifically primed, the child's immune system can develop an adequate protective response of its own and can dispense with the need for the maternal antibodies. Studies on the Gm markers of IgG molecules indicate that the maternal antibodies begin to be replaced during the first 3 months of life and disappear completely by 9–12 months, or even earlier (Grubb, 1970).

Immunoglobulin levels during the early postnatal period

Serum IgG levels normally decrease during the first 2–3 months of life, then rise again owing to the child's own production of this immunoglobulin following antigenic stimulation. The variation seen in IgG levels in individual neonates reflects the differences in their respective mother's serum concentrations. Low levels are seen in infants of hypogammaglobulinaemic mothers and also in premature babies, the latter because of the reduced time for transplacental transmission. Measurements of other classes of immunoglobulins in cord blood or sera of normal infants show that levels of IgM, IgA and IgE are very low, whilst IgD is usually absent (Adinolfi, 1988). Fetal synthesis in utero is the source of these immunoglobulins detected at birth. Following intrauterine infection, however, high levels of IgM, and to a lesser extent of IgA, are detectable in cord and neonatal sera. Fetal synthesis of immunoglobulins, particularly IgM and IgG, is known to occur following maternal infections from at least the 6th month of gestation. On the basis of in vitro studies using fetal tissues it is likely that the spleen and lymph nodes from as early as the 12th week of gestation are able to produce IgM and IgG molecules. This concurs with evidence on the time of development of fetal B lymphocytes.

Manipulation of the fetal immune system

It is worth noting that the levels of the immunoglobulins in the young infant can have an effect on the individual's response to the antigenic challenge of vaccination. The mechanism of such antibody-regulated immune reactivity is not known. There is also a prospect for manipulation of the fetal immune system by maternal vaccination. Sensitization and enhanced antibody responses have been reported against meningococcal polysaccharide and tetanus toxoid in infants born to mothers vaccinated during pregnancy (McCormick et al, 1980; Gill et al, 1983). Although experimental animal studies demonstrate that such procedures can also commonly lead to depression of responsiveness in the offspring (Malley, 1989), it would appear to be worth further investigation for the potential benefits of prophylactic immunization, especially against the human immunodeficiency virus, currently producing a considerable escalation in the reported incidence of perinatal AIDS.

Origin and development of cells of the immune system

The ability of the neonate to respond to antigenic stimulation with both cellular and humoral immunity indicates that all the necessary immunocompetent cells and signalling mechanisms are acquired during fetal development (Table 2). The observed antibody responses to intrauterine infections also demonstrate the immunocompetence of the fetus at certain stages of gestation. Information on the precise ontogeny of these acquired responses has, however, been rather sketchy, but is now becoming clearer, particularly through the availability of highly specific monoclonal antibodies and molecular probes for the identification of the cells and molecules involved.

Table 2. Ontogeny of fetal and neonatal immunity.

Gestational age (weeks)	Developmental events
5	Yolk sac cells (pluripotent)
6	Thymus rudiment; early macrophages?; HLA on fetal cells
7	Lymphopoiesis in liver
8	Pre-B cells
9	T cell progenitors; NK cells; lysozyme
10	Further T cell-surface markers
11	C3 and C4 synthesis; dendritic cells
12	B cells in bone marrow; transmission of maternal IgG
13	Macrophages; reactive T cells
14	Lymphocytes in peripheral blood
15	IgM and IgG synthesis (possibly earlier?)
18	All complement components, except C9
21	Increase in dendritic cell population; cytotoxic T cells
22	Increased rate of maternal IgG transfer
Birth	All immune cells, lymphokines, complement components and non-specific factors present (but immune system normally unprimed)
Suckling	IgA and lysozyme (and immune cells) taken up from breast milk for protection of neonatal gut (and respiratory tract)

The primordial source of lymphoid and erythroid cells is the embryonic yolk sac. The pluripotent yolk sac cells appear by the 5th week of gestation and migrate into the liver and the thymus and subsequently into the bone marrow, spleen and lymph nodes. The details of the sequence and pathways of migration are not yet clarified. It is the microenvironment in which the stem cells become located after migration that determines their major direction of differentiation.

Precursors of B lymphocytes are identifiable in the fetal liver by 8 weeks of gestation. During the next 4 weeks they migrate to the bone marrow and are from then on capable of generating B lymphocytes for export to the peripheral circulation (Wosler and Lawton, 1985). A T lymphocyte-specific surface marker (CD2) is first observed on thymocytes at 8–9 weeks of gestation, whilst T cell-specific responses have been detected at 13 weeks using thymic cells in culture with allogeneic lymphocytes (Stutman, 1985). Dendritic cells, expressing HLA class II molecules and capable of functioning as antigen-presenting cells (APC) for the initiation of immune responses, appear as early as 10 weeks of gestation although not in substantial numbers until some weeks later (Beelen et al, 1990). Populations of natural killer (NK) cells develop in the fetal liver after 9 weeks.

It is clear that the full cell repertoire required for cellular and humoral immune responses arises early in fetal development. Although the precise timing of the differentiation of all the specific T lymphocyte subsets remains to be established, this is undoubtedly completed some time before birth, as all the molecules required for the cellular recognition reactions involved in elicitation of immune responses are expressed on cells in cord blood. On the basis of the limited available data it would also appear likely that all the molecules involved in the regulation of immune cell interactions, particularly those of the interleukin family, are produced during fetal life. All the components of complement, except C9, are present from 18 weeks of gestation and occur at levels between 40 and 70% of normal adult values in cord blood at delivery (Adinolfi, 1988).

Clinical and experimental evidence therefore supports the view that the potential for functional immune competence is achieved by the human fetus some considerable time before birth, providing it with a defence system against those infectious agents that are able to breach the intrauterine barriers. This is supplemented by maternal IgG that can also provide immediate protection for the neonate against environmental pathogens not encountered during its earlier intrauterine existence.

SUMMARY

The antigenic status of the preimplantation embryo is ill-defined and there are no clearly recognized maternal immune reactions against this early stage of development. Following implantation, the pregnant female shows evidence of immune recognition of her intrauterine allogeneic conceptus. In a proportion of pregnancies, particularly in multiparous women, there are maternal cytotoxic antibodies exhibiting specificity for the paternally inherited HLA antigens of the fetus. When these are undetectable there may be other antibodies that are non-complement fixing and non-cytotoxic or antibodies that are not present as free molecules and incapable of identification in conventional assays. Anti-HLA antibodies pose no threat to the fetus, principally owing to their absorption by the placenta and, very likely, the harmless binding of any that do reach the fetal circulation.

No potentially deleterious cytotoxic T lymphocyte generation occurs in most pregnancies. The extent to which this is due to maternal immunoregulatory control processes is not yet established. The fetal trophoblast is able to act as a protective barrier by virtue of unique properties, including a lack of conventional class I and class II HLA molecules, that render it insusceptible to immune attack. The nature and significance of any maternal recognition of non-HLA antigens on trophoblast await elucidation.

Maternal immune cell traffic across the placenta occurs only at a very low level, if at all, in normal pregnancy. This may take place to a greater degree in some of the rare instances of fetal graft-versus-host disease, but this is complicated by the associated fetal immunodeficiency.

Maternal IgG antibodies are transmitted across the placental trophoblast by receptor-dependent mechanisms to provide immediate protection for the neonate against environmental pathogens. Leakage of fetal erythrocytes, leukocytes and platelets into the maternal circulation can elicit IgG isoantibodies that take advantage of the same mechanisms to gain access to the fetus, with pathological consequences. Autoantibodies in women with various disease states may similarly pass into the fetus but these normally produce only mild and transient effects.

The development of the fetal immune system begins at an early stage of gestation. It is competent to respond to intrauterine infections from as early as 12 weeks and has full functional potential at birth. Maternally acquired IgG is available for up to 9 months of life until the infant's own immune system has been adequately primed and activated following first exposure to specific antigens.

The normal fetomaternal immune relationship represents a remarkable harmonious association between two genetically disparate individuals. The full details of the manner in which this is established and maintained throughout the period of gestation remain to be elucidated. In the words of William Wordsworth:

'; there is a dark
Inscrutable workmanship that reconciles
Discordant elements, makes them cling together
In one society.'
(*The Prelude*, 1850)

REFERENCES

Adinolfi M (1988) New and old aspects of the ontogeny of immune responses. In Stern CMM (ed.) *Immunology of Pregnancy and its Disorders*, pp 33–59. London: Kluwer Academic Publishers.

Ammann AJ (1986) Fetal and neonatal graft-vs-host and immunodeficiency diseases. In Clark DA & Croy BA (eds) *Reproductive Immunology 1986*, pp 19–26. Amsterdam: Elsevier Science Publishers.

Antczak DF (1989) Maternal antibody responses in pregnancy. *Current Opinion in Immunology* 1: 1135–1140.

Beelen R, van Rees E, Bos H, Kamperdijk E & Dijkstra C (1990) Ontogeny of antigen-presenting cells. In Chaouat G (ed.) *The Immunology of the Fetus*, pp 33–41. Boca Raton, FL:CRC Press.

Beer AE, Quebbeman JF, Ayers JWT & Haines RF (1981) Major histocompatibility complex antigens, maternal and paternal immune responses, and chronic habitual abortions in humans. *American Journal of Obstetrics and Gynecology* 141: 987–999.

Begley DJ, Firth JA & Hoult JRS (1980) *Human Reproduction and Developmental Biology*, p 78. London: Macmillan Press.

Billington WD (1992a) Transfer of antigens and antibodies between mother and fetus. In Coulam CB, Faulk WP & McIntyre JA (eds) *Immunological Obstetrics*, pp 290–304. New York: WW Norton & Co.

Billington WD (1992b) Immunotherapy of recurrent spontaneous miscarriage. In Stabile I, Grudzinskas JG & Chard T (eds) *Spontaneous Abortion: Diagnosis and Treatment*. London: Springer-Verlag (in press).

Billington WD & Davies M (1987) Maternal antibody to placental syncytiotrophoblast during pregnancy. In Gill TJ & Wegmann TG (eds) *Immunoregulation and Fetal Survival*, pp 15–26. New York: Oxford University Press.

Borelli I, Amoroso A, Richiardi P & Curtoni ES (1982) Evaluation of different technical approaches for the researches of human anti-Ia alloantisera. *Tissue Antigens* 19: 127–140.

Bulmer JN & Johnson PM (1985) Antigen expression by trophoblast populations in the human placenta and their possible immunobiological relevance. *Placenta* 6: 127–140.

Covone A, Kozma R, Johnson PM, Latt SA & Adinolfi M (1988) Analysis of peripheral maternal blood samples for the presence of placenta-derived cells using Y-specific probes and McAb H315. *Prenatal Diagnosis* 8: 591.

Davies M (1986) Blocking factors and human pregnancy: an alternative explanation for the success of lymphocyte transfusion therapy in abortion-prone women. *American Journal of Reproductive Immunology and Microbiology* 10: 58–63.

Davies M & Browne CM (1985a) Identification of selectively solubilised syncytiotrophoblast plasma membrane proteins as potential antigenic targets during normal human pregnancy. *Journal of Reproductive Immunology* 8: 33–44.

Davies M & Browne CM (1985b) Anti-trophoblast antibody responses during normal human pregnancy. *Journal of Reproductive Immunology* 7: 285–297.

Desoye G, Dohr GA, Motter W et al (1988) Lack of HLA Class I and Class II antigens on human preimplantation embryos. *Journal of Immunology* 140: 4157–4159.

Doughty RW & Gelsthorpe K (1976) Some parameters of lymphocyte antibody activity through pregnancy and from eluates of placental material. *Tissue Antigens* 8: 43–48.

Douglas GW, Thomas L, Carr M, Cullen NM & Morris R (1959) Trophoblast in the circulating blood during pregnancy. *American Journal of Obstetrics and Gynecology* 78: 960–973.

Downham MPS, Scott R, Sims DG, Webb JKG & Gardner PS (1976) Breast feeding protects against respiratory syncytial virus infection. *British Medical Journal* 2: 274–276.

Ellis SA, Palmer MS & McMichael AJ (1990) Human trophoblast and the choriocarcinoma cell line BeWo express a truncated HLA Class I molecule. *Journal of Immunology* 144: 731–735.

Gill TJ, Repetti CF, Metlay LA et al (1983) Transplacental immunization of the human fetus to tetanus by immunization of the mother. *Journal of Clinical Investigation* 72: 987–996.

Gilman-Sachs A, Beer AE & Beaman KD (1989) Analysis of anti-lymphocyte antibodies by flow cytometry of microlymphocytotoxicity in women with recurrent spontaneous abortions immunized with paternal lymphocytes. *Journal of Clinical Laboratory Immunology* 30: 53–59.

Goldman AS, Ham Pong AJ & Goldblum RM (1985) Host defenses: development and maternal contributions. *Advances in Pediatrics* 32: 71–100.

Grubb R (1970) *The Genetic Markers of Human Immunoglobulins*. London: Chapman & Hall.

Hanson LA, Ahlstedt S, Andersson B et al (1984) The immune response of the mammary gland and its significance for the neonate. *Annals of Allergy* 53: 576–582.

Head JR (1977) Immunobiology of lactation. *Seminars in Perinatology* 1: 195–210.

Hole N, Cheng HM & Johnson PM (1987) Antibody activity against human trophoblast antigens in the context of normal pregnancy and unexplained recurrent miscarriage? *Colloque INSERM* 154: 213–224.

Hunt JS & Hsi B-L (1990) Evasive strategies of trophoblast cells: selective expression of membrane antigens. *American Journal of Reproductive Immunology* 23: 57–63.

Hunziker RD & Wegmann TG (1986) Placental immunoregulation. *CRC Critical Reviews in Immunology* 6: 245–285.

Iklé FA (1964) Dissemination von Syncytiotrophoblastzellen im mütterlichen Blut während der Gravidität. *Bulletin der Schweizerischen Akademie der Medizinischen Wissenschaften* 20: 62–71.

Iverson GM, Bianchi DW, Cann HM & Herzenberg LA (1981) The detection and isolation of fetal cells from maternal blood using the fluorescence-activated cell sorter (FACS). *Prenatal Diagnosis* 1: 61–73.

Johnson PM, Faulk WP & Wang A-C (1976) Immunological studies of human placenta: the distribution and character of immunoglobulins in chorionic villi. *Clinical and Experimental Immunology* 30: 145–153.

Jones WR & Need JA (1988) Maternal-fetal cell surface antigen incompatibilities. *Baillière's Clinical Immunology and Allergy* 2: 577–605.

King A, Kalra P & Loke YW (1990) Human trophoblast cell resistance to decidual NK lysis is due to lack of NK target structure. *Cellular Immunology* 127: 230–237.

Kovats S, Main EK, Librach C, Stubblebine M, Fisher SJ & DeMars R (1990) A Class I antigen, HLA-G, expressed in human trophoblasts. *Science* 248: 220–223.

Kovats S, Librach C, Fisch P et al (1991) Expression and possible function of the HLA-G α chain in human cytotrophoblasts. *Colloque INSERM* 212: 21–29.

Loke YW (1990) Experimenting with human extravillous trophoblast: a personal view. *American Journal of Reproductive Immunology* 24: 22–28.

McCormick JB, Gusmao HH, Nakamura S et al (1980) Antibody response to serogroup A and C meningococcal polysaccharide vaccines in infants born to mothers vaccinated during pregnancy. *Journal of Clinical Investigation* 65: 1141–1144.

McIntyre JA, Faulk WP, Verhulst SJ & Colliver JA (1984) Human trophoblast lymphocyte cross-reactive (TLX) antigens define a new alloantigen system. *Science* 222: 1135–1137.

Malley M (1989) The immune response of offspring mice from mothers immunized during pregnancy with protein antigens. *Journal of Reproductive Immunology* 16: 173–186.

Menu E, Kaplan L, Andreu G, Denver L & Chaouat G (1989) Immunoactive products of human placenta. I. An immunoregulatory factor obtained from explant cultures of human placenta inhibits CTL generation and cytotoxic effector activity. *Cellular Immunology* 119: 341–352.

Michel M, Underwood J, Clark DA, Mowbray J & Beard RW (1989) Histologic and immunologic study of uterine biopsy tissue of incipiently aborting women. *American Journal of Obstetrics and Gynecology* 161: 409–414.

Mowbray JF, Gibbings C, Liddell H, Reginald PW, Underwood JL & Beard RW (1985) Controlled trial of treatment of recurrent spontaneous abortion by immunization with paternal cells. *Lancet* i: 941–943.

Papadogiannakis N, Johnsen SA & Olding LB (1990) Suppressor cell activity in human cord blood. In Chaouat G (ed.) *The Immunology of the Fetus*, pp 215–227. Boca Raton, FL: CRC Press.

Pitcher-Wilmott RW, Hindocha P & Wood CBS (1980) The placental transfer of IgG subclasses in human pregnancy. *Clinical and Experimental Immunology* 41: 303–308.

Pollack MS, Kirkpatrick D, Kapoor N, Dupont B & O'Reilly RJ (1982) Identification by HLA typing of intra-uterine derived maternal T cells in four patients with severe combined immunodeficiency. *New England Journal of Medicine* 307: 662–666.

Power DA, Catto GRD, Mason RJ, MacLeod AM, Steward KN & Shewan WG (1983) The fetus as an allograft: evidence for protective antibodies to HLA-linked paternal antigens. *Lancet* ii: 701–704.

Pross H, Mitchell H & Werkmeister J (1985) The sensitivity of placental trophoblast cells to intraplacental and allogeneic cytotoxic lymphocytes. *American Journal of Reproductive Immunology and Microbiology* 8: 1–9.

Quayle AJ, Kelly RW, Hargreave TB & James K (1989) Immunosuppression by seminal prostaglandins. *Clinical and Experimental Immunology* **75:** 387–391.

Reed E, Beer AE, Hutcherson H, King DW & Suciu-Foca N (1991) The alloantibody response of pregnant women and its suppression by soluble HLA antigens and anti-idiotypic antibodies. *Journal of Reproductive Immunology* **20:** 115–128.

Regan L & Braude PR (1987) Is antipaternal cytotoxic antibody a valid marker in the management of recurrent abortion? *Lancet* **ii:** 1280.

Roberts JM, Taylor CT, Melling GC, Kingsland CR & Johnson PM (1992) Expression of the CD46 antigen, and absence of Class I MHC antigen on the human oocyte and preimplantation blastocyst. *Immunology* **75:** 202–205.

Sargent IL, Arenas J & Redman CWG (1987) Maternal CMI to paternal HLA may occur but is not a regular event in normal human pregnancy. *Journal of Reproductive Immunology* **10:** 111–120.

Stutman O (1985) Ontogeny of T cells. *Clinical Immunology and Allergy* **5:** 191–234.

Takeuchi S (1990) Is production of blocking antibodies in successful human pregnancy an epiphenomenon? *American Journal of Reproductive Immunology* **24:** 108–119.

Taylor C & Faulk WP (1981) Prevention of recurrent abortion with leucocyte transfusions. *Lancet* **ii:** 68–70.

Taylor PV (1988) Autoimmunity and pregnancy. *Baillière's Clinical Immunology and Allergy* **2:** 665–696.

Tongio MM, Mayer S & Lebec A (1975) Transfer of HLA antibodies from the mother to the child. *Transplantation* **20:** 163–166.

Vives J, Gelabert A & Castillo R (1976) HLA antibodies and period of gestation: decline in frequency of positive sera during last trimester. *Tissue Antigens* **7:** 209–212.

Wild AE (1983) Trophoblast cell surface receptors. In Loke YW & Whyte A (eds) *Biology of Trophoblast*, pp 471–512. Amsterdam: Elsevier.

Wosler LB & Lawton R (1985) Ontogeny of B cells and humoral immune functions. *Clinical Immunology and Allergy* **5:** 235–252.

3

Complement and pregnancy: new insights into the immunobiology of the fetomaternal relationship

CHRISTOPHER H. HOLMES
KAREN L. SIMPSON

Traditionally, complement has been held to comprise a series of proteins that interact effectively and in consort to eliminate micro-organisms. In mammals the system represents a highly sophisticated descendant of an evolutionarily ancient recognition and effector system whose primary function would have been to defend the host from infection. There is evidence to suggest that this ancestral progenitor of the complement system was in place prior to the evolution of an adaptive immune response based on immunoglobulin-dependent antigen recognition. Although antibody-independent access to the effector activity of complement through the alternative pathway has long been recognized, it has nevertheless commonly been assumed that the classical pathway, mediated through antigen–antibody recognition, is of primary importance in activating complement and that the alternative pathway is involved in amplification. Recently, however, the emerging view has been of a complex and subtle complement system that represents much more than an effector for antibody responses. Crucial to these developments has been the discovery of a family of membrane-bound proteins which function to regulate complement activity. These advances have already had considerable impact on reproductive biology not least because several studies have recently documented the presence of complement regulatory proteins on human placental trophoblast. The discovery of a new group of immunologically relevant regulatory proteins on this tissue has implications for our understanding of the immunobiology of the fetomaternal relationship during pregnancy.

THE COMPLEMENT SYSTEM—AN OVERVIEW

An overview of the complement system is schematically presented in Figure 1. The third component of complement, C3, occupies a pivotal position in the system linking components of the activation pathways with the terminal pathway components C5–9 that generate the membrane attack complex (for

Baillière's Clinical Obstetrics and Gynaecology—
Vol. 6, No. 3, September 1992
ISBN 0–7020–1634–9

439

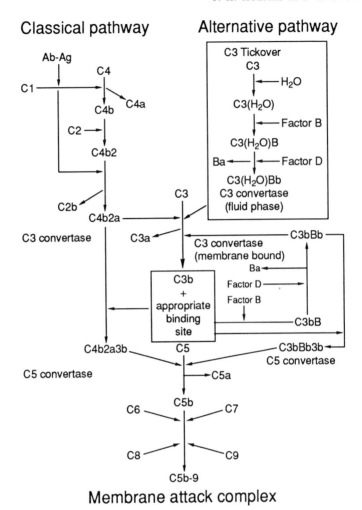

Figure 1. The complement system showing the two activation pathways leading to the formation of convertase enzymes which permit access to the membrane attack complex.

reviews see Campbell et al, 1988; Kinoshita, 1991). C3 possesses an internal thioester bond which is exposed on activation and can form covalent linkages with amino or hydroxyl groups on surfaces (Law et al, 1979). In this way the activated form of C3, C3b, can bind to a variety of surfaces which are potential targets of the complement system. C3b deposited on surfaces can represent a focus for further amplification of the complement cascade and this in turn can unleash the destructive potential of complement on an appropriate target through assembly of the cytolytic membrane attack complex (Muller-Eberhard, 1986). Enzymes known as C3 convertases, which are themselves assembled from complement components, activate C3 to form C3b. The function of the two complement pathways, the alternative and classical pathways, is to generate these C3 activating enzymes. Discrimination within the complement system hinges on the mechanisms that allow these enzymes to be assembled (Atkinson and Farries, 1987).

In the case of the classical pathway, activation is primarily triggered by interaction of subcomponent C1q of the C1 complex with the Fc portion of immunoglobulins (Sim and Reid, 1991). Activated C1 then splits C4 to generate C4a, a pro-inflammatory anaphylatoxin, together with a larger C4b fragment (Schumaker et al, 1987). In common with C3, C4 has a labile internal thioester bond which becomes accessible on cleavage so that C4b has the transient ability to bind to surfaces. The lability of the exposed thioester bond limits C4b binding only to surfaces within the vicinity of the activating C1 complex. C4b can also bind C2, and the C2 component of the resulting C4b2 complex is then also cleaved by the activated C1 complex to generate C4b2a, the classical pathway C3 convertase (Muller-Eberhard, 1988). Since the classical pathway is triggered primarily by immunoglobulin, discrimination within the system is largely dictated by antibody selecting its appropriate target.

It has been known for some time that foreign surfaces exposed to human serum become coated with C3b by a mechanism that is independent of immunoglobulin (Reid and Porter, 1981). This observation encapsulates the dilemma posed by the alternative pathway of complement. How is C3 activated in the absence of classical pathway activators and how is the alternative pathway capable of discriminating between target and host surfaces? The solution to this dilemma appears to lie both in the intrinsic properties of C3 itself and in the identification of a group of regulatory proteins that function to control activated complement components.

Access to complement through the alternative pathway is initially dependent on an unusual biological property of C3 (Law et al, 1980; Lachmann and Hughes-Jones, 1984). The internal thioester bond within the molecule is inherently unstable and, in the absence of any specific activator or convertase enzyme, a small proportion of C3 undergoes spontaneous hydrolysis to form the intermediate $C3(H_2O)$. $C3(H_2O)$ has a C3b-like conformation and can combine with factor B to generate a fluid phase complex, $C3(H_2O)B$. In the presence of factor D, $C3(H_2O)B$ is cleaved to generate a bimolecular complex $C3(H_2O)Bb$, a fluid phase C3 convertase which can cleave C3 to generate C3b (see Figure 1). Through its exposed thioester bond C3b can deposit on surfaces, combine with factor B, and generate the membrane-bound alternative pathway C3 convertase C3bBb. Assembly of a C3 convertase enzyme has the potential to permit the formation of further C3bBb and hence amplification of C3 cleavage and deposition.

The concept of spontaneous hydrolysis of C3, 'C3 tickover', provides a clear picture of how amplification through the alternative pathway is initiated on a foreign surface. On a bacterial cell wall, for example, C3b is at first deposited spontaneously but subsequent assembly of the alternative pathway C3 convertase amplifies C3b deposition and allows the full destructive potential of the complement system to be realized. In particular, C3b combines with either alternative or classical pathway C3 convertases to generate trimolecular C5 convertases (C3bBb3b or C4b2a3b) which split C5 to generate C5b (Figure 1). This initiates the self-assembly of C6 to C9 forming the cytolytic membrane attack complex. In addition, C3b and its split products can bind complement receptors (CR1 and CR3) expressed on phagocytic cells and cleavage of C5, C3 and C4 generates anaphylatoxins, especially C5a and C3a, which activate macrophages, mast cells and basophils. The coordinated response provides an effective attack against the appropriate surface that permits alternative pathway amplification to occur.

The problem has been, however, in understanding how in the alternative pathway the distinction between target and host surfaces is achieved. C3b generated as a result of C3 tickover, or indeed from classical pathway activation, is indiscriminate and will bind to host as well as foreign surfaces. In the classical pathway, deposition occurs primarily in the vicinity of antigen–antibody complexes but in the alternative pathway low level C3b deposition occurs on any autologous cell surface that is exposed to circulating C3. Host cells therefore appeared to be capable in some way of preventing amplification of activated complement components deposited on their surfaces but the mechanism by which this was achieved proved elusive.

The existence of a number of plasma proteins which function to regulate the activity of the complement system in the fluid phase has been known for some time. Not surprisingly in view of their critical role in amplification, C3 convertases represent a primary focus for regulation. Thus, factor H acts as a co-factor for the cleavage of C3b by factor I and similarly, C4 binding protein (C4bp) acts as a co-factor for factor I-mediated cleavage of C4b. However, whereas factor H and C4bp can efficiently control complement activation in the fluid phase, these proteins are generally considered to be ineffective regulators of complement amplification on tissue and cell surfaces. Over the past few years a series of membrane-bound regulatory proteins of the complement system have been discovered which are now accepted to play an essential role in protecting host cells from autologous complement damage (reviewed in Hourcade et al, 1989). The discovery of these proteins has provided an attractive mechanism which accounts for the apparent discriminatory capacity of the alternative pathway; target surfaces such as bacterial cell walls for the most part do not express proteins capable of down-regulating C3b amplification. Host tissues, on the other hand, are equipped with several regulatory proteins that can act rapidly to inhibit C3 convertases, thereby preventing access to the terminal effector functions of complement.

MEMBRANE REGULATORS OF THE COMPLEMENT SYSTEM

The existence of an effector system with the capacity to amplify an initial signal to generate large quantities of activated products brings with it an obligatory requirement for stringent control mechanisms. The importance of control in the complement system in a general sense is indicated by the fact that there are at least as many proteins involved in essential regulatory function as there are components of the pathways themselves. Control

Table 1. Properties of membrane-bound complement regulatory proteins.

Regulator	CD* designation	Membrane linkage	Molecular weight (kDa)	Ligand specificity	Functional activity
DAF	CD55	PI-link	70	C3bBb/C4b2a C3b/C4b	Prevents formation and accelerates decay C3/C5 convertase
MCP	CD46	Transmembrane	45–70	C3b/C4b	Co-factor for factor I
MAC inhibitor	CD59	PI-link	18–20	C5b–8	Prevents assembly of MAC

* Refers to the uniform nomenclature system in which surface markers, originally on lymphocytes, that (a) identify a particular lineage or differentiation stage, (b) have a defined structure and (c) are recognized by a variety of monoclonal antibodies, are assigned a CD or 'cluster of differentiation' number. Complement regulatory proteins all have CD numbers in addition to their more functionally descriptive designations.

proteins act at virtually every stage of the complement system either preventing spontaneous activation or inhibiting or enhancing the action of complement against its target. Thus, while regulation at the level of the C3 convertases is clearly very important, control is also exerted at other levels both proximal and distal to the convergent amplification step. In terms of

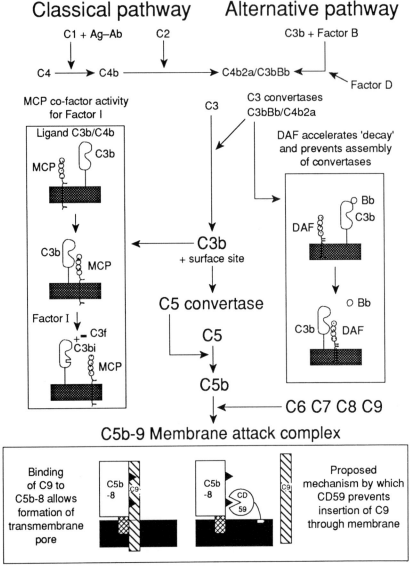

Figure 2. Schematic representation of the mechanism of action of the membrane-bound complement regulatory proteins DAF, MCP, and CD59 (modified from Hourcade et al, 1989; Lublin and Atkinson, 1988; Meri et al, 1990; Rollins et al, 1991).

protection of host cell membranes from complement, attention has focused on three proteins that act at two distinct levels of the complement cascade; the C3 convertases and the membrane attack complex (Figure 2 and Table 1).

C3 convertase regulators

General features

There are two membrane regulators of C3 convertases, decay accelerating factor (DAF, CD55) and membrane co-factor protein (MCP, CD46). These proteins exhibit structural and functional similarities and both are encoded within the so-called regulators of complement activation (RCA) gene cluster which maps to band q32 on chromosome 1 (Carroll et al, 1988; Rey-Campos et al, 1988; Bora et al, 1989). This cluster also encodes several other proteins involved in the control of C3 convertases including CR1, CR2, factor H and C4bp. The linkage group as a whole therefore represents the regulatory counterpart of the MHC class III gene cluster on chromosome 6 which encodes the structural components of the C3 convertases themselves, C4, C2 and factor B (Figure 3).

DAF and MCP, in common with 12 other complement-related proteins (including the RCA cluster proteins and several non-complement products) share a common repeating 60–70 amino acid motif known as a short consensus repeat (SCR) (Campbell et al, 1988; Hourcade et al, 1989). These SCRs appear to represent structural building blocks for the regulatory proteins and possess the C3 and C4 binding domains. DAF and MCP each contain four contiguous SCRs located in the N-terminal region of the

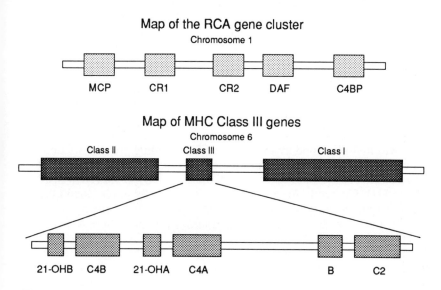

Figure 3. Organization of genes within the MHC class III region and the RCA cluster.

molecule. Despite these similarities and the fact that they both act at the same level of the complement cascade the two regulatory proteins differ in their functional activities and also in the structural properties of their C-terminal domains.

DAF

DAF was originally detected as a complement inhibitory activity present in extracts of human red cells and was subsequently isolated as a 70 kDa glycoprotein (Hoffman, 1969; Nicholson-Weller et al, 1982; Davitz, 1987; Lublin and Atkinson, 1989). The designation refers to its functional activity observed in these studies. C3 convertases are inherently unstable and spontaneously decay to release Bb (alternative pathway convertase) or 2a (classical pathway convertase). DAF was found to accelerate the rate of this decay, a property it shares with CR1, C4bp and factor H. Subsequent studies were to show that DAF also binds to deposited C3b and C4b fragments, thereby inhibiting the formation of both alternative and classical pathway convertases by preventing access of factor B or C2 (Figure 2). This functional activity, inhibition of assembly and acceleration of decay, is co-factor independent and reversible. Thus, following interaction with DAF, the complement components C3b and C4b remain intact. DAF activity is also strictly intrinsic; the molecule can interact only with convertases or activated components assembled or deposited on the same cell on which DAF itself is expressed; unlike CR1, for example, DAF cannot interact with these components on neighbouring cells or foreign surfaces.

Finally, DAF belongs to a family of proteins including acetylcholinesterase, placental alkaline phosphatase, 5'-nucleotidase, and the cell adhesion molecule LFA-3, that are attached to the outer leaflet of the cell membrane by a glycolipid anchor containing phosphatidylinositol (PI). It has been suggested that PI anchorage may facilitate lateral mobility within the lipid bilayer and, more specifically in the case of DAF, this might allow the molecule to move freely and rapidly to encounter complement components deposited randomly on the cell surface (Davitz, 1987; Furguson and Williams, 1988).

MCP

MCP was first identified as a membrane C3b binding protein isolated from human lymphocytes and migrating electrophoretically in the form of two broad bands of 59–68 and 50–58 kDa (Cole et al, 1985; reviewed in Liszewski et al, 1991). Currently there is considerable interest in the possibility that multiple isoforms may be generated from a single MCP gene by alternative splicing and by the use of different cytoplasmic tails, and there is speculation that these different isoforms may be expressed in different tissues (Purcell et al, 1990b). Recently, evidence has been presented to suggest that the two MCP species observed on SDS gels may arise as a result of differential splicing of a single specific exon (exon 13) within the MCP gene. The higher molecular weight electrophoretic variant is also known to contain more sialic acid. Interestingly, there is an inherited variability in the relative quantity of the two components which generates three characteristic patterns on SDS gels. On this basis individuals can be designated either upper band predominant, lower band predominant or equal band predominant (Ballard et al, 1987). These differences are consistent with a co-dominantly inherited expression polymorphism in the protein (Bora et al, 1991).

MCP along with the RCA cluster proteins CR1, C4bp and factor H are all co-factors for the important fluid phase serine protease control protein, factor I (see Holers et al, 1985). Factor I, in the presence of one or other of its co-factors, proteolytically cleaves C3b or C4b to generate the inactive derivatives iC3b or iC4b (Figure 2). This first cleavage exposes a second I-mediated cleavage site which allows further proteolysis to occur, generating degradative products C3c and C3d,g or C4c and C4d. CR1 is a co-factor for both cleavage steps while MCP and factor H are co-factors for only the first cleavage step. By contrast with DAF, therefore, MCP has no decay accelerating activity and its function is co-factor dependent and irreversible. In common with DAF, however, it appears to function as an intrinsic regulator of membrane-bound C3b or C4b.

Because DAF and MCP are almost always co-expressed on cell surfaces, it is likely that their overlapping functional activities (summarized in Table 1) allow them to act synergistically to control complement activation on host tissues (for example, see Seya et al, 1990b).

Regulators of the membrane attack complex (MAC)

Complement-mediated attack against an appropriate target allows formation of C3 and then C5 convertase enzymes which split C5 to C5b. Freshly activated C5b, loosely bound to C3b within a trimolecular C5 convertase, binds C6 and then C7 to generate C5b–7. Binding of C7 induces a conformational change in the C5b–7 complex, releasing it from the C5 convertase and exposing a transient membrane-binding site. At this point, therefore, the C5b–7 complex can bind both to target surfaces and to bystander host cells within their vicinity. Incorporation of C8 into the C5b–7 complex on membranes directs incorporation and polymerization of C9 to generate the cytolytic MAC. C9 within this complex completely traverses the membrane and allows the formation of functional pores which can lead to osmotic cell lysis (see Morgan, 1989, 1990).

Formation of the MAC is strictly regulated and for some time this was thought to be mediated solely by fluid phase proteins, particularly by S-protein which binds to C5b–7, forming an SC5b–7 complex and blocking membrane incorporation. Recently, however, several membrane proteins have been discovered which modulate the activity of the MAC. In experimental systems the inhibitory activity of these proteins can be effectively demonstrated in the absence of activation pathway proteins by reactive lysis; reactive lysis requires only the presence of the terminal complement components C6–9 (Lachmann, 1991). Attention has focused predominantly on the membrane attack inhibitory protein CD59.

CD59

This molecule was discovered independently by several laboratories and has been variously designated as P-18 (Sugita et al, 1988), HRF-20 (Okada et al, 1989), H19 (Groux et al, 1989; Whitlow et al, 1989), MIRL (Holguin et al, 1989), MEM-43 (Stefanova et al, 1989) and CD59 (Davies et al, 1989). It is an 18–20 kDa PI-linked glycoprotein which does not bear a structural resemblance to other complement-related proteins (see Table 1 for comparison with DAF and MCP) but shares structural homology at the primary sequence level with the murine Ly-6 family of antigens. CD59 is encoded on the short arm of chromosome 11.

CD59 acts at the final stages of MAC formation (Meri et al, 1990; Rollins et al, 1991) by binding to an epitope on C8 which is exposed when C8 is incorporated into the C5b–7 complex on membranes (Figure 2). C5b–8 complexes can incorporate one molecule of C9 in the presence of CD59 but insertion of the C9 into the membrane appears to be blocked and, moreover, recruitment of additional C9 molecules to the membrane attack complex also appears to be prevented by CD59.

Tissue distribution of complement regulatory proteins

In the first instance, complement regulatory proteins were studied primarily on red cells (CD59 and DAF) or lymphocytes (MCP). However, in parallel with advances in our understanding of their functional role in controlling complement activity has come the realization that they are not confined solely to circulating blood cells and that they display a very broad tissue distribution. Expression of DAF, MCP and CD59 has now been documented on endothelial cells and at multiple epithelial locations (Asch et al, 1986; Medof et al, 1987; McNearney et al, 1989; Nose et al, 1990; Meri et al, 1991). The three proteins appear frequently to be co-expressed and this, together with their broad expression profile, has been generally interpreted to reflect the importance of their role in providing protection of host tissues from autologous complement-mediated damage.

EXPRESSION OF MEMBRANE-BOUND COMPLEMENT REGULATORY PROTEINS ON TROPHOBLAST

The expression of membrane-bound complement regulatory proteins on human placental trophoblast suggests that these products may play an important role in pregnancy. Trophoblast is an epithelium unique to pregnancy and, in its various anatomically and morphologically defined forms located within the placenta and extra-fetal membranes, provides a continuous intact surface which separates the fetus from the mother throughout gestation. It is primarily over this surface that the maternal immune system is directly and continuously exposed to the semi-allogeneic fetoplacental unit. Although it has long been supposed that trophoblast must hold the key to understanding the fetomaternal relationship in immunological terms, the search for products with immunoregulatory function on this epithelium has proved elusive. Complement regulatory proteins are broadly distributed on many cells and tissues, including those of the pregnant mother, where they function to protect the host from autologous complement-mediated damage. However, their expression on trophoblast may have specific implications in the context of the fetomaternal relationship.

The observation that DAF is expressed on trophoblast emerged unexpectedly from a study originally designed to explore the ontogeny of human blood group antigens (Holmes et al, 1990; Anstee et al, 1992). It was found that antibodies detecting a blood group antigen system known as Cromer consistently bound to trophoblast in human placental tissue sections by immunostaining. A striking feature of this reactivity was its preferential localization to trophoblast surfaces in contact with maternal blood and tissues (Figure 4). This was most evident in first trimester placentae. At this early stage of placental development chorionic villi are covered by two layers of trophoblast: an inner cellular cytotrophoblast cell layer from which an outer acellular syncytiotrophoblast layer arises by differentiation. The apical aspect of the syncytiotrophoblast layer is bathed in maternal blood circulating in the intervillous spaces and is the major component of the fetomaternal interface. Anti-Cromer reactivity was found to be associated predominantly with this apical syncytiotrophoblast brush border; the underlying cytotrophoblast layer, which is not directly exposed to maternal blood, showed little or no reactivity. Similarly, other trophoblast populations in contact with maternal tissues and blood throughout gestation were also reactive. By contrast there appeared to be relatively little anti-Cromer reactivity within the early fetus itself, even in the fetal liver which is a major site of haemopoiesis during mammalian development and which contains large numbers of erythroid precursors whose derivatives in the adult express Cromer-related antigens (Holmes et al, 1990). The significance of the observed expression of a red cell blood group antigen system at the fetomaternal interface during human development was at first unclear.

The Cromer system comprises at least eight high frequency and three low frequency red cell antigens (Daniels, 1989). The designation derives originally from the name of a black antenatal patient who was found to have an antibody which reacted with over 4000 black donors but not with her own cells. The antigens were known to be carried on a 70 kDa red cell glycoprotein (Spring et al, 1987) and, in immunoblotting studies using isolated syncytiotrophoblast membranes as targets, anti-Cromer antibodies were also found to detect a 70 kDa trophoblast component (Figure 5 and Holmes et al, 1990). Thus, the anti-Cromer reactivity appeared to be carried on a similar product on both trophoblast and red cells. At the time, however, the function of this protein was unknown. Subsequent studies carried out by two groups working independently were to reveal that the Cromer antigen system was in fact carried on the 70 kDa complement regulatory protein DAF (Parsons et al, 1988; Telen et al, 1988). Immunostaining studies on the placenta were therefore demonstrating that DAF was expressed at the fetomaternal interface. The well characterized functional activity of DAF in

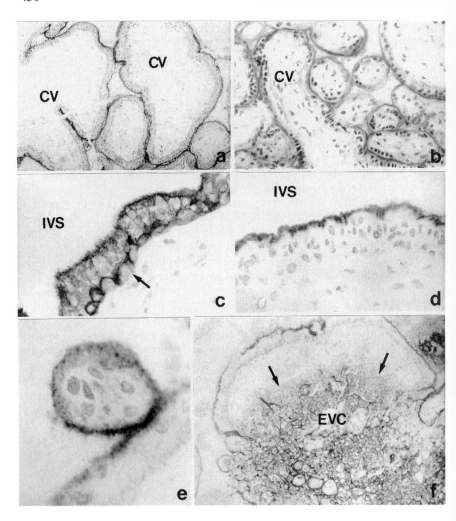

Figure 4. Reactivity of anti-Cromer antibodies by immunoperoxidase staining on the developing human placenta. The antibodies stain the trophoblast epithelium surrounding chorionic villi (CV) in both first trimester (a, × 40, reproduced at 66% of original) and term (b, × 100, reproduced at 66% of original) placental specimens. At higher magnification, in (c), antibody Le61 against cytokeratins reveals the inner cytotrophoblast (arrow) and outer syncytiotrophoblast layers in a first-trimester chorionic villus (× 160, reproduced at 66% of original). Anti-Cromer reactivity shown in (d) (× 160, reproduced at 66% of original), is largely confined to the outer aspect of the syncytiotrophoblast layer in contact with maternal blood circulating in the intervillous spaces (IVS). A similar pattern is evident in (e), where a syncytial sprout is apparently being released from the villous syncytiotrophoblast in a first-trimester specimen (× 320, reproduced at 66% of original). Cytotrophoblast cells are reactive where they have proliferated through the overlying syncytiotrophoblast of a first-trimester chorionic villus to generate extravillous cytotrophoblast cells columns (EVC, f, × 50, reproduced at 66% of original). Cells at the base of the column, proximal to the villus itself are largely unstained. (From Holmes et al, 1990).

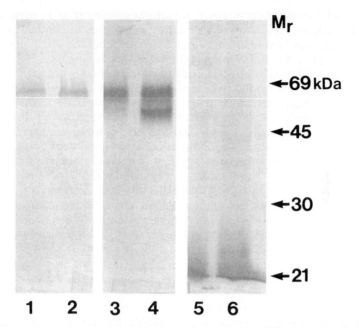

Figure 5. Western analysis of components identified by monoclonal antibodies to DAF (tracks 1 and 2), MCP (tracks 3 and 4) and CD59 (tracks 5 and 6) on syncytiotrophoblast plasma membranes isolated from first-trimester (tracks 1, 3 and 5) and term (tracks 2, 4 and 6) placentae. Non-equivalent quantities of protein were loaded on this gel to maximize the signal from first-trimester membranes. The position of molecular weight markers is indicated by the arrows.

other systems suggested that this molecule could play an important role in protecting the developing semi-allogeneic conceptus from maternal complement. Moreover, these observations also suggested that from an early stage in its development the fetus appeared able to contribute to its own survival in utero by directing expression of this immunoregulatory protein to the fetomaternal interface.

Although the trophoblast epithelium is fetally derived and therefore semi-allogeneic with respect to the mother, there is in fact little evidence to suggest that trophoblast necessarily expresses products that are perceived as immunologically foreign by the mother. For example, trophoblast does not express classically defined polymorphic MHC products which provoke cellular rejection responses in transplants. In terms of its exposure to the maternal complement system, therefore, it is important to consider the extent to which there are factors at work which could suggest that trophoblast is particularly at risk from maternal complement-mediated damage.

From the time of blastocyst implantation, the maternal complement system is directly exposed, *de novo* in primiparous pregnancies, to a rapidly expanding and ultimately very large epithelial surface that is derived entirely from the fetus. Direct deposition of C3b through spontaneous tickover of maternal C3 could allow alternative pathway amplification to occur at this site. In addition, the human placenta is also known to contain maternal immunoglobulin. There has been much debate about the origin of this and about its significance for pregnancy (for review see Billington, 1988; Sargent et al, 1988). Certainly, although trophoblast itself does not express these antigens, maternal antibody responses to fetal HLA and blood group antigens are generated in some pregnancies (particularly in multiparous women) and maternal antibody with these specificities can be eluted from placental tissue. It is also known that the fetus in utero acquires maternal immunoglobulins by transplacental transmission. The precise details remain unclear but it is assumed that placental immunoglobulin, much of it presumably bound to Fc receptors, is associated with this process. Clearly, transport of immunoglobulins with anti-fetal specificities across the placenta could have deleterious consequences and the view has arisen that the placenta can in some way act as an immunoabsorbant or shielding barrier (Head and Billingham, 1984) although, again, the mechanism remains unclear. Notwithstanding this, the possible presence of non-Fc receptor-bound immunoglobulins and immune complexes within the placenta might permit C4b deposition and therefore classical pathway activation at the trophoblast surface. Finally, trophoblast may also be at risk from the deposition, in a bystander fashion, of activated complement components following microbial infection in the mother. Protection against classical pathway activation is not necessarily the most important function of DAF on trophoblast; most likely the molecule could act rapidly and efficiently to restrict the formation of C3 convertases arising as a result of any or all of the above mechanisms.

In other systems where this has been examined, complement regulation on host tissues does not appear to depend solely on the activity of a single regulatory protein but rather reflects an interplay between the two C3 convertase regulators DAF and MCP together with the membrane attack complex inhibitory protein CD59. It has recently become apparent that, in addition to DAF, both MCP and CD59 are also expressed on trophoblast (Figures 5 and 6). Although all three proteins are expressed on trophoblast in contact with maternal blood and tissues, expression of MCP and CD59, unlike that of DAF, is not confined preferentially to this interface. In fact each of the three complement regulatory proteins displays a characteristic reactivity profile in the developing placenta (Holmes et al, 1992).

A 55–65 kDa component expressed by trophoblast throughout gestation was identified some time ago but only recently has it been shown that this represents MCP (Purcell et al, 1990a). The product was originally supposed to represent a member of the so-called TLX family of antigens. TLX is a hypothetical trophoblast–leukocyte cross-reactive (TLX) antigen system that is held to be involved in fetomaternal recognition and immuno-regulation (Faulk et al, 1978; McIntyre et al, 1984). Especially in view of its molecular weight heterogeneity between placentae, the 55–65 kDa component was viewed as a particularly attractive candidate TLX antigen (Stern et al, 1986). It is now clear that this heterogeneity is likely to reflect both inherent differences in glycosylation of the two products as well as the

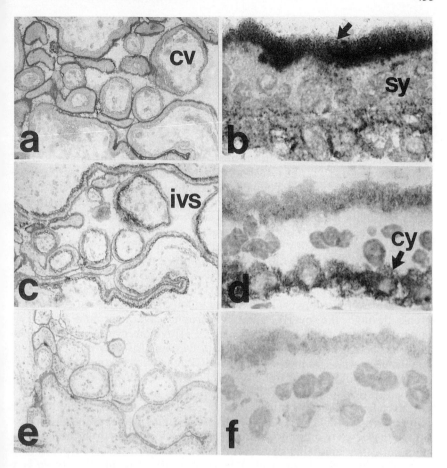

Figure 6. Immunostaining of adjacent sections of first trimester (approximately 7 weeks of gestation) human placenta with monoclonal antibodies to CD59 (a, b), MCP (c, d), and DAF (e, f). The general distribution of staining on chorionic villi (CV) is shown at low magnification in (a), (c) and (e) ($\times 40$, reproduced at 66% of original). IVS, intervillous space. Note the presence of DAF^{+} and DAF^{-} chorionic villi in (e). The distribution of reactivity on villous syncytiotrophoblast (SY) and on underlying villous cytotrophoblast cells (CY) is shown in more detail in (b), (d), and (f) ($\times 400$, reproduced at 66% of original). Arrow in (b) identifies the apical aspect of the syncytiotrophoblast membrane in contact with maternal blood in the intervillous space. Note particularly the differential distribution of anti-MCP and anti-DAF reactivity on villous cytotrophoblast cells in (d) and (f), respectively. (From Holmes et al, 1992).

inherited variability in the relative proportions of the upper and lower MCP components. Even where this expression polymorphism varies between a particular fetomaternal combination (for example, an upper predominant trophoblast pattern in a lower predominant maternal host) there is no evidence that this could be significant in the context of the original TLX concept involving cognate recognition. On the contrary, all individuals express both MCP components and differential tissue expression profiles may reflect a normal distribution of multiple MCP isoforms between different locations. In any case, a maternal anti-fetal antibody response to trophoblast MCP could interfere with what is likely to be the most important function of this product on trophoblast, that of regulating maternal complement by controlling C3b/C4b deposition at the fetomaternal interface.

The different functional activities of the two C3 convertase regulatory proteins are complementary and these two products are normally co-expressed on a variety of normal tissues where they appear to act in consort to control complement activation. In a recent study the distribution of DAF and MCP on the various trophoblast populations present throughout placental development has been directly compared (Figure 6 and Holmes et al, 1992). Both proteins are present on the terminally differentiated syncytiotrophoblast brush border in contact with maternal blood from the earliest stages of gestation (about 6 weeks) examined. However, apparent differences in expression occur on the underlying villous cytotrophoblast cells; these are largely devoid of DAF but appear to contain abundant MCP (Figure 6). Apparent differential expression of the two proteins was also observed on first trimester extravillous cytotrophoblast cell columns. These columns arise following proliferation of villous cytotrophoblast cells which break through the overlying syncytiotrophoblast layer and enter the maternal milieu of the intervillous space. Extravillous cytotrophoblast cells show an increase in anti-DAF reactivity by comparison with their villous counterparts while, in the case of anti-MCP reactivity, the reverse seems to occur—extravillous cytotrophoblast cells show much less reactivity than villous cytotrophoblast cells. One possibility is that this difference, which has also been noted by others (Hsi et al, 1991), may be related to the differentiation status of cells within these columns; changes in the expression of these two regulators according to the maturational or differentiation status of other epithelial or tumour cells have been observed previously (Medof et al, 1987; Seya et al, 1990a). It is also possible that there is a differential requirement for the specific functional activity of a particular product at different locations within the placental epithelium. Further differences in the expression of these proteins have become evident. Thus, levels of DAF appear to be relatively low during early placental development by comparison with MCP and, again in contrast to MCP, both DAF^+ and DAF^- chorionic villi are observed in early placental specimens (Holmes et al, 1992). Clearly, these are areas that merit further investigation.

Expression of CD59 on placental tissue has been noted by Meri et al (1991). Recent studies have also demonstrated that CD59 is ubiquitously expressed both by trophoblast and mesenchymal components throughout placental development (Figure 6 and Holmes et al, 1992). In addition and in line with other systems where this has been explored, there is evidence to suggest that expression of CD59 is higher on trophoblast than that of the C3 convertase regulatory proteins. Thus, trophoblast appears to be protected not only against the formation of C3 convertases of both the classical and alternative pathways but also against the direct cytolytic effects of the membrane attack complex. Finally, levels of DAF, MCP and CD59 have been found to be considerably higher on syncytiotrophoblast plasma membranes than on either red cell or lymphocyte membranes (Holmes et al, 1992). This further supports the contention that these proteins play an important functional role in protection of the developing conceptus from maternal complement.

IMPLICATIONS FOR PREGNANCY PATHOLOGIES

The demonstration of a new family of immunoregulatory molecules on trophoblast raises important questions about the potential involvement of these products in pregnancy pathologies. Over the years there have been many studies where the distribution of complement components has been explored in human placental tissue sections. These studies generally predate the discovery of complement regulatory proteins on trophoblast. Nevertheless they do provide evidence that activated complement components are present not only in various pathological placentae but also in normal placental tissue (for example, Faulk et al, 1980; Sinha et al, 1984; Tedesco et al, 1990). It is interesting to note that, within chorionic villi, these products have often been found to be deposited at the basement membrane. However, it should be emphasized that a more complete assessment of the role of complement regulatory proteins in the maintenance of normal pregnancy is yet required in terms not only of inhibition of C3 convertases and membrane attack complexes but also in preventing release of anaphylatoxins at the fetomaternal interface. This, in turn, must await analysis of the functional activity of the three regulators on isolated trophoblast cells in vitro. It is simply too early to assess properly the likely impact of these new developments on the multiple conditions of pregnancy which are traditionally supposed to have an immune involvement or aetiology. In the past, attempts to interpret these conditions in immunological terms have been compromised because the immunological parameters of normal pregnancy have not been established. Nevertheless, aside from pregnancy, complement regulatory protein deficiency disorders with clinically demonstrable consequences, especially in terms of haemolytic disease, are known to exist and indeed have proved important in establishing the biological role of these proteins in vivo.

Paroxysmal nocturnal haemoglobinuria (PNH) is the most well known of the syndromes resulting from a deficiency in membrane-bound complement regulatory proteins (Rosse, 1986). PNH is a rare acquired disorder in which the red cells are unusually sensitive to complement-mediated lysis; as the name suggests, haemolytic episodes are more frequent at night. The disorder appears to arise following a somatic mutation in a bone marrow stem cell that results in the clonal expansion of abnormal cells (Moore et al, 1985; Rosse, 1986). Erythrocytes from a single PNH patient exhibit different degrees of sensitivity to complement haemolysis and the relative proportion of cells exhibiting these different sensitivities varies between individuals. Originally PNH was thought to represent a DAF deficiency (Nicholson-Weller et al, 1983; Pangburn et al, 1983) but it is now clear that expression of all PI-anchored proteins (Selvaraj, 1987), including CD59, is affected and this suggests that the basic defect is in the biosynthesis of the PI anchor.

Following the discovery that DAF carries the Cromer antigen series, it was realized that red cells from individuals with the rare Cromer null phenotype—the Inab phenotype—completely lack DAF (Telen et al, 1988; Merry et al, 1989; Tate et al, 1989). Although, interestingly, Inab individuals do tend to have various gut disorders, by contrast with PNH they do not have haemolytic anaemia. Thus, absence of DAF alone does not cause haemolytic anaemia and by implication this tends to emphasize the role of CD59 in the PNH phenotype. Recently, a patient has been identified with an inherited deficiency of CD59 but without a deficiency in DAF or other PI-linked proteins and this patient does have PNH-like haemolytic anaemia (Yamashina et al, 1990). Thus, in a system which does not express MCP, CD59 may be more important than DAF in maintaining red cell integrity in vivo. To date, there have been no reports of MCP deficiencies.

By contrast with red cells which express only DAF and CD59, trophoblast expresses relatively high levels of all three complement regulatory proteins and the contribution of the C3 convertase regulators may be important to the overall phenotype in this tissue. The obstetric history of the patient with the inherited CD59 deficiency is unknown but it has been demonstrated that CD59 is absent from skin as well as circulating blood cells in this individual (Yamashina et al, 1990). On this basis it may be speculated that CD59 could also have been absent from trophoblast epithelium during his gestation. If this were indeed the case then it could indicate not only that CD59 expression is not essential for successful pregnancy but, perhaps more importantly, that DAF and MCP can compensate for CD59 deficiency on trophoblast. Functional studies designed to explore the interplay between the three regulatory proteins on isolated trophoblast cells in vitro are now underway. It is possible to manipulate the phenotype of cells for complement regulators in vitro; exogenously added PI-linked proteins will re-incorporate into membranes where they exhibit functional activity. Thus, it should be possible to evaluate not only the importance of individual regulators on trophoblast but also the interplay between these products and the importance of their levels of expression. In terms of the application of this work to pregnancy pathologies, this last parameter is likely to be of particular importance as is the potential opportunity for therapeutic intervention afforded by PI-linked proteins.

SUMMARY

Recent studies have revealed that human trophoblast expresses three membrane-bound proteins which function specifically to regulate the activity of complement. These proteins are already known to be widely distributed in normal adult tissues where they protect host cells from damage resulting from the fortuitous deposition of activated complement components. Their activities are focused at two distinct steps in the complement pathway. Decay accelerating factor (DAF, CD55) and membrane co-factor protein (MCP, CD46) act at the level of the C3 convertase enzymes which activate C3 to C3b. A further protein, CD59, directly regulates the formation and function of the terminal cytolytic membrane attack complex (MAC) by specifically interacting with C8 and C9.

These proteins appear to play an important role in the maintenance of normal human pregnancy. DAF, MCP and CD59 are all expressed where trophoblast surfaces are in contact with maternal blood and tissues and expression occurs from at least 6 weeks of gestation. The semi-allogeneic human conceptus therefore appears to be effectively protected from maternal complement-mediated damage arising either from alternative or classical pathway activation or in a bystander fashion following a response to microbial infection in the mother.

Complement regulatory protein deficiency disorders with clinically demonstrable consequences especially in terms of haemolytic disease are known to exist and have proved valuable in establishing the biological role of these proteins in vivo. The demonstration of this new family of immuno-regulatory proteins on trophoblast raises important questions about the potential involvement of these products in pregnancy pathologies.

Acknowledgements

Work in this laboratory is supported by the Wellcome Trust and the Cancer Research Campaign.

REFERENCES

Anstee DJ, Holmes CH, Judson PA & Tanner MJA (1992) Use of monoclonal antibodies to determine the distribution of red cell surface proteins on human cells and tissues. In Agre P & Cartron J-P (eds) *Biochemistry of the Erythrocyte Polypeptide Blood Group Antigens*, in press. Baltimore: Johns Hopkins University Press.

Asch AS, Kinoshita T, Jaffe EA & Nussenzweig V (1986) Decay accelerating factor is present on cultured human umbilical vein and endothelial cells. *Journal of Experimental Medicine* **63:** 221–226.

Atkinson JP & Farries T (1987) Separation of self from non-self in the complement system. *Immunology Today* **8:** 212–215.

Ballard L, Seya T, Teckman J, Lublin DM & Atkinson JP (1987) A polymorphism of the complement regulatory protein MCP (membrane cofactor protein or gp45-70). *Journal of Immunology* **138:** 3850–3855.

Billington WD (1988) Maternal–fetal interactions in normal human pregnancy. In *Clinical Immunology and Allergy*, Vol. 2 No. 3, pp 527–549. London: Baillière Tindall.

Bora NS, Lublin DM, Kumar BV, Hockett RD, Holers VM & Atkinson JP (1989) Structural gene for human membrane cofactor protein (MCP) of complement maps to within 100 kb of the 3' end of the C3b/C4b receptor gene. *Journal of Experimental Medicine* **169:** 597–603.

Bora NS, Post TW & Atkinson JP (1991) Membrane cofactor protein of the complement system. A HINDIII restriction fragment length polymorphism that correlates with the expression polymorphism. *Journal of Immunology* **146:** 2821–2826.

Campbell RD, Law SKA, Reid KBM & Sim RB (1988) Structure, organization and regulation of the complement genes. *Annual Review of Immunology* **6:** 161–195.

Carroll MC, Alicot EM, Katzman PJ, Lloyd BK, Smith JA & Fearon DT (1988) Organization of the genes encoding complement receptors type 1 and 2, decay-accelerating factor, and C4-binding protein in the RCA locus on human chromosome 1. *Journal of Experimental Medicine* **167:** 1271–1280.

Cole JL, Housley GA, Dykman TR, MacDermott RP & Atkinson JP (1985) Identification of an additional class of C3-binding membrane proteins of human peripheral blood leukocytes and cell lines. *Proceedings of the New York Academy of Sciences (USA)* **82:** 859–863.

Daniels G (1989) Cromer-related antigens—blood group determinants on decay-accelerating factor. *Vox Sanguinis* **56:** 205–211.

Davies A, Simmons DL, Hale G et al (1989) CD59, and Ly-6 like protein expressed in human lymphoid cells, regulates the action of the complement membrane attack complex on homologous cells. *Journal of Experimental Medicine* **170:** 637–654.

Davitz MA (1987) Decay-accelerating factor (DAF): a review of its function and structure. *Acta Medica Scandinavica* **supplement 715:** 111–121.

Faulk WP, Jarret R, Keane M, Johnson PM & Boackle RJ (1980) Immunological studies of human placentae: complement components in immature and mature chorionic villi. *Clinical and Experimental Immunology* **40:** 299–305.

Faulk WP, Temple A, Lovins RE & Smith NC (1978) Antigens of human trophoblast: a working hypothesis for their role in normal and abnormal pregnancies. *Proceedings of the National Academy of Sciences (USA)* **75:** 1947–1951.

Ferguson MAJ & Williams AF (1988) Cell-surface anchoring of proteins via glycosyl-phosphotidylinositol structures. *Annual Review of Biochemistry* **57:** 285–320.

Groux H, Huet S, Aubrit F, Tran HC, Boumsall L & Bernard A (1989) A 19 kDa human erythrocyte molecule H19 involved in rosettes, present on nucleated cells, and required for T-cell activation. Comparison of the roles of H19 and LFA-3 molecules in T cell activation. *Journal of Immunology* **142:** 3013–3020.

Head JR & Billingham RE (1984) Mechanisms of non-rejection of the feto-placental allograft. In Crighton DB (ed.) *Immunological Aspects of Reproduction in Mammals*, pp 133–152. London: Butterworths.

Hoffman EM (1969) Inhibition of complement by a substance isolated from human erythrocytes. Extraction from human erythrocyte stromata. *Immunochemistry* **6:** 391–403.

Holers VM, Cole JL, Lublin DM, Seya T & Atkinson JP (1985) Human C3b- and C4b-regulatory proteins: a new multi-gene family. *Immunology Today* **6:** 188–191.

Holguin MH, Fredrick LR, Bernsham NJ, Wilcox LA & Parker CJ (1989) Isolation and characterization of a membrane protein from normal human erythrocytes that inhibits reactive lysis of the erythrocytes of paroxysmal nocturnal hemoglobinuria. *Journal of Clinical Investigation* **84:** 7–17.

Holmes CH, Simpson KL, Wainwright SD, Tate CG, Houlihan JM, Sawyer IH, Rogers IP, Spring FA, Anstee DJ & Tanner MJ (1990) Preferential expression of the complement regulatory protein decay accelerating factor at the feto-maternal interface during human pregnancy. *Journal of Immunology* **144:** 3099–3105.

Holmes CH, Simpson KL, Okada H et al (1992) Complement regulatory proteins at the feto-maternal interface during human placental development: distribution of CD59 by comparison with membrane cofactor protein (CD46) and decay accelerating factor (CD55). *European Journal of Immunology* **22:** 1579–1585.

Hourcade D, Holers VM & Atkinson JP (1989) The regulators of complement activation (RCA) gene cluster. *Advances in Immunology* **45:** 382–403.

Hsi B-L, Hunt JS & Atkinson JP (1991) Differential expression of complement regulatory proteins on subpopulations of human trophoblast cells. *Journal of Reproductive Immunology* **19:** 209–223.

Kinoshita T (1991) Biology of complement: the overture. *Immunology Today* **12:** 291–295.

Lachmann PJ (1991) The control of homologous lysis. *Immunology Today* **12:** 312–315.

Lachmann PJ & Hughes-Jones NC (1984) Initiation of complement activation. *Springer Seminars in Immunopathology* **7:** 143–162.

Law SK, Lichtenberg NA & Levine RP (1979) Evidence for an ester linkage between the labile binding site of C3b and receptive surfaces. *Journal of Immunology* **123:** 1388–1394.

Law SK, Lichtenberg NA & Levine RP (1980) Covalent binding and haemolytic activity of complement proteins. *Proceedings of the National Academy of Sciences (USA)* **77:** 7194–7198.

Liszewski MK, Post TW & Atkinson JP (1991) Membrane cofactor protein (MCP or CD46): newest member of the regulators of complement activation gene cluster. *Annual Review of Immunology* **9:** 431–455.

Lublin DM & Atkinson JP (1989) Decay-accelerating factor: biochemistry, molecular biology and function. *Annual Review of Immunology* **7:** 35–58.

McIntyre JA, Faulk WP, Verhulst SJ & Colliver A (1984) Human trophoblast—lymphocyte cross-reactive (TLX) antigens define a new alloantigen system. *Science* **222:** 1135–1137.

McNearney T, Ballard L, Seya T & Atkinson JP (1989) Membrane cofactor protein of complement is present on human fibroblast, epithelial and endothelial cells. *Journal of Clinical Investigation* **84:** 538–545.

Medof ME, Walter EI, Rutgers JL, Knowles DM & Nussenzweig V (1987) Identification of the complement decay-accelerating factor (DAF) on epithelium and glandular cells and in body fluids. *Journal of Experimental Medicine* **165:** 848–864.

Meri S, Morgan BP, Davies A et al (1990) Human protectin (CD59), an 18,000–20,000 MW complement lysis restricting factor, inhibits C5b-8 catalysed insertion of C9 into lipid bilayers. *Immunology* **71:** 1–9.

Meri S, Waldmann H & Lachmann PJ (1991) Distribution of protectin (CD59), a complement membrane attack inhibitor, in normal human tissues. *Laboratory Investigation* **65:** 532–537.

Merry AH, Rawlinson VI, Uchikawa M, Daha MR & Simm RB (1989) Studies on the sensitivity to complement-mediated lysis of erythrocytes (Inab phenotype) with a deficiency of DAF (decay accelerating factor). *British Journal of Haematology* **73:** 248–253.

Moore JG, Frank MM, Muller-Eberhard HJ & Young NS (1985) Decay-accelerating factor is present on paroxysmal nocturnal hemoglobinuria erythroid progenitors and lost during erythropoiesis in vitro. *Journal of Experimental Medicine* **162:** 1182–1192.

Morgan BP (1990) *Complement: Clinical Aspects and Relevance to Disease.* London: Academic Press.

Morgan PB (1989) Complement membrane atack on nucleated cells: resistance, recovery and non-lethal effects. *Biochemical Journal* **264:** 1–14.

Muller-Eberhard HJ (1986) The membrane attack complex of complement. *Annual Review of Immunology* **4:** 503–528.

Muller-Eberhard HJ (1988) Molecular organization and function of the complement system. *Annual Review of Biochemistry* **57:** 321–347.

Nicholson-Weller A, Burge J, Fearon DT, Weller PF & Austen KF (1982) Isolation of a human erythrocyte glycoprotein with decay-accelerating activity for C3 convertases of the complement system. *Journal of Immunology* **129:** 184–189.

Nicholson-Weller A, March JP, Rosenfeld SI & Austen KF (1983) Affected erythrocytes of patients with paroxysmal nocturnal hemoglobulinuria are deficient in the complement regulatory protein, decay accelerating factor. *Proceedings of the National Academy of Sciences (USA)* **80:** 5066.

Nose M, Katch M, Okada N, Kyogoko M & Okada H (1990) Tissue distribution of HRF20, a novel factor preventing the membrane attack of homologous complement, and its predominant expression on endothelial cells in vivo. *Immunology* **70:** 145–149.

Okada N, Harada R, Fujita T & Okada H (1989) A novel membrane glycoprotein capable of inhibiting membrane attack by homologous complement. *International Immunology* **1:** 205.

Pangburn MK, Schreiber RD & Muller-Eberhard HJ (1983) Deficiency of an erythrocyte membrane protein with complement regulatory activity in paroxysmal nocturnal hemoglobinuria. *Proceedings of the National Academy of Sciences (USA)* **80:** 5430.

Parsons SF, Spring FA, Merry AH et al (1988) *Proceedings of the 20th Congress of the International Society for Blood Transfusion,* p 116. Plymouth Grove, Manchester, UK: British Blood Transfusion Society.

Purcell DFJ, McKenzie IFC, Lublin DM et al (1990a) The human cell-surface glycoproteins HuLy-m5, membrane cofactor protein (MCP) of the complement system, and trophoblast-leukocyte common (TLX) antigen are CD46. *Immunology* **70:** 155–161.

Purcell DFJ, Russell SM, Deacon NH, Brown MA, Hooker DJ & McKenzie IFC (1990b) Alternatively spliced RNAs encode several isoforms of CD46 (MCP), a regulator of complement activation. *Immunogenetics* **1442:** 2172.

Reid KBM & Porter RP (1981) The proteolytic activation system of complement. *Annual Review of Biochemistry* **50:** 433–464.

Rey-Campos J, Rubinstein P & de Cordoba SR (1988) A physical map of the human regulator of complement activation gene cluster linking the complement genes CR1, CR2, DAF and C4bp. *Journal of Experimental Medicine* **167:** 664–669.

Rollins S, Zhao J, Ninomiya H & Sim PJ (1991) Inhibition of homologous complement by CD59 is mediated by a species-selective recognition conferred through binding to C8 within C5b–8 or C9 within C5b–9. *Journal of Immunology* **146:** 2245–2344.

Rosse WF (1986) The control of complement activation by the blood cells in paroxysmal nocturnal hemoglobinuria. *Blood* **67:** 268–269.

Sargent IL, Wilkins T & Redman CWG (1988) Maternal immune responses to the fetus in early pregnancy and recurrent miscarriage. *Lancet* **ii:** 1099–1101.

Schumaker VN, Zavodoszky PH & Poon PH (1987) Activation of the first component of complement. *Annual Review of Immunology* **5:** 21–42.

Selvaraj P, Dustin ML, Silber R, Low MG & Springer TA (1987) Deficiency of lymphocyte function-associated antigen 3 (LFA-3) in paroxysmal nocturnal hemoglobinuria. Functional correlates and evidence for a phosphotidylinositol anchor. *Journal of Experimental Medicine* **166:** 1011–1025.

Seya T, Hara T, Matsumoto M & Akedo H (1990a) Quantitative analysis of membrane cofactor protein (MCP) of complement: high expression of MCP on human leukemia cell lines, which is down-regulated during cell differentiation. *Journal of Immunology* **145:** 238–245.

Seya T, Hara T, Matsumoto M, Sugita Y & Akedo H (1990b) Complement-mediated tumor cell damage induced by antibodies against membrane cofactor protein (MCP, CD46). *Journal of Experimental Medicine* **172:** 1673–1680.

Sim RB & Reid KMB (1991) C1: molecular interactions with activating systems. *Immunology Today* **12:** 307–311.

Sinha D, Wells M & Faulk PW (1984) Immunological studies of human placentae: complement components in pre-eclamptic chorionic villi. *Clinical and Experimental Immunology* **56:** 175–184.

Spring FA, Judson PA, Daniels GL, Parsons SF, Mallinson G & Anstee DJ (1987) A human cell-surface glycoprotein that carries Cromer-related blood group antigens on erythrocytes and is also expressed on leucocytes and platelets. *Immunology* **62:** 307–313.

Stefanova I, Hilgert I, Kristofova H, Brown R, Low MG & Horejsi V (1989) Characterization of a broadly expressed human leucocyte surface antigen MEM-43 anchored in membrane through phosphatidylinositol. *Molecular Immunology* **26:** 153–161.

Stern PL, Beresford N, Thompson S, Johnson PM, Webb PD & Hole N (1986) Characterization of the human trophoblast-leukocyte antigen molecules defined by a monoclonal antibody. *Journal of Immunology* **137:** 1606–1609.

Sugita Y, Nakano Y & Tomita M (1988) Isolation from human erythrocytes of a new membrane protein which inhibits the formation of complement transmembrane channels. *Journal of Biochemistry* **104:** 633–640.

Tate CG, Uchikawa M, Tanner MJA et al (1989) Studies on the defect which causes absence of decay accelerating factor (DAF) from the peripheral blood cells of an individual with the Inab phenotype. *Biochemical Journal* **261:** 489–493.

Tedesco F, Radillo O, Candussi G, Nazzaro A, Mollnesi TE & Pecorari D (1990) Immuno-histochemical detection of terminal complement complex and S protein in normal and pre-eclamptic placentae. *Clinical and Experimental Immunology* **80:** 236–240.

Telen MJ, Hall SE, Green AM, Moulds JJ & Rosse WF (1988) Identification of human erythrocyte blood group antigens on decay-accelerating factor (DAF) and an erythrocyte phenotype negative for DAF. *Journal of Experimental Medicine* **167:** 1993–1998.

Whitlow MB, Iida K, Bernard A & Nussenzweig NV (1989) H-19, a surface membrane molecule involved in T-cell activation, inhibits channel formation by human complement. *Complement Inflammation* **6:** 415 (abstract).

Yamashina M, Ueda E, Kinoshita T et al (1990) Inherited complete deficiency of 20-kilodalton homologous restriction factor (CD59) as a cause of paroxysmal nocturnal hemoglobinuria. *New England Journal of Medicine* **323:** 1184–1189.

4

Immune aspects of pathology of the placental bed contributing to pregnancy pathology

JUDITH N. BULMER

INTRODUCTION

Studies of the immunopathology of various pregnancy disorders have recently focused on the placental bed as it has become clear that the pathogenic mechanisms may result from disordered maternal–fetal relations at that site. Over the last decade there have been many studies of both maternal and fetal cell types in human uteroplacental tissues leading to considerable advances in our understanding of the complex cellular inter-relationships in the placental bed. Before considering the immunopathology of the placental bed, it is necessary to review briefly recent developments in the immune aspects of the normal placental bed.

NORMAL PLACENTAL BED

Extravillous trophoblast

The chorionic villi which form the definitive placenta are covered by an inner cytotrophoblast and an outer syncytiotrophoblast layer. In early pregnancy, cytotrophoblast cells proliferate from the tips of the chorionic villi, forming columns which extend laterally to form a shell covering the uterine surface. From this cytotrophoblast shell, mononuclear extravillous fetal trophoblast invades maternal decidua basalis, myometrium and spiral arteries, eventually fusing in the placental bed to form syncytial giant cells (Boyd and Hamilton, 1970; Pijnenborg et al, 1980). Interstitial trophoblast invades decidua and the inner third of the myometrium; its abundance has been highlighted with monoclonal antibodies directed against cytokeratins as well as antibodies raised against trophoblast cells (Bulmer and Johnson, 1985). Endovascular trophoblast migrates in a retrograde direction up the spiral arteries, replacing the endothelium (Figure 1a). Decidual vascular invasion is normally completed by 8–10 weeks' gestation and there is a second wave of trophoblast migration into the terminal segments of the radial arteries within the myometrium at 16–20 weeks' gestation (Pijnenborg et al, 1980). Loss of the normal musculoelastic arterial wall and intramural deposition of

Baillière's Clinical Obstetrics and Gynaecology—
Vol. 6, No. 3, September 1992
ISBN 0–7020–1634–9

461

fibrinoid allow the progressive vascular dilatation necessary to accommodate the tenfold increase in uterine blood supply required by the fetoplacental unit during pregnancy.

Controlled invasion of maternal uterine tissues and arteries by fetal trophoblast is an essential feature of normal fetoplacental development. Deficient vascular invasion has been implicated as an aetiological factor in pre-eclampsia, intrauterine growth retardation and spontaneous abortion. Trophoblast invasion of the uterus in placenta accreta appears excessive (see below). The mechanisms which control trophoblastic invasion are not known: extravillous trophoblast may have an inherent ability to limit its invasive potential, or maternal cells within decidua may have a regulatory function. Human decidua contains abundant leukocytes comprising predominantly macrophages, granulated lymphocytes and T lymphocytes. These cells and their potential role in the facilitation and control of trophoblast invasion will be discussed later. The phenotype of villous and extravillous trophoblast has been documented using monoclonal antibodies raised against trophoblast, as well as hormone production, enzyme production and lectin binding (reviewed in Bulmer, 1988). Subpopulations of extravillous trophoblast have been defined which may differ in their invasive potential.

Lectins are proteins or glycoproteins derived from a variety of biological sources which bind to carbohydrates of specific structure and configuration. Alteration of cell surface carbohydrates has been associated with cell transformation and differentiation. Distinctions in lectin binding properties between trophoblast subpopulations may distinguish cells with varying proliferative and invasive potential. For example, lack of reactivity with the lectin, WGA, of trophoblast giant cells may reflect decreased capacity for invasion, in keeping with the observation that syncytial giant cells accumulate in myometrium at the limit of trophoblast invasion (Lalani et al, 1987). Similarly, increased reactivity with another lectin, GSII, of extravillous trophoblast compared with villous trophoblast may define trophoblast capable of invasion (Thrower et al, 1991). The lectin binding of trophoblast in pathological pregnancies has not been extensively studied, although trophoblast in complete molar pregnancy shows more widespread binding of GSII than normal trophoblast (Thrower et al, 1991).

The enzyme content of trophoblast has been investigated by histochemical and immunohistochemical techniques. Proteolytic enzymes play a role in the degradation of the extracellular matrix and basement membrane which occurs during invasion by malignant neoplastic cells: increased production of proteinases such as lysosomal cathepsins, plasminogen activators and metalloproteinases has been linked to the invasive capacity of various types of malignant cell (reviewed in Mullins and Rohrlich, 1983). The proteinase inhibitor α_2-macroglobulin has been demonstrated on the surface of villous syncytiotrophoblast (Johnson et al, 1985) and α_1-antitrypsin and α_1-antichymotrypsin have been localized by immunohistochemistry in endovascular trophoblast (Figure 1b) and syncytiotrophoblast (Earl et al, 1989). Recently, plasminogen activator inhibitors (PAI) 1 and 2 have been demonstrated in trophoblast both in vitro and in vivo,

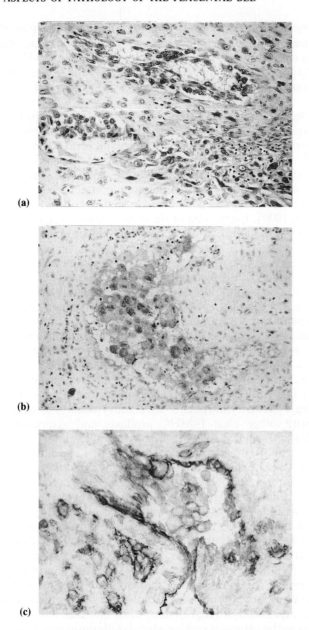

(a)

(b)

(c)

Figure 1. (a) H&E stained section of first trimester placental bed showing normal endovascular and perivascular trophoblast. (b) First trimester placental bed tissue labelled with rabbit anti-α_1-antichymotrypsin showing reactivity with endovascular trophoblast. (c) First trimester placental bed tissue labelled for CD46 with the monoclonal antibody H316 using an indirect immunoperoxidase technique: note reactivity with endovascular and perivascular trophoblast and endothelial cells. Magnification: (a) × 160 (b) × 160 (c) × 250, all reproduced at 65% of original.

PAI-1 predominating in invasive trophoblast cells (Feinberg et al, 1989). Thus, protease and antiprotease production by trophoblast may play a role in regulation of its invasion of uterine tissues, a possibility which has been supported by the failure to detect α_2-macroglobulin in invasive moles and choriocarcinomas which show excessive invasive potential (Saksela et al, 1981).

The complement regulatory protein, membrane co-factor protein (MCP; CD46) is expressed widely by villous and extravillous trophoblast cells, including extravillous trophoblast in the placental bed (Figure 1c) (Bulmer and Johnson, 1985; Purcell et al, 1990). CD46 is an intrinsic-acting protein which binds to C3b attached to other molecules on the same cell surface. A related cell surface complement regulatory protein, decay accelerating factor (DAF), is also expressed by various trophoblast subpopulation (Holmes et al, 1990). Expression of these complement regulatory proteins by extravillous trophoblast would negate complement mediated attack at the fetomaternal interface in the placental bed, arising through either maternal antibody attack or low level complement activation due to local tissue restructuring. This is discussed further in Chapter 3.

Although villous trophoblast does not express class I or class II major histocompatibility complex (MHC) antigens, early immunohistochemical studies with monoclonal antibodies directed against monomorphic determinants indicated that invasive extravillous trophoblast cells express class I MHC antigens (Redman et al, 1984; Wells et al, 1984). Recent serological, biochemical and molecular biological studies have demonstrated that this class I MHC antigen expressed by human extravillous trophoblast is non-classical HLA-G (Ellis et al, 1990; Kovats et al, 1990). The HLA-G gene encodes a non-polymorphic 39 kDa heavy chain which shows close homology with other class I MHC products and associates with β_2-microglobulin at the cell surface. It is a structural homologue of a murine Qa-region gene and expression has not been described on adult human cells. The role of HLA-G expression by extravillous trophoblast is not known. There has been speculation that HLA-G may act as an intercellular recognition molecule in the placental bed, involved in trophoblast invasion or in specific immune responses by specialized decidual leukocytes: HLA-G mediates cell–cell adhesion by CD8 (Sanders et al, 1991), although CD8-positive cells are relatively scanty in decidua (see below). Expression of HLA-G could also protect extravillous trophoblast from attack by maternal natural killer (NK) cells in decidua by acting as a passive non-polymorphic cell surface class I MHC molecule, thus failing to provide a target for a cytotoxic T cell response by lack of expression of a polymorphic class I MHC antigen. The expression of HLA-G at a major interface between maternal and fetal cells in the placental bed has stimulated considerable interest in its function at this site.

Maternal decidua

The decidualized endometrium (decidua) which lines the uterine cavity can be subdivided according to site: decidua basalis forms the implantation site and undergoes invasion by extravillous trophoblast; decidua parietalis (vera) lines the uterine cavity away from the implantation area; and decidua capsularis is attached to the amniochorionic membranes and merges with decidua parietalis in later gestation as the uterine cavity is obliterated. Although the complex cellular relationships within decidua were established by light and electron microscopy, the development of monoclonal antibodies has allowed detailed characterization of the constituent cells at various stages of gestation.

Human decidua contains abundant leukocytes throughout gestation, over 30% of stromal cells in first trimester decidua expressing the leukocyte common antigen (Figure 2a) (Bulmer et al, 1991a). Decidual leukocytes fall into three major groups: macrophages, granulated lymphocytes and T lymphocytes (Table 1); classic natural killer cells expressing the CD16 antigen, B lymphocytes and granulocytes are very scanty.

Granulated lymphocytes

Phenotypically unusual granulated lymphocytes account for up to 75% of leukocytes in first trimester human decidua. After mid-gestation they decrease in number and are scanty at term. Immunohistochemical studies of paraffin-embedded sections and cell suspensions have established that these cells are analogous to the cells which have previously been termed 'endometrial stromal granulocytes', 'Körnchenzellen' or 'K cells' (Figure 2b) (Bulmer et al, 1987). Endometrial granulated lymphocytes (EGL) have an unusual antigenic phenotype: they do not express the T cell antigens CD3, CD4 and CD8, nor the peripheral blood natural killer (NK) cell antigens, CD16 and CD57. However, they are intensely positive for CD56, another antigen which is expressed by NK cells. They are also positive for CD38, an antigen expressed on immature and activated cells, and a proportion express the E-rosette receptor, CD2 (Bulmer et al, 1991a). This phenotype CD56++ CD16− CD3− is similar to that of a small subset (less than 1%) of peripheral blood large granular lymphocytes (Nagler et al, 1989).

The role of EGL in normal pregnancy is not known. The detection of a small granulated non-T non-B lymphocyte in murine decidua, which mediates immunosuppression by secretion of a transforming growth factor β_2 (TGF-β_2) (Clark et al, 1990), led to suggestions that EGL may function as suppressor cells in early pregnancy. However, evidence to date does not support the suggestion that EGL are the major suppressor cell population in first trimester human decidua since supernatants from decidual explants and unfractionated decidual cell suspensions produced higher levels of suppression of mitogen-induced lymphoproliferation than supernatants from enriched EGL (Bulmer et al, 1991b).

Large granular lymphocytes in peripheral blood can mediate non-MHC restricted cytotoxicity (natural killer or NK cell activity). Endometrial granulated lymphocytes have been purified from first trimester decidua using a variety of techniques, including density gradient centrifugation, fluorescence-activated cell sorting and panning for CD56-positive cells onto immunoglobulin-coated plates. The cells have consistently been shown to

Table 1. Leukocyte populations in human decidua.

Cell type	Phenotype	Distribution	In vitro function and potential in vivo roles
Granulated lymphocyte	CD2±, CD3−, CD4−, CD7±, CD8−, CD16−, CD38+, CD56+, CD57−, CD69+	Endometrium throughout menstrual cycle, dramatic increase in late luteal phase and early pregnancy, forming the major leukocyte population, decline in number in second half of pregnancy	NK cell activity: control of trophoblast invasion Immunosuppression: suppression of maternal antifetal immune response Cytokine production: stimulation and control of trophoblast proliferation and differentiation Non-specific antiviral defence mechanism[1]
Macrophage	CD4±, CD11b±, CD14+, class II MHC+, CD68+, α₁AT+, α₁ACT+, NSE+, ACP+	Endometrium throughout menstrual cycle, increase premenstrually and in early pregnancy, persist into third trimester	Antigen presentation: presentation of fetal antigens to maternal immune system Immunosuppression: as above Cytokine production: as above Phagocytosis: removal of tissue debris following trophoblast invasion
T lymphocyte	CD2+, CD3+, CD4± (25%), CD8± (75%)	Low proportion of endometrial leukocytes, little change during menstrual cycle and pregnancy	Immunosuppression: as above[2] Cytokine production: as above[2] Interaction with HLA-G-positive extravillous trophoblast[1]

[1] No relevant in vitro studies to date to support a possible in vivo role.
[2] No relevant in vitro studies in human but in vitro evidence in murine pregnancy.
α₁AT, α₁-antitrypsin; α₁ACT; α₁-antichymotrypsin; NSE, non-specific esterase; ACP, acid phosphatase.

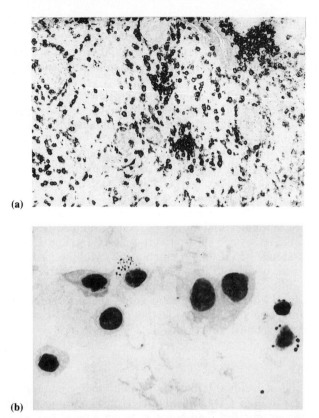

Figure 2. (a) Cryostat section of first trimester decidua labelled for CD45 using an indirect immunoperoxidase technique showing abundant leukocytes. **(b)** Imprint preparation of first trimester decidua stained with Giemsa showing endometrial granulated lymphocytes. Magnification: **(a)** × 160 **(b)** × 1000, reproduced at 65% of original.

lyse the NK target cell line, K562, although they are poor effectors compared with peripheral blood lymphocytes (King et al, 1989; Manaseki and Searle, 1989; Ritson and Bulmer, 1989; Ferry et al, 1990). Non-activated EGL do not lyse isolated trophoblast cells (King et al, 1989): human trophoblast does not appear to be susceptible to decidual NK cells, although it can be lysed by lymphokine-activated killer (LAK) cells (King and Loke, 1990; Ferry et al, 1991).

The consistent detection of NK activity in in vitro studies and their abundance at the implantation site in early pregnancy has led to the suggestion that EGL in human decidua may play a role in the control of trophoblastic invasion of maternal tissues. The proposed cellular analogues in rat and mouse, the granulated metrial gland (GMG) cells, have been shown to be capable of direct lysis of labyrinthine trophoblast in vitro and there is electron microscope evidence of a functional interaction in the labyrinth between GMG cells in maternal vascular channels and layer I trophoblast (Stewart and Mukhtar, 1988; Peel and Adam, 1991). Despite the lack of evidence for direct lysis of trophoblast by human EGL in vivo in uteroplacental tissue sections, it is possible that these cells are able to detect and lyse occasional individual trophoblast cells with excessive invasive potential.

Cytokines are polypeptide regulatory factors with various immune and non-immune functions. The 'immunotropism' theory has proposed that cytokines produced by T lymphocytes in maternal decidua are essential for normal trophoblast development (Wegmann, 1988). Human placenta expresses receptors for M-CSF, G-CSF, GM-CSF, TNF and IFN-γ, amongst others, although the expression of cytokine receptors by extravillous trophoblast in the placental bed has not been thoroughly investigated (Hoshina et al, 1985; Eades et al, 1988; Uzumaki et al, 1989; Calderon et al, 1988; Gearing et al, 1989). Natural killer cells are capable of producing a wide variety of cytokines and clones of EGL produced from normal first trimester decidua have been shown to produce TGF-β and TNF (Christmas et al, 1990). Hence, EGL may function as cytokine producers at the implantation site, and could thus play a role in the control of trophoblast proliferation, differentiation and invasion as well as in immunosuppression.

Finally, natural killer cells represent a non-specific defence mechanism against viral infection and it is possible that the role of EGL is to protect the fetoplacental unit against infection.

Macrophages

The second major decidual leukocyte population are macrophages which account for 35–40% of CD45-positive cells in first trimester decidua. In contrast to the granulated lymphocytes, macrophages persist in decidua throughout pregnancy. Decidual macrophages express the tissue macrophage antigens CD14 and CD68 and most are class II MHC antigen-positive (Bulmer et al, 1988a). Macrophages in decidua basalis are often closely associated with extravillous trophoblast (Bulmer et al, 1988b). The function of macrophages in human decidua is not known, although in vitro studies have led to suggested in vivo roles.

Antigen presenting cells have been detected in first trimester human decidua (Oksenberg et al, 1986; Dorman and Searle, 1988). Although the cell type responsible has not been throughly characterized apart from expression of class II MHC antigens, macrophages are prime candidates as decidual antigen presenting cells. However, Dorman and Searle (1988) noted low numbers of CD14-positive cells in cell suspensions prepared from first trimester together with small numbers of CD1-positive cells. Scanty CD1-positive cells have also been detected by immunohistochemistry in both non-pregnant endometrium (Kamat and Isaacson, 1987) and early pregnancy decidua (Bulmer and Sunderland, 1984).

Decidual macrophages have also been implicated as suppressor cells, by secretion of prostaglandin E_2. Such immunosuppression has been reported to block lytic activity of cells in decidua with potential antitrophoblast activity (Parhar et al, 1989). However, decidualized stromal cells have also been reported to mediate immunosuppression by secretion of PGE_2 and the relative in vivo importance of the various local suppressor mechanisms in human pregnancy has not been established. Decidualized endometrial stromal cells have also been reported to mediate immunosuppression by secretion of a 43–67 kDa soluble factor (Matsui et al, 1990) and supernatants produced by epithelial cells purified and cultured from secretory endometrium also suppress mixed lymphocyte reactions in vitro (Johnson et al, 1987).

Macrophages are able to produce a variety of cytokines, including M-CSF, G-CSF and TNF, for which receptors have been detected in human placenta. Decidual macrophages also possess lysosomal enzyme activity including acid phosphatase, non-specific esterase, α_1-antitrypsin and α_1-antichymotrypsin (Earl et al, 1989); the in vivo role of decidual macrophages may thus be in the phagocytosis of tissue debris consequent on trophoblast invasion of uterine tissue. However, Mues et al (1989) studied the phenotype of macrophages in term decidua basalis: expression of an antigen associated with downregulatory stages of inflammation was considered to provide support for an immunoregulatory, non-inflammatory role for macrophages in human decidua.

T lymphocytes

T cells account for only 15–20% of leukocytes in first trimester human decidua, although they form a higher proportion at term when CD56-positive granulated lymphocytes have declined in number. They are scattered throughout decidua basalis and decidua parietalis as well as in an intraepithelial position and over 75% are CD8-positive suppressor/cytotoxic T cells (Bulmer et al, 1991a; Pace et al, 1991). Although lack of expression of either $\alpha\beta$ or $\gamma\delta$ heterodimer of the T cell receptor has been reported (Dietl et al, 1990), others have detected expression of the $\alpha\beta$ heterodimer on the large majority of T cells in human decidua using a different panel of antibodies (Yeh et al, 1990; Bulmer et al, 1991c). The specific function of the T cell population in human decidua has not been investigated, probably partly because of the difficulty in separating this relatively small population from other leukocyte types. However, a large hormone-dependent suppressor cell in murine decidua expresses surface markers of a suppressor T cell and it is possible that CD8-positive cells in human decidua may also have this function, although there is little variation in the number of T cells in endometrium according to menstrual cycle stage (Bulmer et al, 1991a; Klentzeris et al, 1992). CD8-positive cells in peripheral blood in pregnancy have been reported to express progesterone receptors (Szekeres-Bartho et al, 1983), although Tabibzadeh and Satyaswaroop (1989) failed to detect progesterone receptor on T cells in non-pregnant human endometrium.

T cells are also able to produce a variety of cytokines including GM-CSF for which a role in the control of placental cell proliferation has been proposed (Wegmann, 1988). Although the immunotropism theory was developed in a murine pregnancy model, both macrophages and T lymphocytes are virtually absent in the mesometrial decidua in murine pregnancy, the predominant leukocyte in decidua basalis being the granulated metrial gland cell (Redline and Lu, 1989). Furthermore, recent studies have indicated that epithelial cells are the major source of GM-CSF in the mouse reproductive tract (Robertson and Seamark, 1990).

Decidualized endometrial stromal cells

In early pregnancy endometrial stromal cells accumulate cytoplasmic glycogen and lipid, becoming large and polygonal with a pale vesicular nucleus: nutritional, endocrine and immunological roles have been proposed. The immunosuppressive activity of decidual cells has been documented and the proposed mechanisms include secretion of 43–67 kDa soluble produce (Matsui et al, 1989) and production of prostaglandin E_2 (Parhar et al, 1988).

Decidual cells appear to produce laminin which may play a role in facilitating and controlling the extent of trophoblast invasion: expression of laminin receptors by extravillous trophoblast may facilitate invasion through the laminin-producing decidual cells (Loke et al, 1989). Although it is clear that decidual cells do not form a distinct barrier separating maternal and fetal cells in uteroplacental tissues, a role in the limitation of trophoblastic invasion within the uterus may be indicated by the frequent absence of decidua in placenta accreta in which trophoblast can invade through the entire thickness of the myometrium. Decidual cells also produce various hormones, pregnancy proteins and growth factors, including insulin-like growth factor binding protein-1 (Bell, 1991). The role of these various factors at the implantation site is not certain.

Uterine spiral arteries

Endovascular trophoblast migrates in a retrograde direction up uterine spiral arteries in early pregnancy. The mechanisms which facilitate and control the invasion of maternal uterine vessels are not known, although localization of α_1-antitrypsin and α_1-antichymotrypsin in endovascular trophoblast may reflect production of specific products by this subpopulation required for the facilitation and control of invasion of spiral arteries (Earl et al, 1989). During the third trimester, spiral arteries are normally re-endothelialized and involution of the uteroplacental arteries normally occurs within a few days of delivery.

Defective trophoblastic invasion into myometrial segments of spiral arteries and consequent inadequate development of 'physiological changes' has been implicated in the pathogenesis of pre-eclampsia and intrauterine growth retardation (see later). Although several investigators have considered localization of complement components and immunoglobulins in spiral artery walls to be evidence of immune-mediated damage in various pregnancy disorders, others have detected deposits of C3 in uteroplacental arteries in normal pregnancy (Weir, 1981; Hustin et al, 1983; Wells et al, 1987). The additional detection of C1q, C4, C6 and C9 provides support for an immune basis for such complement deposition (Wells et al, 1987). Lichtig et al (1985) reported heavy deposition of C3 in 14.6% of primiparae in a series of 110 first trimester placental bed specimens obtained from termination of apparently healthy pregnancy: it was suggested that the high frequency of spiral artery complement deposits in primiparae may represent early pre-eclamptic lesions. Thus, several studies indicate that deposition of complement components in spiral arteries is a feature of normal pregnancy and the value of this observation as a manifestation of pregnancy immunopathology is doubtful.

PATHOLOGICAL PREGNANCY

Although the concept that various pregnancy disorders are a consequence of immune-mediated damage is attractive, concrete evidence of immunopathology is often elusive. The clarification of immunological interactions between maternal and fetal cells in the placental bed in normal pregnancy will provide a basis for more meaningful studies of the placental bed in pathological pregnancy with more rational interpretation of results. However, a significant problem remains: namely that the pathogenic lesion in an abnormal pregnancy most probably occurs several weeks or months before delivery of the fetus and placenta and subsequent immunological and histological examination of uteroplacental tissues. A further problem is that while the delivered placenta may show associated abnormalities, the pathogenic lesion may lie in the placental bed, accessible only by placental bed biopsy.

Primary unexplained infertility

The role played both by the various cell types in decidua and by the extravillous trophoblast in successful implantation and early development of the placenta has not yet been established. Investigation of pathological tissues may provide additional information regarding cell function in normal pregnancy. Soffer et al (1983) reported a deficiency of E-rosette bearing cells (presumed to be T lymphocytes) in cell suspensions prepared from luteal phase endometrium from infertile women. Although there have been several immunohistochemical studies of stromal leukocyte populations in normal non-pregnant human endometrium, many lack precise dating of samples and definition of normal subjects. Klentzeris et al (1991) compared leukocyte populations in luteal phase endometrial biopsies, precisely timed from the luteinizing hormone (LH) surge, between normal fertile women and women with primary unexplained infertility. Around the time of implantation at day LH+7, the endometrial leukocyte population comprised 41% CD56-positive (granulated lymphocytes), 32% CD3-positive (T lymphocytes) and 28% CD68-positive (macrophages) cells. Endometrium from infertile women contained fewer CD8-positive suppressor/cytotoxic T cells and CD56-positive granulated lymphocytes and more CD4-positive helper/inducer T cells than normal endometrium. Furthermore, throughout the luteal phase a lower proportion of CD56-positive cells co-expressed CD2 in infertile endometrium compared with normal samples. This deficiency of CD56-positive cells and additional lack of CD2 expression may reflect the decreased number of E-rosette receptor bearing cells noted by Soffer et al (1983) in endometrial cell suspensions. These studies raise further questions regarding the role of decidual granulated lymphocytes and T cells in early pregnancy and demonstrate the use of carefully controlled studies of normal and pathological tissues to provide insight into the function of cells in normal implantation and placentation.

Spontaneous abortion

The concept that spontaneous abortion can be explained by maternal rejection of the fetal semiallograft is attractive. Reports of successful immunotherapy with paternal or third party leukocytes for recurrent miscarriage (Taylor and Faulk, 1981; Mowbray et al, 1985) have stimulated further interest in this proposal. Recurrent miscarriage patients form a relatively homogeneous group but to date there have been few studies of their uteroplacental tissues. However, specimens suitable for histological and immunological studies can be difficult to obtain since abortion may occur at home so that tissues are lost; furthermore, fetal death may occur several days or even weeks before clinical presentation, thus allowing secondary inflammatory changes to develop within decidua.

Khong et al (1987) suggested that defective haemochorial placentation may play a role in spontaneous abortion: a deficiency of vascular trophoblast was noted in placental bed tissues from two of seven first trimester and five of five second trimester miscarriages. Defective invasion of spiral arteries by extravillous trophoblast has thus been reported in pre-eclampsia, small-for-gestational age infants (SGA) and spontaneous abortion raising the question of a common defect in placentation with diverse pathogenic mechanisms. The mechanisms underlying the inadequate trophoblast invasion will, however, remain elusive until the mechanisms facilitating and controlling this migration in normal pregnancy are elucidated.

Studies in the mouse have provided evidence that decidual leukocyte populations play a role in spontaneous pregnancy loss in this species. In the CBA/J × DBA/2 mouse model, pregnancy resorption rates can be decreased by treatment with anti-asialo GM1 antibody and increased by enhancement of NK activity (de Fougerolles and Baines, 1987). Furthermore, the implantation site of resorbing pregnancies is infiltrated by asialo GM1-positive cells (Gendron and Baines, 1988). Pregnancy resorption in the SCID mouse, which is deficient in T and B lymphocytes, shows infiltration of the resorption site by granulocytes, macrophages and large granular lymphocytes (Crepeau and Croy, 1988). Murine trophoblast is normally not susceptible to lysis by NK cells or cytotoxic T cells (CTL) but can be killed by lymphokine (IL-2) activated killer (LAK) cells or CTL cultured in GIBCO-Opti-MEM medium (Head, 1989). Local blocking of interleukin 2 has been considered to be an important immunosuppressive mechanism in normal murine pregnancy, possibly mediated by a transforming growth factor β (Clark et al, 1990) and it is possible that loss of normal

IL-2 blocking leads to generation of LAK cells and hence direct cytotoxic attack on trophoblast.

In contrast, decidual leukocytes in spontaneous abortion in humans have received little study. In common with the mouse system, human trophoblast appears to be resistant to lysis by NK cells but is susceptible to LAK cells (King and Loke, 1990; Ferry et al, 1991). Nebel et al (1986) investigated early clinical abortions occurring 22–30 days after embryo transfer on an in vitro fertilization–embryo transfer programme: although dense lymphocyte infiltrates were identified in deep decidua and around blood vessels, the cells were not characterized phenotypically, nor was comment made concerning cytoplasmic granularity. Clark et al (1987) reported deficiency of mono-nuclear cells with large cytoplasmic granules and the additional presence of large granular lymphocytes with small cytoplasmic granules in decidua from pregnancies aborting between 8 and 21 weeks' gestation. Michel et al (1989) subsequently expanded this study and reported that lymphocytes with granules $< 1 \mu m$ diameter were associated with pregnancies destined to abort, whereas lymphocytes with $> 1 \mu m$ diameter granules were a feature of normal pregnancy. Michel et al (1990) subsequently reported a deficiency of decidual suppressor cell activity, attributed in the study to lymphocytes with large granules, in aborting pregnancies compared with normal controls.

The few studies of placental bed leukocytes in human spontaneous abortion reported to date, together with evidence from murine models of pregnancy resorption, raises the possibility that decidual leukocytes play a role in pregnancy loss via non-MHC-restricted lytic mechanisms. Consider-able scope for future investigation remains, although it will be necessary to ensure that studies are performed on well defined clinical subgroups and that confounding factors such as secondary inflammatory changes are avoided.

Pre-eclampsia

The placenta is of central importance in the pathogenesis of pre-eclampsia. Pre-eclampsia occurs in the absence of a fetus in molar pregnancy and the incidence also correlates with placental mass, being higher in twin pregnancy, molar pregnancy and hydrops fetalis (Fox, 1978): placental removal is curative.

Although there have been reports of pathology and immunopathology affecting chorionic villi in pre-eclampsia, most studies have focused on placental bed lesions. In pregnancies complicated by pre-eclampsia the previously noted physiological vascular changes are restricted to the decidua, the myometrial segments of spiral arteries retaining their musculo-elastic wall and hence responding to vasomotor influences (Robertson et al, 1986). Furthermore, Khong et al (1986) demonstrated absence of physio-logical changes throughout the entire length of the spiral arteries in some pre-eclamptic pregnancies, an abnormality which can easily be detected by histological examination of the maternal facing surface of the placenta after delivery. The same authors also observed endovascular trophoblast in third trimester placental bed tissues from pre-eclampsia pregnancies, whereas spiral arteries in normal pregnancy re-endothelialize after the second trimester.

The maternal vascular response is therefore inadequate and abnormal in pre-eclampsia, raising the possibility of defective interactions between maternal and fetal cells in the placental bed. Since the mechanisms which facilitate and control trophoblast invasion in normal pregnancy remain unknown, the pathogenesis of defective invasion in pre-eclampsia is difficult to determine. Khong (1987) noted no difference in the type or quantity of decidual leukocytes in an immunohistochemical study of placental bed biopsies from normal and pre-eclamptic pregnancies. However, Tatarova et al (1989) quantitated 'endometrial stromal granulocytes' (now known to be granulated lymphocytes) in decidua parietalis attached to the amniochorionic membranes in normal pregnancy, mild pre-eclampsia and severe pre-eclampsia: the number of granulated cells showed a progressive increase in numbers in mild and severe pre-eclampsia compared with normal pregnancy.

Spiral arteries in pre-eclampsia may show 'acute atherosis' which is characterized by fibrinoid necrosis and lipophage infiltration of the vessel wall, together with a perivascular mononuclear inflammatory cell infiltrate (Robertson et al, 1986). Acute atherosis is most clearly seen in decidua parietalis where the vessels do not show changes induced by trophoblast invasion. Although originally considered pathognomonic of pregnancy-induced hypertension (Robertson et al, 1986), similar decidual vascular changes have also been reported in pregnancies complicated by intrauterine growth retardation, systemic lupus erythematosus and normotensive diabetes mellitus (Sheppard and Bonnar, 1981; Robertson et al, 1986).

The resemblance of acute atherosis to the vascular changes observed in renal and cardiac allograft rejection led to speculation of an immune pathogenesis and complement (C3), IgG and fibrin have been localized in placental bed vessels in pre-eclampsia (Kitzmiller and Benirschke, 1973). More recently detection of C3 and IgM in association with fibrinoid necrosis and acute atherosis in decidual vessels in pre-eclampsia, stable chronic hypertension and normotensive diabetes led to the suggestion that immuno-protein deposition may reflect local intravascular coagulation and fibrino-genesis rather than an immune reaction (Kitzmiller et al, 1981). However, Hustin et al (1983) reported C3 and IgG in decidual portions of utero-placental arteries in pre-eclampsia, C3 only being observed in association with IgG. Nevertheless, the significance of immunoglobulin and comple-ment deposition in vascular lesions in pre-eclampsia is doubtful since fibrin and C3 have been localized in normal placental bed vessels and their deposition may have an immune basis (Weir, 1981; Wells et al, 1987).

A major difficulty in the investigation of pregnancy disorders such as pre-eclampsia is that the pathogenic lesion is likely to occur early in gestation, often long before clinical presentation and several months before tissues are available for immunopathological examination. Lichtig et al (1985) reported the morphological changes of atherosis and C3 deposition in spiral arteries in first trimester placental bed tissues from therapeutic termi-nations of apparently normal pregnancy. These lesions were significantly more common in primiparae and the possibility was raised that they may represent early pre-eclamptic lesions. Although the causative lesion may arise in the first half of pregnancy, it is not possible to predict which pregnancies will develop pre-eclampsia. Deported trophoblast elements in maternal peripheral blood appear to be more numerous in pre-eclampsia than normal pregnancy (Chua et al, 1991). Recent reports indicate that trophoblast can be identified and separated from maternal blood using a trophoblast-specific monoclonal antibody (Mueller et al, 1990) or antibodies to low molecular weight cytokeratins (Chua et al, 1991): quantitation of deported trophoblast cells in maternal blood may therefore provide a potential predictive technique for the early diagnosis of pre-eclampsia.

Intrauterine growth retardation

There are many established causes of small-for-gestational age (SGA) infants including infection, congenital malformations and cigarette smoking but most cases remain unexplained. Acute atherosis in spiral arteries was initially described in, and considered specific for, pre-eclampsia arising *de novo* or superimposed on essential hypertension, renal disease, diabetes mellitus or systemic lupus erythematosus (SLE). However, acute atherosis has also been reported in severe intrauterine growth retardation (IUGR) independent of the level of blood pressure (Sheppard and Bonnar, 1981; De Wolf et al, 1980; Althabe et al, 1985; Labarrere et al, 1985), although whether lesions are confined to small superficial vessels in basal decidua or whether they extend into intramyometrial segments as in pre-eclampsia is disputed (Robertson et al, 1986). In albuminuric pre-eclampsia, acute atherosis is best observed in decidual and myometrial vessels which have not been subject to physiological changes. Labarrere et al (1985) reported deposition of C3, C1q and IgM in acute atherosis lesions associated with normotensive IUGR.

Inadequate trophoblastic invasion and resultant defective spiral artery physiological changes have also been reported in normotensive IUGR with a deficiency of endovascular trophoblast in myometrial vessels and sometimes throughout the length of the artery (Brosens et al, 1977; De Wolf et al, 1980; Gerretsen et al, 1981; Khong et al, 1986). However, retardation of fetal growth cannot be entirely attributed to restricted physiological vascular changes since similar vascular abnormalities have been noted in pre-eclampsia with and without associated IUGR (Khong et al, 1986).

Chronic villitis of unknown aetiology has also been strongly associated with IUGR: Labarrere et al (1982) reported chronic focal villitis in placentas from 26% controls and 86% SGA neonates, with more severe lesions in SGA compared with controls. Russell (1980) also noted correlation between the severity of chronic villitis and the degree of intrauterine growth retardation. Infection has been considered to be the most likely aetiological factor for chronic villitis, but others have favoured an immune pathogenesis resulting from maternal immune attack on fetal tissues (Labarrere et al, 1982). Chronic villitis lesions in the placenta have also been reported in association with placental bed vascular lesions, including acute atherosis and defective physiological changes, in pregnancies complicated by sustained chronic hypertension and pre-eclampsia unassociated with SGA. The possibility has been raised that the villitis represents a fetal response within chorionic villi to a maternal immune attack which itself causes defective placentation (Labarrere and Althabe, 1985).

Systemic lupus erythematosus

Systemic lupus erythematosus (SLE) is associated with a high incidence of spontaneous abortion, prematurity and perinatal death. Poor fetal outcome has been attributed to trophoblast injury but there is little convincing morphological evidence of such injury at both light and electron microscope levels. Granular deposits of C3, IgG and fibrinogen in trophoblast basement membrane (Grennan et al, 1978) are of uncertain significance since similar deposits have been reported in normal placentas (Faulk and Johnson, 1977). Villitis of unknown aetiology has also been reported (Labarrere et al, 1986).

Placental infarcts are also a feature of SLE and can be attributed to a necrotizing decidual vasculopathy (Abramowsky et al, 1980). Spiral arteries in the placental bed may show fibrinoid necrosis and a mononuclear or polymorphonuclear inflammatory cell infiltrate; acute atherosis has also been reported with deposition of IgM, C3, C1q and fibrin within involved vessels (Abramowsky et al, 1980; Labarrere et al, 1986). Defective physiological changes in spiral arteries have also been noted in placentas from women suffering from SLE (Labarrere et al, 1986). Both maternal vascular lesions and chronic villitis have also been noted in other autoimmune diseases, but patients with SLE appear to show more severe placental vascular damage which has been related to poor fetal outcome (Labarrere et al, 1986).

Diabetes mellitus

Documented morphological changes in the villous placenta in diabetes mellitus include cytotrophoblast hyperplasia, trophoblast basement membrane thickening and focal syncytial necrosis: these lesions all represent a response to trophoblast damage the pathogenesis of which is not clear, evidence for hypoxia or immune complex deposition being absent. Abnormal glucose metabolism may play a role but trophoblast damage must be at least partly independent of hyperglycaemia, similar features having been noted in both overt diabetes and well controlled gestational diabetes (Fox and Jones, 1983).

Although placentation generally proceeds normally (Robertson, 1979), acute atherosis and fibrinoid necrosis of spiral arteries have been reported: arterial lesions, often associated with IgM and C3 deposits, were reported to be present in decidua basalis and decidua parietalis in one third of 41 normotensive diabetes (Kitzmiller et al, 1981). Thus, abnormalities in uterine spiral arteries appear morphologically and immunopathologically similar in pre-eclampsia, SGA, SLE and normotensive diabetes mellitus, although the pathogenic mechanisms leading to the lesions is likely to vary.

Placenta accreta

The term placenta accreta includes conditions in which chorionic villi adhere to (accreta), invade into (increta) or penetrate through (percreta) the myometrium. The histological diagnosis is made when there is opposition of chorionic villi directly onto myometrium with no intervening decidua. Placental adherence may be focal in association with focal decidual loss, and the degree of penetration of the myometrium may not be uniform (Fox, 1972; Hutton et al, 1983).

The pathogenesis of placenta accreta is not known. Previous surgical manipulation leading to decidual deficiency, such as uterine curettage or caesarean section, has been implicated (Hutton et al, 1983). However, the possibility of a disordered fetomaternal relationship in the placental bed has also been raised (Khong and Robertson, 1987), defective interactions between migratory extravillous trophoblast and maternal uterine tissues resulting in undue adherence and penetration of trophoblast. In a study of uteroplacental tissues from placenta accreta, focal accreta sites were some-times identified adjacent to morphologically normal decidua basalis, and decidua parietalis was plentiful. Mononuclear and binucleate extravillous trophoblast accumulated at the junction of chorionic villi and decidua and the multinucleate trophoblast characteristically detected in normal third trimester placental bed tissues was absent. Physiological changes were absent in some vessels but in others extended more deeply than normal, sometimes reaching the arcuate system. The abnormalities of extravillous trophoblast, hyalinization of myometrium and the presence of interstitial mononuclear inflammatory cell infiltrate were considered to represent varying degrees of destruction of both maternal and fetal tissues in the placental bed resulting from loss of the normal balanced interaction between migratory trophoblast and maternal decidua. Defective physiological changes in some spiral arteries may lead to excessive migration of tropho-blast in others as an attempted compensatory mechanism (Khong and Robertson, 1987).

The possibility of an abnormal interaction between maternal and fetal cells in the placental bed as a cause of placenta accreta is intriguing and may also be partly in keeping with previous suggestions of a deficiency of decidua as the pathogenic mechanism: loss of normal controlling mechanisms in decidua could allow excessive trophoblast migration into uterine tissues. The antigenic phenotype of trophoblast in placenta accreta is comparable with that of normal third trimester placental tissue (Earl et al, 1987), although the lack of fresh tissue limits the scope of immunohistochemical studies. Leukocyte populations in the residual decidua have not been investigated. The possibility of abnormal maternal–fetal interactions is difficult to assess at clinical presentation postpartum, although there have been reports of placenta accreta occurring in early pregnancy (Hutton et al, 1983). The pathogenesis of the abnormal trophoblast invasion and placental adherence in placenta accreta is unlikely to be established until normal regulatory mechanisms are fully understood.

Subinvolution of the uteroplacental arteries

Although physiological vascular changes in the placental bed in normal pregnancy have been thoroughly documented, the precise sequence of events in involution of the placental site are not clearly defined. Uteroplacental arteries undergo thrombosis and organization and the placental site subsequently shrinks and the endometrium regenerates. Subinvolution of the uteroplacental arteries is a well recognized cause of haemorrhage in the postpartum period: regression of the uterine musculature and vasculature occurs at all sites except the placental bed where there is failure of physiological obliteration of the large vessels underlying the placental site (Lee et al, 1986). The clinical presentation is of abrupt haemorrhage occurring 1 week to several months after delivery with maximal incidence in the second postpartum week. Reported antecedent factors are multiparity and early ambulation; subinvolution may recur in subsequent pregnancies.

In a recent study of curettage and hysterectomy specimens from 22 cases of subinvolution of uteroplacental arteries presenting with postpartum haemorrhage, the possibility of a disordered maternofetal relationship in the placental bed was raised (Andrew et al, 1989). Non-involuted vessels contained thrombus and had no endothelial lining, whereas uteroplacental arteries normally re-endothelialize in the third trimester. In contrast with adjacent normally involuted vessels, interstitial and occasionally endovascular trophoblast persisted in subinvoluted vessels. In an immunohistochemical study of the same cases, C1q, C3d, C4 and C9 deposits detected within the walls of normally involuted vessels, but were virtually absent in subinvoluted vessels (Figure 3a,b). Deposition of IgG, IgA and IgM mirrored that of the complement components (Andrew et al, 1992). The possibility of a disordered relationship between maternal uterine decidual and endothelial cells and migratory endovascular and perivascular trophoblast requires further investigation.

Maternal infection

Placental infection arises via blood or from the endometrium and takes the form of a villitis. There has been relatively little investigation of placental bed tissues in maternal infection during pregnancy. Studies of the histological abnormalities in uteroplacental tissues associated with listeriosis in pregnant mice have led to the suggestion that the deficiency of maternal T cells and macrophages in murine decidua basalis causes increased susceptibility of uteroplacental tissues to *Listeria* infection (Redline and Lu, 1989).

Plasmodium falciparum malaria is much commoner in pregnant women than in their non-pregnant counterparts: this effect is most prominent in primigravidae, resistance being regained with increasing multiparity (McGregor et al, 1983). Parasites are more numerous and persistent in placental compared with peripheral blood. Congenital malaria is extremely uncommon but maternal infection with *Plasmodium falciparum* is associated with a high incidence of intrauterine growth retardation, and hence with increased neonatal morbidity and mortality. Reduced birth weight in

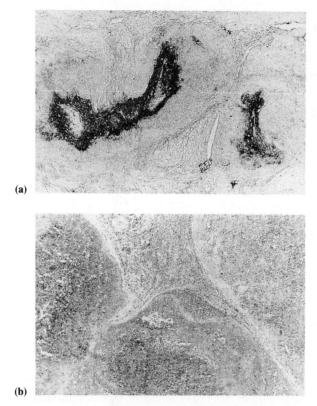

Figure 3. Term placental bed tissue labelled for C1q: (**a**) shows normally involuted utero-placental arteries with intimal deposition of C1q; (**b**) shows absence of complement deposition in subinvoluted arteries. Magnification: (**a**) × 160 (**b**) × 63, reproduced at 65% of original.

malaria has been attributed to immune-mediated damage to the placenta, supported by detection of fibrinoid necrosis and increased deposition of C1q, C3, C4, C9, fibrinogen and plasminogen in chorionic villi (Galbraith et al, 1980).

The mechanisms which underlie the apparent selective retention of parasites in the placenta are not known. *Plasmodium falciparum* adheres to endothelial cells by means of specific adhesion molecules, some of which have been defined (Hommel and Semoff, 1988) but adherence of parasites to villous syncytiotrophoblast in the delivered placenta has not been demonstrated in electron microscope studies (Bray and Sinden, 1979). The development of antibodies to the malarial adhesion molecules ICAM-1 (CD54), CD36 and thrombospondin will allow investigation of expression of these molecules by human uteroplacental tissues in first and subsequent pregnancies. Although not expressed by villous trophoblast, expression of CD54 and, to a lesser extent, CD36 by decidualized stromal cells, leukocytes and vascular endothelial cells within decidua basalis may partly account for accumulation of malarial parasites within the intervillous spaces of the placenta (Bulmer et al, 1991c). Hence, study of placental bed tissues, including decidua basalis attached to the delivered placenta, may help to elucidate the mechanisms underlying both the high incidence of malaria in human pregnancy and its association with small-for-gestational age infants.

Trophoblast tumours

The clinical and immunological features of gestational trophoblastic neoplasia are discussed elsewhere (Chapter 7). Complete hydatidiform moles are diploid, usually 46XX, and androgenetic in origin; hence, complete moles are fully allogeneic with the maternal host. Partial moles are triploid with an extra paternal chromosome component. The mechanisms underlying the increased trophoblast proliferation in molar pregnancy are not yet known. Investigations of molar placental bed tissues have predominantly focused on two areas: phenotypic analysis of extravillous trophoblast populations and characterization of decidual leukocytes. The expression of trophoblast and MHC antigens by villous and extravillous molar trophoblast is similar to that in normal pregnancy of matched gestational age (Figure 4a) (Sunderland et al, 1985a; Bulmer et al, 1988c). While villous trophoblast lacks class I MHC antigens, extravillous molar trophoblast expresses an antigen with comparable immunoreactivity with extravillous trophoblast in normal pregnancy (Sunderland et al, 1985a). MHC antigen expression appears to be similar in partial, complete and invasive moles (Sasagawa et al, 1987).

There are few reported studies of the maternal host response in molar pregnancy. Berkowitz et al (1982) failed to detect complement (C3) and immunoglobulin at the implantation site in ten complete molar pregnancies. Kabawat et al (1985) characterized leukocytes in decidua basalis in ten complete molar pregnancies and reported a fourfold increase in CD3-positive T cells compared with decidua in normal pregnancy, with CD4-positive cells contributing over two thirds of the total T cell population. This contrasts with normal gestation in which over 75% of decidual T cells are CD8-positive suppressor/cytotoxic cells (Bulmer et al, 1991a). CD56-positive, CD3-negative cells have also been detected in frozen sections of molar pregnancy decidua and correspond to the granulated cells which can be detected in paraffin-embedded sections of decidua (Bulmer et al, 1988c). Macrophages also form a major leukocyte population at the molar implantation site and, in common with normal decidua basalis, may be closely associated with extravillous fetal trophoblast (Figure 4b, c).

The immunotropism hypothesis suggests that maternal T cells in decidua secrete cytokines which promote placental growth (Wegmann, 1988). Evidence is accumulating that human decidua is a source of a wide variety of cytokines and that human trophoblast expresses several cytokine receptors. Rigorous comparative studies of decidual leukocyte populations and cytokine production between normal and molar pregnancy may be an important first step in elucidating possible decidual influences on the abnormal trophoblast proliferation in hydatidiform moles.

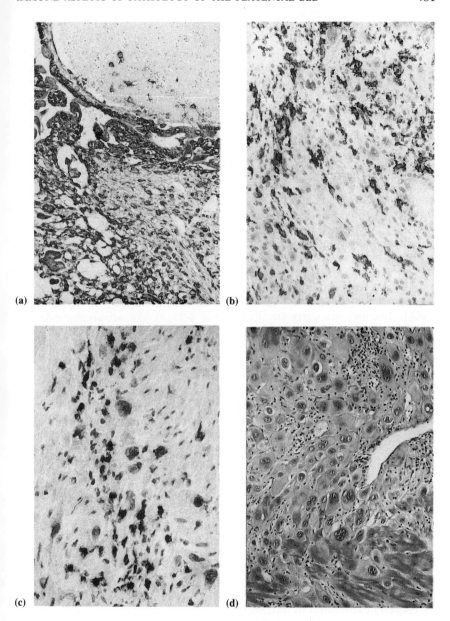

Figure 4. (a) Complete molar pregnancy implantation site labelled with CAM 5.2 (low molecular weight cytokeratins): note extensive invasion of uterine tissues by extravillous trophoblast. (b) Decidua basalis from partial molar pregnancy labelled for HLA-DR and (c) CD2 showing macrophages and T cells, respectively, associated with extravillous trophoblast. (d) Placental site trophoblastic tumour stained with H&E. Magnification: (a) ×63 (b) ×160 (c) ×250 (d) ×160, all reproduced at 65% of original.

Choriocarcinoma is considered to arise from villous trophoblast and in the United Kingdom approximately equal numbers follow normal term delivery, molar pregnancy and non-molar abortion. Trophoblast in choriocarcinoma shows uncontrolled proliferation and invasion. Experimental studies have been limited by the extreme rarity of this tumour, although several chorio-carcinoma cell lines have been developed. Choriocarcinoma shows differen-tial expression of class I MHC antigens: syncytial elements and small cytotrophoblast cells are negative while other cytotrophoblast cells, accounting for 40–70% of total cell numbers, show similar immunoreactivity for class I MHC antigens to normal extravillous trophoblast (Sunderland et al, 1985b; Bulmer et al, 1988c). Recent serological, biochemical and molecular studies have confirmed expression of HLA-G by the BeWo choriocarcinoma cell line (Risk and Johnson, 1990), an observation which is discrepant from its proposed origin from the villous placenta which does not normally express HLA-G. The demonstration of HLA-G expression by choriocarcinoma cells raises further questions regarding the role of this molecule in the regulation of normal trophoblast proliferation and invasion.

The absence of α_2-macroglobulin from invasive moles and chorio-carcinomas has been suggested to reflect involvement of this antiprotease in the control of trophoblast invasion in normal pregnancy (Saksela et al, 1981). Intense reactivity for hyaluronic acid at the advancing edge of choriocarcinomas may reflect disruption of cellular matrices by hyaluronic acid and consequent facilitation of trophoblast invasion (Sunderland et al, 1985c). Macrophages and T cells are commonly identified associated with choriocarcinomas but the lack of fresh tissue has limited the scope of immunohistochemical studies (Bulmer et al, 1988c).

Placental site trophoblastic tumour (PSTT) is an extremely rare tumour with variable clinical behaviour, which usually follows a normal pregnancy and is considered to arise from extravillous trophoblast (Figure 4d). PSTT shows consistent immunoreactivity for human placental lactogen (hPL) reflecting its origin from extravillous trophoblast (Kurman et al, 1984). Despite interest in PSTT as a tumour of extravillous trophoblast cells, its extreme rarity limits the potential for future investigations.

CONCLUSIONS

Considerable advances have been made in understanding of the complex inter-relationships between maternal and fetal cells in the human placental bed. Current research effort is directed towards elucidation of the function of HLA-G expression by extravillous trophoblast populations and the role of the various decidual leukocytes in normal implantation and early placentation. Morphological and immunohistochemical studies have raised the possibility that a variety of pregnancy disorders, most notably pre-eclampsia, may be caused by an abnormality of the mechanisms controlling trophoblast migration into uterine tissues. The pathogenic role of both extravillous trophoblast and decidual leukocytes will be easier to elucidate as the normal regulatory mechanisms are unravelled. Meanwhile, careful, well controlled studies will continue to provide valuable information to cast light on the pathogenesis of abnormalities of pregnancy which continue to cause considerable morbidity and mortality of the mother and her fetus.

SUMMARY

Interest has recently focused on the role of the placental bed in the pathogenesis of a variety of pregnancy disorders. Considerable advances have been made in the understanding of the complex relationships between maternal and fetal trophoblast in the placental bed in normal pregnancy. Invasion of uterine spiral arteries by extravillous trophoblast effects the physiological changes required to accommodate increased blood flow to the fetoplacental unit. Control of trophoblast invasion may depend on intrinsic properties, such as production of proteolytic enzymes and expression of a non-classical class I MHC antigen, but maternal cells within decidua may also play a role. Leukocytes form a major component of human decidualized endometrium and in the first trimester consist of granulated lymphocytes, macrophages and T lymphocytes. Suggested roles for decidualized leukocytes include natural killer cell activity, cytokine secretion, antigen presentation and immunosuppression.

Several pregnancy disorders, including pre-eclampsia and intrauterine growth retardation, may be due to abnormal maternofetal cellular relationships within the placental bed causing inadequate invasion of spiral arteries and acute atherosis. However, the role of immunological factors in the pathogenesis of these disorders is uncertain since deposition of immunoglobulins and complement has also been detected in spiral arteries in normal pregnancy. Placenta accreta may reflect undue invasiveness of trophoblast and immunohistochemical studies of subinvolution of uteroplacental arteries also suggest an abnormal maternofetal relationship in the placental bed. Although the in vivo role of decidual leukocytes is not known, studies of infertile endometrium have reported a deficiency of granulated lymphocytes, suggesting a possible role in early implantation and placentation. Granulated lymphocytes may also play a role in pregnancy loss.

There have been considerable advances in understanding of the abnormal maternofetal relationships in the placental bed which can lead to pregnancy disorders. However, the aetiology and pathogenesis of the various clinical conditions is unlikely to be fully established until regulatory mechanisms in normal pregnancy are elucidated.

REFERENCES

Abramowsky CR, Vegas ME, Swinehart G & Gyves MT (1980) Decidual vasculopathy of the placenta in lupus erythematosus. *New England Journal of Medicine* **303:** 668–672.

Althabe O, Labarrere C & Telenta M (1985) Maternal vascular lesions in placentae of small-for-gestational-age infants. *Placenta* **6:** 265–276.

Andrew AC, Bulmer JN, Wells M, Morrison L & Buckley CH (1989) Subinvolution of the uteroplacental arteries in the human placental bed. *Histopathology* **15:** 395–405.

Andrew A, Bulmer JN, Morrison L, Wells M & Buckley CH (1992) Subinvolution of the uteroplacental arteries: an immunohistochemical study. *International Journal of Gynecological Pathology* (in press).

Bell SC (1991) The insulin-like growth factor binding proteins—the endometrium and decidua. *Annals of the New York Academy of Sciences* **622:** 120–137.

Berkowitz RS, Mostoufi-Zadeh M, Kabawat SE, Goldstein DP & Driscoll SG (1982) Immunopathologic study of the implantation site in molar pregnancy. *American Journal of Obstetrics and Gynecology* **144:** 925–930.

Boyd JD & Hamilton WJ (1970) *The Human Placenta.* Cambridge: W. Heffer.

Bray RS & Sinden RE (1979) The sequestration of *Plasmodium falciparum* infected erythrocytes in the placenta. *Transactions of the Royal Society of Tropical Medicine and Hygiene* **73:** 716–719.

Brosens I, Dixon HG & Robertson WB (1977) Fetal growth retardation and the arteries of the placental bed. *British Journal of Obstetrics and Gynaecology* **84:** 656–663.

Bulmer JN (1988) Immunopathology of pregnancy. *Baillière's Clinical Immunology and Allergy* **2:** 697–734.

Bulmer JN & Johnson PM (1985) Antigen expression by trophoblast populations in the human placenta and their possible immunobiological relevance. *Placenta* **6:** 127–140.

Bulmer JN & Sunderland CA (1984) Immunohistological characterisation of lymphoid cell populations in the early human placental bed. *Immunology* **52:** 349–357.

Bulmer JN, Hollings D & Ritson A (1987) Immunocytochemical evidence that endometrial stromal granulocytes are granulated lymphocytes. *Journal of Pathology* **153:** 281–287.

Bulmer JN, Smith JC & Morrison L (1988a) Expression of class II MHC gene products by macrophages in human uteroplacental tissues. *Immunology* **63:** 707–714.

Bulmer JN, Smith JC, Morrison L & Wells M (1988b) Maternal and fetal cellular relationships in the human placental basal plate. *Placenta* **9:** 237–246.

Bulmer JN, Johnson PM, Sasagawa M & Takeuchi S (1988c) Immunohistochemical studies of fetal trophoblast and maternal decidua in hydatidiform mole and choriocarcinoma. *Placenta* **9:** 183–200.

Bulmer JN, Morrison L, Longfellow M, Ritson A & Pace D (1991a) Granulated lymphocytes in human endometrium: histochemical and immunohistochemical studies. *Human Reproduction* **6:** 791–798.

Bulmer JN, Longfellow M & Ritson A (1991b) Leukocytes and resident blood cells in endometrium. *Annals of the New York Academy of Sciences* **622:** 57–68.

Bulmer JN, Morrison L, Longfellow M & Ritson A (1991c) Leucocyte markers in human decidua: investigation of surface markers and function. *Colloque INSERM* **212:** 189–196.

Calderon J, Sheehan KCF, Chance C, Thomas ML & Schreiber RD (1988) Purification and characterization of the human interferon-gamma receptor from placenta. *Proceedings of the National Academy of Sciences (USA)* **85:** 4837–4841.

Christmas SE, Bulmer JN, Meager A & Johnson PM (1990) Phenotypic and functional analysis of human CD3− decidual leucocyte clones. *Immunology* **71:** 182–189.

Chua S, Wilkins T, Sargent I & Redman C (1991) Trophoblast deportation in pre-eclamptic pregnancy. *British Journal of Obstetrics and Gynaecology* **98:** 973–979.

Clark DA, Mowbray J, Underwood J & Lidell H (1987) Histopathologic alterations in the decidua in human spontaneous abortion: loss of cells with large cytoplasmic granules. *American Journal of Reproductive Immunology and Microbiology* **13:** 19–22.

Clark DA, Flanders KC, Banwatt D et al (1990) Murine pregnancy decidua produces a unique immunosuppressive molecule related to transforming growth factor β-2. *Journal of Immunology* **144:** 3008–3014.

Crepeau MA & Croy BA (1988) Evidence that specific cellular immunity cannot account for death of *Mus caroli* embryos transferred to *Mus musculis* with severe combined immunodeficiency disease. *Transplantation* **45:** 1104–1110.

de Fougerolles AR & Baines MG (1987) Modulation of the natural killer cell activity in pregnant mice alters the spontaneous abortion rate. *Journal of Reproductive Immunology* **11:** 147–153.

De Wolf F, Brosens I & Renaer M (1980) Fetal growth retardation and the maternal arterial supply of the human placenta in the absence of sustained hypertension. *British Journal of Obstetrics and Gynaecology* **87:** 678–685.

Dietl J, Horny HP, Ruck P et al (1990) Intradecidual T lymphocytes lack immunohistochemically detectable T-cell receptors. *American Journal of Reproductive Immunology* **24:** 33–36.

Dorman PJ & Searle RF (1988) Alloantigen presenting capacity of human decidual tissue. *Journal of Reproductive Immunology* **13:** 101–112.

Eades DK, Cornelius P & Pekala PH (1988) Characterization of the tumour necrosis factor receptor in human placenta. *Placenta* **9:** 247–251.

Earl U, Bulmer JN & Briones A (1987) Placenta accreta: an immunohistological study of trophoblast populations. *Placenta* **8:** 273–282.

Earl U, Morrison L, Gray C & Bulmer JN (1989) Proteinase and proteinase inhibitor localization in the human placenta. *International Journal of Gynecological Pathology* **8:** 114–124.

Ellis SA, Palmer MS & McMichael A (1990) Human trophoblasts and the choriocarcinoma cell line BeWo express a truncated HLA class I molecule. *Journal of Immunology* **144:** 731–735.

Faulk WP & Johnson PM (1977) Immunological studies of human placentae: identification and distribution of proteins in mature chorionic villi. *Clinical and Experimental Immunology* **27:** 365–375.

Feinberg RF, Kao L-C, Haimowitz JE et al (1989) Plasminogen activator inhibitor types 1 and 2 in human trophoblasts. *Laboratory Investigation* **61:** 20–26.

Ferry BL, Starkey PM, Sargent IL et al (1990) Cell populations in the human early pregnancy decidua; natural killer activity and response to interleukin-2 of CD56-positive larger granular lymphocytes. *Immunology* **70:** 446–452.

Ferry BL, Sargent IL, Starkey PM & Redman CWG (1991) Cytotoxic activity against trophoblast and choriocarcinoma cells of large granular lymphocytes from human early pregnancy decidua. *Cellular Immunology* **132:** 140–149.

Fox H (1972) Placenta accreta, 1945–1969. *Obstetrical and Gynaecological Survey* **27:** 475–490.

Fox H (1978) *Pathology of the Placenta.* London: Philadelphia and Toronto: WB Saunders.

Fox H & Jones CJP (1983) Pathology of trophoblast. In Loke YW & Whyte A (eds) *Biology of Trophoblast*, pp 137–185. Amsterdam: Elsevier Science Publishers.

Galbraith RM, Fox H, Hsi B-L et al (1980) The human materno-foetal relationship in malaria. II. Histological, ultrastructural and immunopathological studies of the placenta. *Transactions of the Royal Society of Tropical Medicine and Hygiene* **74:** 61–72.

Gearing DP, King JA, Gough NM & Nicola NA (1989) Expression cloning of a receptor for human granulocyte-macrophage colony-stimulating factor. *EMBO Journal* **8:** 3667–3676.

Gendron RL & Baines MG (1988) Infiltrating decidual natural killer cells are associated with spontaneous abortion in mice. *Cellular Immunology* **113:** 261–267.

Gerretsen G, Huisjes HJ & Elema JD (1981) Morphological changes of the spiral arteries in the placental bed in relation to pre-eclampsia and fetal growth retardation. *British Journal of Obstetrics and Gynaecology* **88:** 876–881.

Grennan DM, McCormick JN, Wojtacha D, Carty M & Behan W (1978) Immunological studies of the placenta in systemic lupus erythematosus. *Annals of the Rheumatic Diseases* **37:** 129–134.

Head JR (1989) Can trophoblast be killed by cytotoxic cells? In vitro evidence and in vivo possibilities. *American Journal of Reproductive Immunology* **15:** 12–18.

Holmes CH, Simpson KL, Wainwright SD et al (1990) Preferential expression of the complement regulatory protein decay accelerating factor at the fetomaternal interface during human pregnancy. *Journal of Immunology* **144:** 3099–3105.

Hommel M & Semoff S (1988) Expression and function of erythrocyte-associated surface antigens in malaria. *Biology of the Cell* **64:** 183–203.

Hoshina M, Nishio A, Bo M, Boime I & Mochizuki M (1985) Expression of the oncogene fms in human chorionic tissue. *Acta Obstetrica Gynaecologia Japonica* **37:** 2791–2798.

Hustin J, Foidart JM & Lambotte R (1983) Maternal vascular lesions in pre-eclampsia and intrauterine growth retardation: light microscopy and immunofluorescence. *Placenta* **4:** 489–498.

Hutton L, Yang SS & Bernstein J (1983) Placenta accreta: a 26-year old clinicopathologic review (1956–1981). *New York State Journal of Medicine* **6:** 857–866.

Johnson PM, Arnaud P, Werner P & Galbraith RM (1985) Native α_2-macroglobulin binds to a surface component of human placental trophoblast. *Placenta* **6:** 323–328.

Johnson PM, Risk JM, Bulmer JN, Niewola Z & Kimber I (1987) Antigen expression at human maternofetal interfaces. In Gill TJ III & Wegmann TG (eds) *Immunoregulation and Fetal Survival*, pp 181–196. New York: Oxford University Press.

Kabawat SE, Mostoufi-Zadeh M, Berkowitz RS et al (1985) Implantation site in complete molar pregnancy: a study of immunologically competent cells with monoclonal antibodies. *American Journal of Obstetrics and Gynecology* **152:** 97–99.

Kamat BR & Isaacson PG (1987) The immunocytochemical distribution of leukocytic subpopulations in human endometrium. *American Journal of Pathology* **127:** 66–73.

Khong TY (1987) Immunohistologic study of the leukocytic infiltrate in maternal uterine tissues in normal and pre-eclamptic pregnancies at term. *American Journal of Reproductive Immunology and Microbiology* **15:** 1–8.

Khong TY & Robertson WB (1987) Placenta creta and placenta praevia creta. *Placenta* **8:** 399–409.

Khong TY, De Wolf F, Robertson WB & Brozens I (1986) Inadequate maternal vascular response to placentation in pregnancies complicated by pre-eclampsia and by small-for-gestational age infants. *British Journal of Obstetrics and Gynaecology* **93:** 1049–1059.

Khong TY, Liddell HS & Robertson WB (1987) Defective haemochorial placentation as a cause of miscarriage: a preliminary study. *British Journal of Obstetrics and Gynaecology* **94:** 649–655.

King A & Loke YW (1990) Human trophoblast and JEG choriocarcinoma cells are sensitive to lysis by IL2-stimulated decidual NK cells. *Cellular Immunology* **129:** 435–448.

King A, Birkby C & Loke YW (1989) Early human decidual cells exhibit NK activity against the K562 cell line but not against first trimester trophoblast. *Cellular Immunology* **118:** 337–344.

Kitzmiller JL & Benirschke K (1973) Immunofluorescent study of placental bed vessels in pre-eclampsia of pregnancy. *American Journal of Obstetrics and Gynecology* **115:** 248–251.

Kitzmiller JL, Watt N & Benirshke K (1981) Decidual arteriopathy in hypertension and diabetes in pregnancy: immunofluorescent studies. *American Journal of Obstetrics and Gynecology* **141:** 773–779.

Klentzeris LD, Bulmer JN, Morrison L et al (1991) The endometrial lymphoid tissue in women with unexplained infertility. *Human Reproduction* **6(supplement 1):** 8.

Klentzeris LD, Bulmer JN, Warren A et al (1992) Endometrial lymphoid tissue in the timed endometrial biopsy: morphometric and immunohistochemical aspects. *American Journal of Obstetrics and Gynecology* (in press).

Kovats S, Main EK, Librach C et al (1990) A class I antigen, HLA-G, expressed in human trophoblasts. *Science* **248:** 220–223.

Kurman RJ, Young RH, Norris HJ et al (1984) Immunocytochemical localization of placental lactogen and chorionic gonadotrophin in the normal placenta and trophoblastic tumors, with emphasis on intermediate trophoblast and the placental site trophoblastic tumor. *International Journal of Gynecological Pathology* **3:** 101–121.

Labarrere C & Althabe O (1985) Chronic villitis of unknown etiology and maternal arterial lesions in pre-eclamptic pregnancies. *European Journal of Obstetrics, Gynecology and Reproductive Biology* **20:** 1–11.

Labarrere C, Althabe O & Telenta M (1982) Chronic villitis of unknown aetiology in placentae of idiopathic small-for-gestational-age infants. *Placenta* **3:** 309–318.

Labarrere C, Alonso J, Manni J, Domenichini E & Althabe O (1985) Immunohistochemical findings in acute atherosis associated with intrauterine growth retardation. *American Journal of Reproductive Immunology and Microbiology* **7:** 149–155.

Labarrere CA, Catoggio LJ, Mullen EG & Althabe OH (1986) Placental lesions in maternal autoimmune diseases. *American Journal of Reproductive Immunology and Microbiology* **12:** 78–86.

Lalani E-NMA, Bulmer JN & Wells M (1987) Peroxidase-labelled lectin binding of human extravillous trophoblast. *Placenta* **8:** 15–26.

Lee ETC, Marley NJE & Bevan JR (1986) A rare late complication of first trimester induced abortion requiring hysterectomy—subinvolution of the placental bed. *British Journal of Obstetrics and Gynaecology* **93:** 777–781.

Lichtig C, Deutsch M & Brandes J (1985) Immunofluorescent studies of the endometrial arteries in the first trimester of pregnancy. *American Journal of Clinical Pathology* **38:** 633–636.

Loke YW, Gardner L, Burland K & King A (1989) Laminin in human trophoblast–decidua interaction. *Human Reproduction* **4**: 457–463.

McGregor IA, Wilson ME & Billewicz WZ (1983) Malaria infection of the placenta in The Gambia, West Africa: its incidence and relationship to stillbirth, birth weight and placental weight. *Transactions of the Royal Society of Tropical Medicine and Hygiene* **77**: 232–244.

Manaseki S & Searle RF (1989) NK cell activity of first trimester human decidua. *Cellular Immunology* **121**: 166–173.

Matsui S, Yoshimura N & Oka T (1989) Characterization and analysis of soluble suppressor factor from early human decidual cells. *Transplantation* **47**: 678–683.

Michel M, Underwood J, Clark DA et al (1989) Histologic and immunologic study of uterine biopsy tissue of women with incipient abortion. *American Journal of Obstetrics and Gynecology* **161**: 409–414.

Michel MZ, Khong TY, Clark DA & Beard RN (1990) A morphological and immunological study of human placental bed biopsies in miscarriages. *British Journal of Obstetrics and Gynaecology* **97**: 984–988.

Mowbray JF, Gibbings C, Lidell H et al (1985) Controlled trial of treatment of recurrent spontaneous abortion by immunisation with paternal cells. *Lancet* **i**: 941–943.

Mueller UW, Hawes CS, Wright AE et al (1990) Isolation of fetal trophoblast cells from peripheral blood of pregnant women. *Lancet* **336**: 197–200.

Mues B, Langer D, Zwadlo G & Sorg G (1989) Phenotypic characterization of macrophages in human term placenta. *Immunology* **67**: 303–307.

Mullins DE & Rohrlich ST (1983) The role of proteinases in cellular invasiveness. *Biochimica et Biophysica Acta* **695**: 177–214.

Nagler A, Lanier LL, Cwirla S & Phillips JH (1989) Comparative studies of human FCR III positive and negative natural killer cells. *Journal of Immunology* **143**: 3183–3191.

Nebel L, Fein A, Rudak E et al (1986) Structural aspects of embryo failure following in vitro fertilization and embryo transfer; immune rejection or malimplantation. In Clark DA & Croy BA (eds) *Reproductive Immunology 1986*, pp 227–235. Amsterdam: Elsevier Science Publishers.

Oksenberg JR, Mor Yosef S, Persitz E et al (1986) Antigen presenting cells in human decidual tissue. *American Journal of Reproductive Immunology and Microbiology* **11**: 82–88.

Pace DP, Longfellow M & Bulmer JN (1991) Intraepithelial lymphocytes in human endometrium. *Journal of Reproduction and Fertility* **91**: 165–174.

Parhar RS, Kennedy TG & Lala PK (1988) Suppression of lymphocyte alloreactivity by early gestational human decidua. I. Characterization of suppressor cells and suppressor molecules. *Cellular Immunology* **116**: 392–410.

Parhar RS, Yagel S & Lala PK (1989) PGE$_2$-mediated immunosuppression by first trimester human decidual cells blocks activation of maternal leukocytes with potential anti-trophoblast activity. *Cellular Immunology* **120**: 61–74.

Peel S & Adam E (1991) The killing of rat placental cells by rat and mouse granulated metrial gland cells in vitro. *Placenta* **12**: 161–171.

Pijnenborg R, Dixon G, Robertson WB & Brosens I (1980) Trophoblast invasion of human decidua from 8–18 weeks of pregnancy. *Placenta* **1**: 3–19.

Purcell DFJ, McKenzie IFC, Lublin DM et al (1990) The human cell-surface glycoproteins HuLy-m5, membrane co-factor protein (MCP) of the complement system, and trophoblast leucocyte-common (TLX) antigen are CD46. *Immunology* **70**: 155–161.

Redline RW & Lu CY (1989) Localization of fetal major histocompatibility complex antigens and maternal leukocytes in murine placenta. *Laboratory Investigation* **61**: 27–36.

Redman CWG, McMichael AJ, Stirrat GM, Sunderland GA & Ting A (1984) Class I major histocompatibility complex antigens on human extravillous trophoblast. *Immunology* **52**: 457–468.

Risk JM & Johnson PM (1990) Northern blot analysis of HLA-G expression by BeWo human choriocarcinoma cells. *Journal of Reproductive Immunology* **18**: 199–203.

Ritson A & Bulmer JN (1989) Isolation and functional studies of granulated lymphocytes in first trimester human decidua. *Clinical and Experimental Immunology* **77**: 263–268.

Robertson SA & Seamark RF (1990) Granulocyte-macrophage colony stimulating factor (GM-CSF) in the murine reproductive tract; stimulation by seminal factors. *Reproduction, Fertility and Development* **2**: 359–368.

Robertson WB (1979) Uteroplacental blood flow in maternal diabetes. In Sutherland HW &

Stowers JM (eds) *Carbohydrate Metabolism in Pregnancy and the Newborn, 1978*, pp 63–75. Berlin, Heidelberg and New York: Springer-Verlag.

Robertson WB, Khong TY, Brosens I et al (1986) The placental bed biopsy: review from three European centers. *American Journal of Obstetrics and Gynecology* **155:** 401–412.

Russell P (1980) Inflammatory lesions of the human placenta. III. The histopathology of villitis of unknown aetiology. *Placenta* **1:** 227–244.

Saksela O, Wahlstrom T, Lehtovirta P, Seppala M & Vaheri A (1981) Presence of α_2 macro-globulin in normal but not malignant human syncytiotrophoblast. *Cancer Research* **41:** 2507–2513.

Sanders SK, Giblin PA & Kavathas P (1991) Cell–cell adhesion mediated by CD8 and human histocompatibility leukocyte antigen G, a non-classical major histocompatibility complex class I molecule on cytotrophoblasts. *Journal of Experimental Medicine* **174:** 737–740.

Sasagawa M, Ohmomo Y, Kanazawa K & Takeuchi S (1987) HLA expression by trophoblast of invasive moles. *Placenta* **8:** 111–118.

Sheppard BL & Bonnar J (1981) An ultrastructural study of uteroplacental spiral arteries in hypertensive and normotensive pregnancy and fetal growth retardation. *British Journal of Obstetrics and Gynaecology* **88:** 695–705.

Soffer Y, Caspi E & Weinstein Y (1983) Endometrial cell-mediated immunity and contraception: new perspectives. In Dondero F (ed.) *Immunological Factors in Human Contraception*, pp 161–167. Rome: Field Educational Italia Acta Medica.

Stewart I & Mukhtar DDY (1988) The killing of mouse trophoblast cells by granulated metrial gland cells in vitro. *Placenta* **9:** 417–426.

Sunderland CA, Redman CWG & Stirrat GM (1985a) Characterization and localization of HLA antigens on hydatidiform mole. *American Journal of Obstetrics and Gynecology* **151:** 130–135.

Sunderland CA, Sasagawa M, Kanazawa K, Stirrat GM & Takeuchi S (1985b) An immuno-histochemical study of HLA antigen expression by gestational choriocarcinoma. *British Journal of Cancer* **51:** 809–814.

Sunderland CA, Bulmer JN, Luscombe M, Redman CWG & Stirrat GM (1985c) Immuno-histochemical and biochemical evidence for a role for hyaluronic acid in the growth and development of the placenta. *Journal of Reproductive Immunology* **8:** 197–212.

Szekeres-Bartho J, Csernus V, Hadnagy I & Pasca AS (1983) Immunosuppressive effect of serum progesterone during pregnancy depends on the progesterone binding capacity of the lymphocytes. *Journal of Reproductive Immunology* **5:** 81–88.

Tabibzadeh S & Satyaswaroop PG (1989) Sex steroid receptors in lymphoid cells of human endometrium. *American Journal of Clinical Pathology* **91:** 656–663.

Tatarova NA, Susloparov LA, Bistrova DA & Mikhailor VM (1989) Changes in the cellular stroma of decidual tissue in physiologically developing pregnancy and rising toxicosis (Russian). *Archiv Anatomii Gistologii I Embriologii (Leningrad)* **97:** 76–82.

Taylor C & Faulk WP (1981) Prevention of recurrent abortions with leucocyte transfusions. *Lancet* **ii:** 68–70.

Thrower S, Bulmer JN, Griffin N & Wells M (1991) Further studies of lectin binding by villous and extravillous trophoblast in normal and pathological pregnancy. *International Journal of Gynecological Pathology* **10:** 238–251.

Uzumaki H, Okabe T, Sasaki N et al (1989) Identification and characterization of receptors for granulocyte colony-stimulating factor on human placenta and trophoblastic cells. *Proceedings of the National Academy of Sciences (USA)* **86:** 9323–9326.

Wegmann TG (1988) Maternal T cells promote placental growth and prevent spontaneous abortion. *Immunology Letters* **17:** 297–302.

Weir PE (1981) Immunofluorescent studies of the uteroplacental arteries in normal pregnancy. *British Journal of Obstetrics and Gynaecology* **88:** 301–307.

Wells M, Hsi B-L & Faulk WP (1984) Class I antigens of the major histocompatibility complex on cytotrophoblast of the human placental basal plate. *American Journal of Reproductive Immunology* **6:** 167–174.

Wells M, Bennett J, Bulmer JN, Jackson P & Holgate CS (1987) Complement component deposition in uteroplacental (spiral) arteries in normal human pregnancy. *Journal of Reproductive Immunology* **12:** 125–135.

Yeh C-JG, Bulmer JN, Hsi B-L et al (1990) Monoclonal antibodies to T cell receptor δ complex react with human endometrial glandular cells. *Placenta* **11:** 253–261.

5

Immunological contributions to recurrent pregnancy loss

JOSEPH A. HILL

Recurrent pregnancy loss is a catastrophic malady affecting 1–3% of couples during pregnancy (Roth, 1963; Warburton and Fraser, 1963). In the United States, recurrent spontaneous abortion is defined as the occurrence of three or more clinically detectable pregnancy losses prior to the 20th week of gestation. In the United Kingdom, this definition extends to the 24th week from the first day of the last menstrual period, while the definition proposed by the World Health Organisation is repetitive loss of an embryo or fetus weighing less than or equal to 500 g which is approximately 24 weeks' gestation. These definitions should be changed from three to two prior losses to allow search for causation especially when the woman is older than 35 years, the couple is having difficulty conceiving or for couples anxious to initiate investigation of potential causes (Stirrat, 1990).

It is incumbent on clinicians to be aware of tabulated miscarriage recurrence risks not only for purposes of patient counselling but also to enable a more informed view of the literature, since the more pessimistic the figures, the more optimistic potential therapeutic modalities for recurrent abortion will appear. Based on both prospective and retrospective epidemiological surveys, after three consecutive pregnancy losses the chance for a fourth miscarriage is between 32% and 47% (Warburton and Fraser, 1961; Alberman, 1988).

Many potential causes of recurrent abortion have been proposed (reviewed in Hill and Ravnikar, 1989) but the majority of cases (60%) are unexplained by conventional genetic, anatomical and endocrinological diagnostic criteria (Stray-Pedersen and Stray-Pedersen, 1984; Hill et al, 1992). Immunological theories have been proposed for many of these otherwise unexplained losses (reviewed in Hill, 1990) since the developing embryo and trophoblast are natural immunological targets due to their paternally inherited gene products and tissue-specific differentiation antigens (Hill and Anderson, 1988a). Based on these theories speculation has arisen that unexplained recurrent abortion may be due to impaired maternal immune tolerance to the semi-allogenic conceptus. This speculation has given rise to many investigative procedures and diverse immunotherapies, often with little substantive data regarding their rationale and efficacy. The purpose of this chapter is to present the immunological contributions to

Table 1. Immunological theories of recurrent pregnancy loss.

Antiphospholipid antibodies
Suppressor cell and factor deficiency
Major histocompatibility antigen expression
Blocking antibody deficiency
Immunodystrophism
Cytokine and growth factor deficiency

recurrent pregnancy loss including a discussion of their possible mechanisms of action, evaluative measures and proposed therapies for immunological recurrent abortion. The major immunological theories proposed for recurrent pregnancy loss are presented in Table 1. Antiphospholipid antibodies are discussed in Chapter 6 and therefore will not be explored here except to include them among the theories proposed for recurrent pregnancy loss.

SUPPRESSOR CELL AND FACTOR DEFICIENCY

The decidua in human pregnancy has been proposed to constitute a distinct immunological microenvironment (Dudley et al, 1990). One mechanism proposed for immunological pregnancy loss is based on the finding of suppressor immune cell deficiency in the decidua of mice prior to spontaneous abortion (Clark et al, 1986). Extrapolation of animal data to humans should be cautiously interpreted due to inherent anatomical, morphological, endocrinological, and immunological differences between species. Support for this theory, however, has been advanced by the observation of decidual suppressor cell deficiency in biopsies from women with failing chemical pregnancies following in vitro fertilization and embryo transfer (Nabel, 1984). Suppressor cell deficiency has also been observed in the decidua of three women with a missed abortion between 10 and 11 weeks of gestation (Daya et al, 1985). In this same study the decidua of three out of fifteen women undergoing elective pregnancy termination between 10 and 16 weeks' gestation also had evidence of suppressor cell deficiency (Daya et al, 1985). Therefore, it is not possible to conclude from these limited data that recurrent pregnancy loss is due to suppressor cell deficiency. Macrophage activation and function, which are normally suppressed in human pregnancy, have been observed to be enhanced in the decidua from women with spontaneous abortion as compared with macrophages isolated from the decidua of women having elective pregnancy termination (Hill, submitted). Causal relationships are difficult to ascribe since these observations could be the result of spontaneous abortion rather than their cause. The factors responsible for suppressor cell recruitment and function, or the lack of same, have never been isolated nor has their specificity been determined. This theory, although intriguing, cannot be substantiated until larger studies are reported that determine and compare immune cellular and functional differences within the decidua of women experiencing: (1) their first spontaneous abortion; (2) recurrent abortion of both unexplained and presumed aetiology; and (3) those having elective pregnancy termination.

INDUCTION OF MAJOR HISTOCOMPATIBILITY (MHC) ANTIGEN EXPRESSION

As reviewed in Chapter 2, syncytiotrophoblast does not normally express MHC class I or class II antigens except for an atypical form of class I MHC antigens on cytotrophoblast termed HLA-G (Kovats et al, 1990). Due to the absence of typical class I MHC determinants and class II MHC antigen expression, trophoblast cannot serve as a classical immunogen for maternal sensitization or as a target for MHC-directed cytotoxic T cells. In some circumstances MHC antigen expression can be induced on trophoblast in response to the T cell cytokine, interferon-γ (IFN-γ) (Anderson and Berkowitz, 1985; Feinman et al, 1987). T cells have been observed in human endometrium as discussed in Chapter 4. Upon T cell activation either by alloimmunity to reproductive antigens or non-specifically due to infection, IFN-γ may be released inducing aberrant class I MHC expression in trophoblast. Cytotoxic T cell attack could then ensue and further helper T cell activation inducing immunity to trophoblast culminating in spontaneous absortion. Further work is needed to determine if this theory can be validated.

BLOCKING ANTIBODY DEFICIENCY

The theory that maternal blocking antibody deficiency is a cause of recurrent spontaneous abortion is based on three suppositions: (1) there is an antifetal, maternal cell-mediated immune response that develops in all pregnancies that must be blocked; (2) blocking antibodies develop in all successful pregnancies that prevent the maternal, antifetal cell-mediated immune response; and (3) in the absence of blocking antibodies, abortion of the fetus occurs (Sargent et al, 1988). These suppositions, although widely believed, have not been scientifically validated. To begin with, there is no direct pathological evidence that an antifetal, maternal immune response occurs in all pregnancies either with or without blocking antibodies. Secondly, there is little evidence that an immunoglobulin effector occurs in all successful pregnancies to block this presumed antifetal immune response. In fact, there is no direct immunoglobulin assay available to assess whether purported blocking antibodies exist. Investigators have assumed that lack of serum blocking activity as assessed by maternal responder, paternal stimulator, mixed lymphocyte culture (MLC) reactivity is due to absence of an immunoglobulin effector. However, the serum factors responsible for MLC inhibition have never been thoroughly characterized. Lack of blocking activity as assessed by MLC inhibition has been reported in women with recurrent pregnancy loss (Rocklin et al, 1976; Beer et al, 1981). However, not all women with presumed immunological recurrent abortion have evidence of aberrant MLC responses (Sargent et al, 1988). Similarly, not all women with successful pregnancies produce serum factors capable of inhibiting MLC reactions (Rocklin et al, 1982) and not all pregnant women make antibodies directed against paternal human leukocyte antigens (HLA)

(Amos and Kostyn, 1980). Therefore, neither the presence nor the absence of MLC inhibition nor antipaternal cytotoxic antibodies are helpful in the management of recurrent aborting couples (Regan and Braude, 1987). The theory that blocking antibody deficiency is a cause of pregnancy loss is further challenged by the fact that B lymphocyte-deficient agammaglobulinaemic mice and women can achieve successful pregnancy (Rodger, 1985).

A novel HLA-linked antigen system has been proposed, based on rabbit polyclonal antisera that was cross-reactive with both trophoblast and lymphocytes, termed the trophoblast–lymphocyte cross-reactivity (TLX) antigen system (McIntyre et al, 1983). HLA sharing was proposed as a marker for TLX antigen sharing and it was suggested that TLX homozygosity caused inhibition of blocking antibodies believed essential for normal pregnancy (McIntyre and Faulk, 1983). Direct evidence that TLX heterozygosity induces an antibody or any factor essential to pregnancy maintenance has never been causally demonstrated. The recent finding that TLX is identical to CD46, a receptor for complement (Purcell et al, 1990), implies that its function is to bind complement, thus preventing complement-mediated attack of the developing trophoblast. This complement receptor is found on a wide variety of cells including leukocytes and spermatozoa (Anderson et al, 1989), thus explaining the cross-reactive nature of the antisera that originally defined TLX and contributed to the misconception that TLX defined a new alloantigen system.

IMMUNODYSTROPHISM

Female reproductive tissues contain diverse lymphocyte and macrophage populations capable of mediating cellular immunity through the secretion of their activated soluble immune/inflammatory products called cytokines (Hill and Anderson, 1990). Recent data indicate that certain cytokines have toxic or deregulating effects on fetal–placental tissues if present during specific intervals of development. This concept has been termed immunodystrophism in pregnancy (Hill, 1990; Anderson et al, 1991).

The hypothesis involving immunodystrophism is based on the finding that certain cytokines can exert cytotoxic effects either directly or indirectly in a non-paternal/fetal–MHC restricted manner, since macrophages do not require MHC antigens for activation, and T helper/inducer lymphocytes can become activated without target cell MHC antigen involvement if they are stimulated by activated macrophages (Goodman, 1991). In susceptible women, macrophages may become activated by reproductive (sperm, trophoblast, endometriosis) or microbial antigens (Hill and Anderson, 1988b). The macrophage cytokines, interleukin 1 (IL-1), tumour necrosis factor α (TNF-α) and other soluble factors like free oxygen radicals, prostaglandins and hydrogen peroxide can be released as a result of activation and have direct detrimental effects on reproductive processes (Anderson and Hill, 1988). Macrophages play a pivotal role in initiating an immune response via the secretion of IL-1 which can stimulate the release of interleukin 2 (IL-2) by IL-1 activated T helper/inducer lymphocytes. IL-2 in turn stimulates the proliferation and differentiation of other IL-2-responsive lymphocytes, causing the secretion of other cytokines in a process known as the cytokine cascade. Some of these cytokines either directly or indirectly through activation of additional cytocidal mediators (natural killer cells, cytotoxic cells, and antibodies) may be detrimental to pregnancy maintenance (Hill and Anderson, 1988b).

Certain cytokines have been demonstrated over a wide concentration to adversely affect embryo development (Hill et al, 1987b), implantation events (Haimovici et al, 1991) and trophoblast proliferation in vitro (Berkowitz et al, 1988). Other cytokines, including growth factors and differentiation-inducing factors, may interfere with gestation by causing inappropriate growth or differentiation signals (Anderson et al, 1991). In addition, the maternal immune response to reproductive antigens themselves (sperm and trophoblast) can lead in some women to local (within the reproductive environment) immune activation causing the production of embryo/trophoblast-toxic factors (Hill et al, 1992). Ectopic endometrial implants such as occur in endometriosis may also elicit in susceptible women immunodystrophic reactions culminating in reproductive failure (reviewed in Hill, 1992). Finally, since the effects of cytokines are neither MHC-restricted nor antigen-specific, the reproductive tissues themselves (reviewed in Tabibzadeh, 1991), the conceptus (reviewed in Hill and Anderson, 1988b) and placental membranes (Romero et al, 1989) could be nonspecifically damaged (innocent bystander effect) in regions of immune activation such as can occur in response to infection caused by bacterial and viral antigens.

Clinical studies are needed to verify the significance of this theory of immunological recurrent abortion. There are currently no commercially available assays to test for this potential new mechanism of immunological recurrent abortion. However, recent data from our laboratory, using bioassays involving mouse embryo development and human trophoblast cell line proliferation, indicate that immune cells from some women with recurrent abortion can be activated by trophoblast or sperm antigens to secrete soluble factors that are detrimental to either embryo development and/or trophoblast proliferation in vitro (Hill et al, 1992). Preliminary characterization experiments suggest that at least one of the factors responsible for embryo toxicity involves the T lymphocyte cytokine, IFN-γ (Hill et al, 1992). Further studies are needed to determine both the clinical relevance and the other factors responsible for these immunodystrophic effects. More efficient and less complicated assays also need to be developed, although the embryotoxic factors bioassay may be useful in predicting pregnancy outcome in women with a history of recurrent abortion, as it has recently been demonstrated to have a positive and negative predictive value of 0.76 and 0.86, respectively (Ecker et al, 1992).

Growth factor, oncogene and cytokine deficiency

Peptide growth factors and proto-oncogenes are involved in mammalian development (reviewed in Hamilton, 1983; Simmen and Simmen, 1991).

Certain macrophage and T cell cytokines are also proposed to be involved in the establishment of mammalian pregnancy (reviewed in Clark, 1989; Hunt, 1989; Wegmann, 1989). The absence of certain growth factors such as epidermal growth factor and transforming growth factor β (TGF-β) have been shown to cause abortion in mice (Tsutsumi and Oka, 1987; Clark et al, 1988). The absence of colony stimulating factor cytokines in mice has been theorized to contribute to embryonic loss (reviewed in Wegmann, 1988). However, colony stimulating factor-1 has been demonstrated not to prevent abortion but rather to induce early embryonic loss in certain mouse strains (Tartakovsky, 1989). Growth factors, oncogenes and cytokines, specifically colony stimulating factor and transforming growth factor β, have also been identified in human pregnancy (Wu and Yunis, 1980; Frolik et al, 1983). The absence of these factors has been theorized to lead to maternal rejection by the developing conceptus (Kauma et al, 1990, 1991; Anderson et al, 1991). Further work is needed to validate this new theory for immunological recurrent pregnancy loss and to identify responsible factors.

EVALUATION OF RECURRENT SPONTANEOUS ABORTION

Before considering an immunological aetiology for recurrent abortion, parental chromosomal, anatomical and endocrinological aetiologies should be investigated (Hill and Ravnikar, 1989) (Table 2). Potential immunological mechanisms for pregnancy loss are more difficult to evaluate. Current

Table 2. Investigative procedures useful in the evaluation of recurrent pregnancy loss.

Peripheral blood karyotype of both partners
Hysterosalpingogram (followed by hysteroscopy/laparoscopy, if indicated)
Luteal phase endometrial biopsy
Thyroid function studies (thyroid stimulating hormone, free thyroxin)
Anticardiolipin antibody
Lupus anticoagulant (activated partial thromboplastin time or Russell viper venom)

evidence supports the rationale for testing for antiphospholipid antibodies (anticardiolipin antibody and lupus anticoagulant) as discussed in Chapter 6. Current evidence does not support a rationale for screening for antinuclear antibodies (ANA), antipaternal cytotoxic antibodies, MLC reactivities, or parental HLA profiles. Since many clinicians continue to refer many of their patients with pregnancy loss for these tests, a brief discussion as to why they should not be obtained is in order.

Antinuclear antibodies

A positive correlation between pregnancy loss and frequency of antinuclear antibody-positive sera has been demonstrated (Cowchock et al, 1984; Xu et al, 1990) although not by all investigators (Petri et al, 1987). Similarly, there is no demonstrative difference in antinuclear antibody-positive sera between women with unknown and presumed aetiologies for their recurrent abortions (Cowchock et al, 1984; Xu et al, 1990). Serum autoantibodies commonly and non-specifically occur in the general population. Their association with particular clinical conditions varies depending on the titre considered positive. Antinuclear antibodies are heterogeneous with many different staining patterns and may even be a transitory phenomena. The clinical significance of antinuclear antibody profiles in reproduction have never been established. Thus, it appears unlikely that antinuclear antibodies are helpful in determining aetiology as they could simply be a consequence of abortion rather than a contributing cause.

Antipaternal cytotoxic antibodies

In a retrospective study of 12 women with either stillbirth or repetitive pregnancy loss, McConnachie and McIntyre (1984) reported that the majority of these women exhibited antipaternal cytotoxic antibodies and speculated that this represented an inappropriate maternal immune response to fetal extra-embryonic antigens resulting in fetal demise. In a larger, prospective study, Regan et al (1981) observed that 32% of 256 women achieving a successful pregnancy had evidence of antipaternal cytotoxic antibodies in their serum as compared with only 10% of 50 women whose pregnancy ended in spontaneous abortion. The difference in the occurrence of these antibodies between these two groups of women was related to gestation as antipaternal cytotoxic antibodies were rarely demonstrable prior to 28 weeks' gestational age and a positive value during pregnancy usually disappeared between pregnancies (Regan et al, 1981). Thus, these investigators demonstrated that antipaternal cytotoxic antibody determinations were not a useful screening test for either the diagnosis or the prognosis of recurrent pregnancy loss (Regan et al, 1981; Regan and Braude, 1987).

Parental HLA profiles

Observations in animals that reproductive performance was enhanced when there were mating pair differences in MHC antigens (Beer and Billingham, 1977) prompted investigation into possible parental HLA sharing as a cause of recurrent abortion. Parental HLA homozygosity with corresponding fetal homozygosity was believed to cause an inability of the maternal immune system to generate blocking antibodies, thus causing abortion. Initial reports based on limited sample sizes appeared to support this association; however, more recent HLA typing studies from many study groups have been unable to identify a clear association between parental sharing of specific HLA alleles and pregnancy loss (reviewed in Johnson, 1991). The association between parental HLA sharing continues to be controversial. Most reports regarding HLA sharing were retrospective and without population-based controls. However, prospective, population-based studies in Hutterites (a human isolate with extensive HLA homozygosity) have conclusively demonstrated that parental HLA heterogeneity is not an essential requirement for successful pregnancy (Ober et al, 1983, 1985).

Similarly, animal studies do not support the concept that MHC heterozygosity is required for successful gestation since inbred animal strains have been maintained for generations. Therefore, the association of recurrent abortion with parental HLA sharing should no longer be considered controversial as HLA tissue typing of couples experiencing recurrent abortion is of no diagnostic or prognostic significance (Johnson et al, 1988a,b).

MLC reactivities

As previously mentioned, MLC reactivities do not appear to be helpful in the management of recurrent aborting couples, because not every woman with presumed immunological pregnancy loss has evidence of suppressed MLC reactivity with her husband's cells (Sargent et al, 1988) and not all women with successful pregnancies produce serum factors capable of inhibiting MLC reactions (Rocklin et al, 1982). Investigators reporting MLC hyporesponsiveness between couples with recurrent abortion as compared with couples experiencing multiple livebirths have not satisfactorily addressed causal relationships, as MLC hyporesponsiveness may represent an effect of abortion or represent differences resulting from multiple livebirths rather than being the cause of recurrent abortion (Sargent et al, 1988). The clinical relevance of this test has also been questioned because interpretation of 'blocking' activity in maternal serum depends on the equation used for calculation of MLC results (Park et al, 1990). Since viable pregnancies can occur in the absence of blocking activity and spontaneous abortion can occur in the presence of blocking activity, the ascertainment of MLC reactivities are clinically irrelevant and should not be obtained.

IMMUNOTHERAPIES

Both immunostimulating and immunosuppressive therapies (Table 3) have been proposed for recurrent pregnancy loss depending on whether the maternal immune system is believed to be either hypo- or hyper-responsive to paternal–fetal antigens.

Table 3. Immunotherapies proposed for recurrent pregnancy loss.

Immunostimulation
Leukocyte transfusions
Trophoblast vesicle fluid transfusions
Seminal plasma suppositories
Immunoglobulin transfusions
Immunosuppression
Corticosteroids
Aspirin
Heparin
Progesterone
Pentoxifylline (Oxpentifylline)
Cyclosporine
Nifedipine

Immunostimulation in the form of immunization with leukocytes (Taylor and Faulk, 1981; Beer et al, 1985; Mowbray et al, 1985), trophoblast membrane vesicle extracts (Johnson et al, 1988a, 1991) and seminal plasma (Coulam, 1988) has arisen from belief in the theory concerning blocking antibody deficiency as a cause of recurrent pregnancy loss. As previously discussed, this theory is less tenable today than when it was initially proposed. Nevertheless, immunization continues to be recommended by many practitioners to recurrent aborting couples. Four tenets (Table 4) have been proposed as the rationale for leukocyte immunization (Hill, 1991). The scientific validity of the first three tenets—HLA homozygosity, MLC hyporesponsiveness and absence of antipaternal lymphocytotoxic antibodies—has been disputed as discussed earlier in this chapter. Although it is important to exclude women possessing antipaternal cytotoxic antibodies before immunizing them with paternal cells, data indicate that neither the presence nor the absence of such antibodies is relevant in the management of women experiencing recurrent pregnancy loss.

Table 4. Rationale for leukocyte immunization.

Parental HLA sharing
Maternal MLC hyporesponsiveness
Maternal lack of antipaternal lymphocytotoxic antibodies
Efficacious

Many practitioners are unconcerned that the scientific rationale for leukocyte immunization has been invalidated or that the theory of blocking antibody deficiency is disputed, because they are convinced that this form of therapy is efficacious in preventing a subsequent miscarriage. This belief in efficacy has become the latest rationale for leukocyte immunization in women with recurrent abortion. This belief is based on many anecdotal series suggesting a therapeutic benefit with leukocyte immunization for recurrent pregnancy loss. These series were publicized (Taylor and Faulk, 1981; Beer et al, 1985; Unander et al, 1985; Cowchuck et al, 1990) before adequately controlled studies were performed. Therapeutic efficacy can only be demonstrated in prospective, double-blind, randomized, appropriately controlled trials. Despite the many individuals offering leukocyte immunization and their claims of efficacy, only three published studies have reported that they were prospective, double-blind, randomized and placebo controlled (Mowbray et al, 1985; Cauchi et al, 1991; Ho et al, 1991). The first of these three published studies claimed therapeutic efficacy for leukocyte immunization as compared with placebo (77% versus 37% viable births, respectively, a statistically significant difference) (Mowbray et al, 1985). Statistical significance alone, however, does not justify scientific confidence in data reliability, as it is imperative that a significant finding be replicated by independent observers for verification before clinical implementation can be advised. The Mowbray study has been critically examined, and concerns have been expressed including how the patients in this study were randomized and whether the study was indeed double-blind (Hill, 1991; Johnson, 1991) because of the very low term pregnancy rate in the placebo group

(37%) as compared with what is known from epidemiological surveys (Warburton and Fraser, 1961; Polard et al, 1977; Vlaanderen and Treffers, 1987; Alberman, 1988; Stirrat, 1990) and the other double-blind control studies indicating a placebo success rate of nearly 60% (Cauchi et al, 1991; Ho et al, 1991; Johnson et al, 1991). The results of the two other published, prospective, randomized, double-blind, placebo-controlled trials were unable to distinguish a significant difference in subsequent reproductive performance between women immunized with donor leukocytes and their own (Cauchi et al, 1991; Ho et al, 1991). Importantly, the (background) term pregnancy success rate in the placebo-treated group confirmed the nearly 60% incidence indicated from epidemiological studies (Warburton and Fraser, 1961; Polard et al, 1977; Vlaanderen and Treffers, 1987; Alberman, 1988; Parazzini et al, 1988; Regan et al, 1989; Stirrat, 1990): The significance of the placebo effect should not be underestimated as supportive psychotherapy (tender loving care) has claimed high pregnancy success rates in women suffering repetitive reproductive loss (Stray-Pedersen and Stray-Pedersen, 1988).

Immunization with trophoblast membrane preparations have also not demonstrated a therapeutic benefit over placebo when prospectively tested in a double-blind randomized clinical trial (Johnson et al, 1991). This study also demonstrated a 60% pregnancy success rate with placebo and the authors have emphasized that it is against this background (60% placebo success) that studies of other immunotherapies for recurrent abortion have to be assessed (Johnson et al, 1991).

The results of a prospective, randomized, double-blind, placebo-controlled trial with seminal plasma have not been published. However, verbal presentations at scientific meetings have stated that there has been no significant difference between seminal plasma treated and placebo groups. (C.B. Coulam, Fourth International Congress, Reproductive Immunology 1989 and 46th Annual Meeting, American Fertility Society, 1990). The rationale behind seminal plasma suppositories involved the TLX/blocking antibody deficiency hypothesis since substances reacting with the polyclonal antisera defining TLX were reported to be present in seminal plasma (Kajino et al, 1988). This observation has been challenged by the finding that the TLX common antigen (H316) is found not in seminal plasma but on spermatozoa (Anderson et al, 1989).

Regrettably, none of the studies addressing immunization therapy has included in its study design an irrelevant antigen as an additional control to determine whether any observed therapeutic benefit could be due to the immunological phenomenon known as antigenic competition (Roitt, 1980). If non-specific immunopotentiation, such as occurs with antigenic competition, was found to be therapeutically efficacious then perhaps more innocuous immunization regimens could be devised (Hill, 1990). This point is highlighted by the finding that complete Freund's adjuvant was capable of reversing fetal resorption in a murine abortion model (Toder et al, 1989).

The recent discovery that many immunological reactions can often be dramatically modified by intravenous administration of large amounts of immunoglobulin G (IgG) (reviewed in Dwyer, 1992) has prompted its use for many autoimmune disorders in pregnancy (reviewed in Sacher and King, 1988). The rationale for IgG use in women with recurrent abortion other than in those with documented autoimmunity awaits elucidation. Until the dosage, frequency of administration and potential efficacy in prospectively randomized, double-blind, placebo-controlled trials have been determined, the routine clinical use of IgG should not be advised.

Immunosuppressive therapy (Table 3) has also been advocated for women suffering recurrent pregnancy loss believed due to adverse humoral or cellular maternal immune responses to the developing conceptus. The rationale and potential efficacy of glucocorticosteroids, aspirin and heparin for treating women with antiphospholipid antibodies are discussed in Chapter 6. The empiric use of these agents in cases where antiphospholipid antibodies are not involved in pregnancy loss cannot be condoned due to their potential for adverse side-effects and the unsubstantiated rationale for their use. Even their use in the treatment of antiphospholipid antibodies remains controversial since the optimal dosage, timing of administration, and efficacy have not been fully determined.

The 21-carbon molecule, progesterone, is essential for pregnancy maintenance (Csapo et al, 1973). Progesterone has been called 'nature's immunosuppressant' (Siiteri et al, 1977), since concentrations attained at the maternal–fetal interface (10^{-5} M) are capable of inhibiting immune function including: macrophage phagocytosis; lymphocyte proliferation; and cytotoxic activity (Siiteri and Stites, 1982; Clemens et al, 1979; Szekeres-Bartho et al, 1985; Hill et al, 1987a). Progesterone may also mediate the release of immunosuppressive factors during pregnancy (Szekeres-Bartho et al, 1989). Increased concentrations of progesterone may be required to suppress interleukin-activated mononuclear cell cytotoxicity (Feinberg et al, 1991). Progesterone production can also be modulated by macrophage supernatants and cytokines (Fineberg et al, 1992). Progesterone or one of its synthetic derivatives has been used since the 1950s for a variety of pregnancy-related disorders including as an antiabortifacient agent (reviewed in Yazigi et al, 1991). The use of progesterone during pregnancy was based on the potential endocrinological benefits it may afford. Meta-analysis of the data obtained from trials of progestational agents in pregnancy have not revealed a therapeutic benefit for their use (Goldstein et al, 1989). Meta-analysis of data is retrospective by nature and dependent on the results obtained from individual studies no matter how adequately or inadequately designed. Use of progesterone as an immunosuppressive agent has never been tested in a prospective, randomized, double-blind trial for the treatment of pregnancy loss believed due to maternal immune activation to the developing conceptus and therefore cannot be clinically recommended at this time.

Newer agents with immunosuppressive capabilities such as pentoxifylline (oxpentifylline), cyclosporine and the calcium channel blocker, nifedipine, offer therapeutic possibilities. However, their use cannot be clinically advocated until the scientific rationale for immunosuppression is validated and adequately controlled studies are published documenting both their safety and efficacy.

CONCLUSIONS

Recurrent pregnancy loss is a devastating experience for couples desiring children. Feelings of helplessness, hopelessness and even worthlessness are rife among many of these couples, often rendering them susceptible to well intentioned practitioners who may be tempted to recommend expensive, unwarranted testing and unsubstantiated therapies. Before entertaining an immunological diagnosis for recurrent pregnancy loss, it is incumbent on the clinician to ascertain and, where applicable, eliminate chromosomal, anatomical and endocrinological aetiologies. Scientific evidence currently supports the rationale for obtaining antiphospholipid antibodies but not antinuclear antibodies, antipaternal cytotoxic antibodies, parental HLA profiles or MLC reactivities. Further work is needed before suppressor cell/factor determination, embryo-toxic/trophoblast-toxic (immunodystrophic factors) or cytokine and growth factor assessment can be clinically justified and available.

Safe and effective treatment modalities are needed for couples experiencing recurrent pregnancy loss. The rationale for therapy, however, must be scientifically well founded and more innocuous than the disease (Hill and Anderson, 1986). More basic research and testing in adequately controlled clinical trials are needed before any treatment modality for immunological pregnancy loss can be promoted. Otherwise, we run the risk of adding more unsubstantiated remedies to an already cumbersome therapeutic armamentarium.

Acknowledgements

This work was supported by Grants HD23547 and HD00815 from the National Institutes of Health and the Fearing Laboratory Endowment.

REFERENCES

Alberman E (1988) The epidemiology of repeated abortion. In Sharp F & Beard RW (eds) *Early Pregnancy Loss: Mechanisms and Treatment*, pp 9–17. New York: Springer-Verlag.
Amos DB & Kostyn DD (1980) HLA-A central immunological agency of man. *Advances in Human Genetics* **10**: 137–141.
Anderson DJ & Berkowitz RS (1985) Gamma-interferon enhances expression of class I MHC antigens in the early HLA(+) human choriocarcinoma cell line BeWo but does not induce MHC expression in the HLA(−) choriocarcinoma cell line Jar. *Journal of Immunology* **135**: 2498.
Anderson DJ & Hill JA (1988) Cell-mediated immunity in infertility. *American Journal of Reproductive Immunology and Microbiology* **17**: 22–30.
Anderson DJ, Michaelson JS & Johnson PM (1989) Trophoblast/leukocyte common antigen is expressed by human testicular germ cells and appears on the surface of acrosome-reacted sperm. *Biology of Reproduction* **41**: 285–293.
Anderson DJ, Hill JA, Haimovici F & Berkowitz RS (1991). Adverse effects of immune cell products in pregnancy. In Gill T & Wegman T (eds) *Molecular and Cellular Immunobiology of the Maternal Fetal Interface*, pp 207–218. New York: Oxford Press.
Beer AE & Billingham RE (1977) Histocompatibility gene polymorphisms and maternal–fetal interaction. *Transplantation Proceedings* **9**: 1393–1401.

Beer AE, Quebbeman JF, Ayers JWI & Haines F-RF (1981) Major histocompatibility complex antigens, maternal and paternal immune responses and chronic habitual abortion in humans. *American Journal of Obstetrics and Gynecology* **141:** 987–999.

Beer AE, Semprini AE, Ziaoyu Z & Quebbeman JF (1985) Pregnancy outcome in human couples with recurrent spontaneous abortions: HLA antigen profiles; HLA antigen sharing; female serum MLR blocking factors; and paternal leukocyte immunization. *Experimental and Clinical Immunogenetics* **2:** 137–183.

Berkowitz RS, Hill JA, Jurtz CB & Anderson DJ (1988) Effects of products of activated leukocytes (lymphokines and monokines) on the growth of malignant trophoblast cells in vitro. *American Journal of Obstetrics and Gynecology* **158:** 199–203.

Cauchi MN, Lim D, Young DE, Kloss M & Pepperell RJ (1991) The treatment of recurrent aborters by immunization with paternal cells: controlled trial. *American Journal of Reproductive Immunology* **25:** 16–17.

Clark DA (1989) Cytokines and pregnancy. *Current Opinion in Immunology* **1:** 1148–1152.

Clark DA, Chaput A & Tutton O (1986) Active suppression of host-versus-graft reaction in pregnant mice: spontaneous abortion of allogenic CBA/J, DBA/Z fetuses in the uterus of CBA/J mice correlates with deficient non-T cell suppressor cell activity. *Journal of Immunology* **136:** 1668–1675.

Clark DA, Falbo M, Rowley RB, Banwatt D & Stedronska-Clark J (1988) Active suppression of host vs graft reaction in pregnant mice: soluble suppressor activity obtained from allopregnant mouse decidua that blocks the cytolytic effector response to IL-2 is related to transforming growth factor-beta. *Journal of Immunology* **145:** 3833–3840.

Clemens LE, Siiteri PK & Stites DP (1979) Mechanism of immunosuppression of progesterone on maternal lymphocyte activation during pregnancy. *Journal of Immunology* **122:** 1978–1985.

Coulam CD (1988) Treatment of recurrent spontaneous abortion. *American Journal of Reproductive Immunology and Microbiology* **17:** 149.

Cowchock S, Dehoratius RO, Wapmer RJ & Jackson LG (1984) Subclinical autoimmune disease and unexplained abortion. *American Journal of Obstetrics and Gynecology* **150:** 367–371.

Cowchock FS, Smith JB, David S, Scher J, Batzer F & Corson S (1990) Paternal mononuclear cell immunization therapy for repeated miscarriage: predictive variables for pregnancy success. *American Journal of Reproductive Immunology* **22:** 12–17.

Csapo AL, Pulkkinen MO & Wiest WG (1973) Effects of luteectomy and progesterone replacement in early pregnant patients. *American Journal of Obstetrics and Gynecology* **115:** 759.

Daya S, Clark DA, Devlin C & Jarrell J (1985) Preliminary characterization of two types of suppressor cells in the human uterus. *Fertility and Sterility* **44:** 778–785.

Dudley DJ, Mitchell MD, Creighton K & Branch DW (1990) Lymphokine production during term human pregnancy: differences between peripheral leukocytes and decidual cells. *American Journal of Obstetrics and Gynecology* **163:** 1890–1893.

Dwyer JM (1992) Manipulating the immune system with immune globulin. *New England Journal of Medicine* **326:** 107–116.

Ecker JL, Laufer MR & Hill JA (1992) Measurement of embryotoxic factors is predictive of pregnancy outcome in women with a history of recurrent abortion (Abstract). *Pacific Coast Fertility Society 40th Annual Meeting, April 8–12*.

Feinberg BB, Tan NS, Gonik B, Brath PC & Walsh SW (1991) Increased progesterone concentrations are necessary to suppress interleukin-2-activated human mononuclear cell cytotoxicity. *American Journal of Obstetrics and Gynecology* **165:** 1872–1876.

Feinberg BB, Steller MA, Fulop V, Walsh SW, Berkowitz RS, Anderson DJ & Hill JA (1992) Cytokine regulation of trophoblast steroidogenesis. *Abstracts of the 39th Annual Meeting of the Society for Gynecological Investigation*.

Feinman MA, Kliman JH & Main EK (1987) HLA antigen expression and induction by γ-interferon in cultured human trophoblast. *American Journal of Obstetrics and Gynecology* **157:** 1429–1434.

Frolik CA, Cart LL, Meyers CA, Smith DM & Sporn MB (1983) Purification and characterization of a type beta transforming growth factor from human placenta. *Proceedings of the National Academy of Sciences (USA)* **80:** 3676–3680.

Goldstein P, Berrier J, Rosen S, Sacks HS & Chalmers TC (1989) A meta-analysis of randomized clinical trials of progestational agents in pregnancy. *British Journal of Obstetrics and Gynaecology* **96:** 265.

Goodman JW (1991) The immune response. In Stites DP & Terr AI (eds) *Basic and Clinical Immunology*. Norwalk: Appleton and Lange.

Haimovici F, Hill JA & Anderson DJ (1991) The effects of soluble products of activated lymphocytes and macrophages on blastocyst implantation events in vitro. *Biology of Reproduction* **44:** 69–75.

Hamilton MS (1983) Maternal immune responses to oncofetal antigens. *Journal of Reproductive Immunology* **5:** 249–264.

Hill JA (1990) Immunological mechanisms of pregnancy maintenance and failure: a critique of theories and therapy. *American Journal of Reproductive Immunology* **22:** 33–42.

Hill JA (1991) The rationale for leukocyte immunization in women with recurrent spontaneous abortion: fact or fiction? In Chauat G & Mowbray J (eds) *Cellular and Molecular Biology of the Maternal–fetal Relationship*. INSERM John Libbey Eurotext **212:** 263–275.

Hill JA (1992) Immunological factors in endometriosis and endometriosis-associated reproductive failure. *Infertility and Reproductive Medicine Clinics of North America* **3**.

Hill JA (1989) Macrophage phagocytic function in normal pregnancy and spontaneous abortion. Abstracts of the 39th Annual Meeting of the Society for Gynaecological Investigation.

Hill JA & Anderson DJ (1986) Blood transfusions for recurrent abortion: is the treatment worse than the disease? *Fertility and Sterility* **46:** 152–153.

Hill JA & Anderson DJ (1988a) The embryo as an immunologic target in infertility and recurrent abortion. In Mathur S & Fredericks CM (eds) *Perspectives in Immunoreproduction: Conception and Contraception*, pp 261–277. New York, Hemisphere Publishing Corporation.

Hill JA & Anderson DJ (1988b) Cell-mediated immune mechanisms in recurrent spontaneous abortion. In Talwar GP (ed) *Contraceptive Research for Today and the Nineties*, pp 171–180. New York: Springer-Verlag.

Hill JA & Anderson DJ (1990) Evidence for the existence and significance of immune cells and their soluble products in reproductive tissues. *Immunology Allergy Clinics of North America* **10:** 1.

Hill JA & Ravnikar VA (1989) Recurrent abortion. In Ryan KJ, Barbieri RL & Berkowitz, RS (eds) *Kistner's Gynecology: Principles and Practice*, pp 406–430. New York: Year Book Medical Publishers.

Hill JA, Barbieri RL & Anderson DJ (1987a) Immunosuppressive effects of danazol in vitro. *Fertility and Sterility* **48:** 414–418.

Hill JA, Haimovici F & Anderson DJ (1987b) Products of activated lymphocytes and macrophages inhibit mouse embryo development in vitro. *Journal of Immunology* **139:** 2250–2254.

Hill JA, Anderson DJ, Polgar K & Harlow BL (1992) Evidence of embryo and trophoblast toxic cellular immune response(s) in women with recurrent spontaneous abortion. *American Journal of Obstetrics and Gynecology* **166:** 1044–1052.

Ho HN, Gill TJ, Itsieh HJ, Jimmy JJ, Lee TY & Itsieh CY (1991) Immunotherapy for recurrent spontaneous abortions in a Chinese population. *American Journal of Reproductive Immunology* **25:** 10–15.

Hunt JS (1989) Cytokine networks in the uteroplacental unit: macrophages as pivotal regulatory cells. *Journal of Reproductive Immunology* **16:** 1–17.

Johnson PM (1991) MHC region genetics and trophoblast antigen expression in human pregnancy. In Gill T & Wegman T (eds) *Molecular and Cellular Immunobiology of the Maternal Fetal Interface*. New York: Oxford Press.

Johnson PM, Chia KV, Hart, CA, Griffith HB, Francis WJA (1988a) Trophoblast membrane infusion for unexplained recurrent miscarriage. *British Journal of Obstetrics and Gynaecology* **95:** 342–347.

Johnson PM, Chia KV, Risk JM, Barnes RMR & Woodrow JC (1988b) Immunological and immunogenetic investigation of recurrent spontaneous abortion. *Disease Markers* **6:** 163–171.

Johnson PM, Ramsden GH, Chia KV, Hart CA, Farquharson RG & Francis WJA (1991) A combined randomized double-blind and open study of trophoblast membrane infusion (TMI) in unexplained recurrent miscarriage. In Chaouat G & Mowbray J (eds). *Cellular* and *Molecular Biology of the Maternal–fetal Relationship*. INSERM John Libbey Eurotext **212:** 272–284.

Kajino T, Torry DS, McIntyre JA & Faulk WP (1988) Trophoblast antigens in human seminal plasma. *American Journal of Reproductive Immunology and Microbiology* **17:** 91.

Kauma S, Matt D, Strom S, Eierman D & Turner T (1990) Interleukin-1 beta, human leukocyte antigen HLA-DR alpha, and transforming growth factor-beta expression in endometrium, placenta and placental membranes. *American Journal of Obstetrics and Gynecology* **163:** 1430–1437.

Kauma SW, Aukerman SL, Eierman D & Turner T (1991) Colony stimulating factor-1 and c-fms expression in human endometrial tissues and placenta during the menstrual cycle and early pregnancy. *Journal of Clinical Endocrinology and Metabolism* **73:** 746–751.

Kovats S, Main EK, Librach C, Stubblebine M, Fisher SJ & DeMarrs R (1990) A class I antigen, HLA-G, expressed in human trophoblasts. *Science* **248:** 220–223.

McConnachie PR & McIntyre JA (1984) Maternal antipaternal immunity in couples predisposed to repeated pregnancy losses. *American Journal of Reproductive Immunology* **5:** 145–150.

McIntyre JA & Faulk WP (1983) Recurrent spontaneous abortion in human pregnancy: results of immunogenetical, cellular and humoral studies. *American Journal of Reproductive Immunology and Microbiology* **4:** 165.

McIntyre JA, Faulk WP, Verhulst SJ & Colliver JA (1983) Human trophoblast-lymphocyte cross-reactive (TLX) antigens define a new alloantigen system. *Science* **222:** 1135–1137.

Mowbray JF, Gibbings C, Liddell H, Reginald PW, Underwood JL & Benard RW (1985) Controlled trial of treatment of recurrent spontaneous abortion by immunostimulation with paternal cells. *Lancet* **i:** 941–943.

Nabel C (1984) Malimplantation—a cause of failure after IVF and GT. *American Journal of Reproductive Immunology* **6:** 56–57.

Ober CL, Martin AO, Simpson JL et al (1983) Shared HLA antigens and reproductive performance among Hutterites. *American Journal of Human Genetics* **35:** 994–1004.

Ober CL, Hauck WW, Kostyn DD et al (1985) Adverse effects of human leukocyte antigen DR sharing on fertility: a cohort study in a human isolate. *Fertility and Sterility* **44:** 227–232.

Parazzini F, Acaia B, Ricciardiello O, Fedelle L & Liati P (1988) Short-term reproductive prognosis when no cause can be found for recurrent miscarriage. *British Journal of Obstetrics and Gynaecology* **95:** 654–658.

Park MI, Edwin SS, Scott JR & Branch DW (1990) Interpretation of blocking activity in maternal serum depends on the equation used for calculation of mixed lymphocyte culture results. *Clinical and Experimental Immunology* **82:** 363–368.

Petri M, Golbus M, Anderson R, Whiting-O'Keefe Q, Corah L & Hellman D (1987) Antinuclear antibody lupus anticoagulant and anticardiolipin antibody in women with idiopathic habitual abortion: a controlled, prospective study of forty-four women. *Arthritis and Rheumatism* **30:** 601–606.

Polard BJ, Miller JR, Jones DC et al (1977) Reproductive counseling in patients who have had a spontaneous abortion. *American Journal of Obstetrics and Gynecology* **127:** 685–691.

Purcell DFJ, McKenzie IFC, Lublin DM, Johnson PM, Atkinson JP & Oglesby TJ (1990) The human cell surface glycoproteins Huly-MJ, membrane co-factor protein (MCP) of the complement system, and trophoblast leukocyte common (TLX) antigen, are CD 46. *Immunology* **70:** 155–161.

Regan L & Braude PR (1987) Is antipaternal cytotoxic antibody a valid marker in the management of recurrent abortion? *Lancet* **ii:** 1280–1282.

Regan L, Braude PR & Hill DP (1981) A prospective study of the incidence, time of appearance and significance of anti-paternal lymphocytotoxic antibodies in human pregnancy. *Human Reproduction* **6:** 294–298.

Regan L, Braude PR & Trenbath PL (1989) Influence of past reproductive performance on risk of spontaneous abortion. *British Medical Journal* **299:** 541–545.

Rocklin RE, Kitsmiller JL, Carpenter CB, Garvey MR & David JR (1976) Maternal–fetal relations: absence of an immunologic blocking factor from the serum of women with chronic abortions. *New England Journal of Medicine* **295:** 1209–1213.

Rocklin RE, Kitzmiller JL & Garvey MR (1982) Maternal–fetal relation: further characterization of an immunologic blocking factor that develops during pregnancy. *Clinical Immunology and Immunopathology* **22:** 305–315.

Rodger JC (1985) Lack of a requirement for a maternal humoral immune response to establish and maintain successful allogenic pregnancy. *Transplantation* **40:** 372–375.

Roitt IM (1980) *Essential Immunology*, p 102. Boston: Blackwell Scientific Publications.

Romero R, Manogue KR, Mitchell MD et al (1989) Cachectin-tumor necrosis factor in the amniotic fluid of women with intraamniotic infection and preterm labor. *American Journal of Obstetrics and Gynecology* **161:** 336–341.

Roth DB (1963) The frequency of spontaneous abortion. *International Journal of Fertility* **8:** 431.

Sacher RA & King JC (1988) Intravenous gamma-globulin in pregnancy: a review. *Obstetrical and Gynecological Survey* **44:** 25–34.

Sargent IL, Wilkins T & Redman CWG (1988) Maternal immune responses to the fetus in early pregnancy and recurrent miscarriage. *Lancet* **ii:** 1099–1104.

Siiteri PK & Stites DP (1982) Immunologic and endocrine interrelationships in pregnancy. *Biology of Reproduction* **26:** 1.

Siiteri PK, Febres F, Clemens LE, Chang RJ, Gondo B & Stites D (1977) Progesterone and maintenance of pregnancy. Is progesterone nature's immunosuppressant. *Annals of the New York Academy of Sciences* **286:** 384.

Simmen FA & Simmen RCM (1991) Peptide growth factors and proto-oncogenes in mammalian conceptus development. *Biology of Reproduction* **44:** 1–5.

Smith JB & Cowchuck S (1988) Immunological studies in recurrent spontaneous abortion: effects of immunization of women with paternal mononuclear cells in lymphocytotoxic and mixed lymphocyte reaction blocking antibodies and correlation with sharing of HLA and pregnancy outcome. *Journal of Reproductive Immunology* **14:** 99–115.

Stirrat GM (1990) Recurrent miscarriage—Definition and epidemiology. *Lancet* **336:** 673–675.

Stray-Pedersen B & Stray-Pedersen S (1984) Etiological factors and subsequent reproductive performance in 195 couples with a prior history of habitual abortion. *American Journal of Obstetrics and Gynecology* **148:** 140–146.

Stray-Pedersen B & Stray-Pedersen S (1988) Recurrent abortion: the role of psychotherapy. In Beard RW & Ship F (eds). *Early Pregnancy Loss: Mechanisms and Treatment*, pp 433–440. New York: Springer-Verlag.

Szekeres-Bartho J, Kilar F, Falkay G, Csernus V, Torok A & Pacsa AS (1985) The mechanism of the inhibitory effect of progesterone on lymphocyte cytotoxicity. *American Journal of Reproductive Immunology and Microbiology* **9:** 15–18.

Szekeres-Bartho J, Autran B, Debre P, Andrew G, Denver L & Chaouat G (1989) Immunoregulatory effects of a suppressor factor from healthy pregnant women's lymphocytes after progesterone induction. *Cellular Immunology* **122:** 289–294.

Tabibzadeh S (1991) Human endometrium: an active site of cytokine production an action. *Endocrine Review* **12:** 272–290.

Tartakovsky B (1989) CSF-1 induces resorption of embryos in mice. *Immunology Letters* **23:** 65–70.

Taylor C & Faulk WP (1981) Prevention of recurrent abortion with leukocyte transfusions. *Lancet* **ii:** 68–70.

Toder V, Strassburger D, Irlin Y et al (1989) Complete Freund's adjuvant reverses high fetal resorption rate in CBA/JX, DBA/ZJ mouse combination. *Journal of Reproductive Immunology* **124 (Supplement):** 1989.

Tsutsumi O & Oka T (1987) Epidermal growth factor deviency during pregnancy causes abortion in mice. *American Journal of Obstetrics and Gynecology* **156:** 241–244.

Unander AM, Lindholm A & Olding LB (1985) Blood transfusions generate/increase previously absent blocking antibody in women with habitual abortion. *Fertility and Sterility* **44:** 766–771.

Vlaanderen W & Treffers PE (1987) Prognosis of subsequent pregnancies after recurrent abortion in first trimester. *British Medical Journal* **295:** 92–93.

Warburton D & Fraser FC (1961) On the probability that a women who has had a spontaneous abortion will abort in subsequent pregnancies. *British Journal of Obstetrics and Gynaecology* **68:** 784–787.

Warburton D & Fraser FC (1963) Spontaneous abortion rate in man: data from reproductive histories collected in a medical genetics unit. *American Journal of Human Genetics* **16:** 1.

Wegmann TG (1988) Maternal T cells promote placental trophoblast growth and prevent spontaneous abortion. *Immunology Letters* **17:** 297–302.

Wegmann TG (1989) The cytokine basis for cross-talk between the maternal immune and reproductive systems. *Current Opinion in Immunology* **2:** 765–769.

Wu M & Yunis AA (1980) Common pattern of two distinct types of colony stimulating factor in human tissue and cultured cells. *Journal of Clinical Investigation* **66:** 772–775.

Xu L, Chang V, Murphy A et al (1990) Antinuclear antibodies in sera of patients with recurrent pregnancy wastage. *American Journal of Obstetrics and Gynecology* **163:** 1453–1457.

Yazigi RA, Saunders EK & Gast MJ (1991) Hormonal therapy during early pregnancy. *Contemporary Ob-Gyn.* **35:** 61–78.

6

Obstetrical implications of antiphospholipid antibodies

DOUGLAS A. TRIPLETT

INTRODUCTION AND HISTORICAL PERSPECTIVES

Antiphospholipid antibodies (APA) are a family of related antibodies which have historically been defined by laboratory tests (Triplett, 1989a). The first APA was identified by the Wassermann test for syphilis (Wassermann et al, 1906). Subsequently, it became evident that some patients who did not have syphilis had a biologically false positive test for syphilis (BFP-STS). Patients with a chronic BFP-STS were frequently found to have an underlying autoimmune disease such as systemic lupus erythematosus (SLE) (Moore and Mohr, 1952). The presence of a BFP-STS identified a subset of SLE patients who had a greater risk of thrombosis, thrombocytopenia or fetal loss (Berglund and Carlsson, 1966; Love and Santoro, 1990).

In 1952, Conley and Hartmann described a circulating anticoagulant in two patients with SLE. Although the title of the original article suggested their patients were predisposed to haemorrhage, subsequent publications emphasized the paradoxical lack of bleeding and apparent increased thrombotic risk (Bowie et al, 1963). In 1972, Feinstein and Rapaport proposed the term 'lupus anticoagulant' (LA) to define this coagulation inhibitor. This designation is unfortunate since many patients with LA do not have SLE. In most clinical settings, the vast majority of patients with LA will be found to have conditions other than autoimmune disease (Triplett and Brandt, 1988). LA may be defined as an immunoglobulin(s) which interferes with one or more of the in vitro phospholipid dependent tests of coagulation (e.g. activated partial thromboplastin time [APTT]; prothrombin time [PT]; dilute Russell viper venom time [dRVVT]).

Harris and colleagues pursued a different approach to identifying APA. Recognizing the clinically interesting subset of SLE patients with chronic BFP-STS, they designed a solid phase RIA to enhance the sensitivity and specificity to detect anticardiolipin antibodies (ACA) (Harris et al, 1983). In contrast to the Venereal Disease Research Laboratory (VDRL) reagent which is composed of cholesterol, cardiolipin and phosphatidylcholine, they used cardiolipin only. The RIA was 200–400 times more sensitive than the old flocculation test systems. Recently, an ELISA test has replaced the RIA for ACA detection (Loizou et al, 1985).

Baillière's Clinical Obstetrics and Gynaecology—
Vol. 6, No. 3, September 1992
ISBN 0–7020–1634–9

Table 1. Antiphospholipid antibody family.

	ACA	LA	VDRL
Antigen	Cardiolipin	Phospholipids Animal or vegetable	Cardiolipin Phosphatidylcholine Cholesterol
Physical state	Lamellar, micellar on a solid surface	Suspension of micelles	Suspension of liposomes
Co-factor	B_2 Glycoprotein I	Prothrombin	None
Isotypes	All isotypes	IgG/IgM	Primarily IgM
Sensitivity	+++	++	+
Assay	ELISA	Coagulation (fibrin end point)	Agglutination
Test variability	++	+++	++
Reagent variability	++	++++	+
Technical difficulty	++	+++	+
Predictive of clinical complications	No (?)	No	No

The evaluation of APA has been facilitated by three different types of laboratory tests. Because of methodological, specificity and sensitivity differences, the three different tests are often not concordant in a given patient (Triplett et al, 1988). Recent work suggests varying dependence of the ACA and LA on plasma cofactors (Galli et al, 1990; McNeil et al, 1990; Matsuura et al, 1990). Consequently, it is appropriate to regard APA as a family of antibodies which have different specificities and co-factor requirements (Table 1).

Hughes (1983) was the first to propose the concept of an antiphospholipid antibody syndrome (APAS). Subsequently, criteria to define this syndrome were proposed by Harris in 1987 (Table 2). The APAS in many patients is not associated with clinical or serological evidence of SLE (primary APAS) (Alarcon-Segovia and Sanchez-Guerrero, 1989; Asherson et al, 1989).

Table 2. Proposed criteria for antiphospholipid antibody syndrome.

Clinical	Laboratory
Venous thrombosis	IgG anticardiolipin antibody (> 10 GPL units)
Arterial thrombosis	Positive lupus anticoagulant test
Recurrent fetal loss	IgM anticardiolipin antibody (> 10 MPL units) and positive LA test
Thrombocytopenia	

Taken from Harris (1987). Patients with the antiphospholipid antibody syndrome should have at least one clinical and one laboratory finding during their disease. The laboratory test results should be positive on at least two occasions more than 8 weeks apart. The lupus anticoagulant should be confirmed by correction of the prolonged clotting studies with freeze-thawed platelets (platelet neutralization procedure) or hexagonal phase phospholipid neutralization.

GPL and MPL refer to IgG and IgM phospholipid antibodies. The units are referenced to standards proposed by Harris et al (1987).

OBSTETRICAL IMPLICATIONS OF APA

The presence of APA has been associated with a variety of obstetrical and gynaecological problems including infertility (Taylor et al, 1989), chorea gravidarum (Lubbe and Walker, 1983), early pre-eclampsia (Branch et al, 1989), intrauterine fetal growth retardation (Triplett, 1989a) and endometriosis (Gleicher et al, 1987). Most studies have focused on the association of recurrent fetal loss and/or first trimester abortions (Triplett, 1989a; Out et al, 1991a). The studies of APA and recurrent pregnancy loss have in most cases been retrospective (Derue et al, 1985; Barbui et al, 1987).

Beaumont (1954) probably described the first case of recurrent pregnancy loss and a circulating anticoagulant. However, Laurell and Nilsson (1957) usually receive credit for the first identification of an association between a chronic BFP-STS, circulating anticoagulant and recurrent pregnancy loss. Subsequent case reports in the 1960s and 1970s continued to report an apparent association between LA and pregnancy loss (Lubbe and Liggins, 1988; Triplett, 1989a). In 1980 Soulier and Boffa reported a series of three women with histories of recurrent spontaneous abortion and previous thromboembolic events. Each of these patients also had a circulating LA. The triad of recurrent fetal loss, thromboembolic episodes and LA is called the Soulier–Boffa syndrome.

The association of ACA with pregnancy loss was first reported by Derue et al (1985) and Lockshin et al (1985). Lockshin and colleagues suggested the ACA was a more sensitive test than LA to identify women with increased risk of pregnancy loss. However, Derksen et al (1988) and Petri et al (1987) have suggested LA has greater specificity in identifying a patient at risk while the ACA is more sensitive. There seems to be good agreement regarding the titre of ACA and relative risk of obstetrical complications. High titre ACA is associated with an increased risk of pregnancy loss while low titres are usually of no clinical significance (Harris et al, 1986; Lockshin et al, 1989). No attempts have been made to correlate the degree of prolongation of coagulation tests and pregnancy loss. This lack of data is due to the marked variability of test reagents used to detect LA (Brandt et al, 1987; Brandt and Triplett, 1989).

Previous pregnancy history is of importance in determining the significance of a positive laboratory test for APA. If there is no history of previous pregnancy loss, the presence of a positive test for LA or ACA is not an accurate predictor of pregnancy outcome (Triplett, 1989a; Out et al, 1991a). A firm relationship between pregnancy loss and APA is only established in patients with SLE, 'lupus-like conditions' and patients with clinical findings of the APAS (Love and Santoro, 1990; Out et al, 1991a).

The association of APA and pregnancy loss has gained widespread recognition among obstetricians (Branch, 1990; Cowchock, 1991; Out et al, 1991a). As a result, many questions have been asked regarding the need to test for these antibodies and the proper interpretation of laboratory results. Physicians are in many cases defensive because of medical legal implications and as a result feel a need to order APA tests. There is no need to order APA testing as a routine in healthy pregnant women (Harris and Spinnato, 1991).

The incidence of APA positivity in normal pregnancy is relatively low, varying from 1.2 to 12% (Triplett, 1989a). In most incidental cases the titre of the ACA will be low and often of IgM isotype. Indications for ordering APA testing include: recurrent unexplained pregnancy loss, history of deep vein thrombosis or arterial thromboembolic events, and diagnosis of SLE or 'lupus-like conditions' (Out et al, 1991a).

POSTULATED MECHANISM OF APA-INDUCED PREGNANCY LOSS

The question of whether APA are causative, coincidental or a consequence of pregnancy loss and thromboembolic events has not been resolved. Initial reports of placental pathology stressed the frequent association of placental infarction in patients with positive tests for LA or ACA (Nilsson et al, 1975; DeWolf et al, 1982; Out et al, 1991b). However, subsequent reports stressed a lack of correlation between degree of infarction and pregnancy loss (Lockshin et al, 1985; Hanly et al, 1988). In the later reports, the placentae were most often small for gestational age.

Various potential mechanisms to explain the pathogenicity of APA have been presented. The most frequently quoted hypothesis was first reported by Carreras et al (1981). They found sera from selected patients with LA inhibited production of prostacyclin (PGI_2) by endothelial cells or human myometrium. Since PGI_2 is a potent inhibitor of platelet aggregation and a vasodilator, impaired PGI_2 production offered an attractive explanation for placental infarction and resulting pregnancy loss. Subsequent studies have not confirmed the original work (Hasselaar et al, 1988; Dudley et al, 1990).

Several investigators have focused on the protein C system. Protein C is a vitamin K-dependent protein which requires a co-factor, protein S, to inhibit coagulation by proteolytic degradation of factors Va and VIIIa (Cariou et al, 1986; Freyssinet and Cazenave, 1987). Decreased activation of protein C will result in a thrombotic predisposition. Since the thrombomodulin–thrombin mediated activation of protein C is a phospholipid-dependent reaction, this is an attractive hypothesis to explain the pathophysiology of APA.

Various other proposals have received some attention including inhibition of fibrinolysis (Tsakiris et al, 1989), platelet activation (Weiner et al, 1991) and decreased functional antithrombin III (Cosgriff and Martin, 1981).

Recently two reports have described animal models which suggest a causative effect of APA in the induction of recurrent fetal loss (Branch et al, 1990; Blank et al, 1991). Branch and colleagues (1990) injected pregnant mice intraperitoneally with purified IgG from women with a history of recurrent pregnancy loss and positive APA tests. The mice which received the IgG from the patient group had recurrent miscarriages while control IgG or saline had no effect. Histologically, the uteroplacental interface showed prominent intravascular decidual IgG and fibrin deposition. Blank and co-workers (1991) used two sources of ACA to evaluate their effects on fecundity, fetal loss, and weight of placentae in a mouse model. Both a mouse monoclonal ACA and polyclonal IgG and IgM ACA obtained from a patient with primary APAS resulted in decreased fecundity, fetal loss, and decreased weight of embryos and placentae.

LABORATORY DIAGNOSIS

Prior to the observation of clinical complications in patients with positive APA, these antibodies were regarded as a laboratory nuisance (Triplett and Brandt, 1988). This was particularly true in the case of LA. The description of the APAS and the availability of specific tests for ACA have increased the demands on the laboratory to screen and quantitate APA. As discussed earlier, ACA and LA appear to be separate although related antibodies (McNeil et al, 1989). Thus, when a physician requests a study for LA or an ACA, it is important to perform *both* fibrin based assays to identify LA and solid phase assays to identify and quantitate ACA. The most efficient approach requires a panel which includes both types of tests.

The diagnosis of LA is variable from laboratory to laboratory. Consequently, there is a strong need for recommended criteria to establish the diagnosis of LA. Recently, the SSC Subcommittee for the Standardization of Lupus Anticoagulants has proposed a set of criteria (Exner et al, 1991). Also the LA Working Party of the BCSH Haemostasis and Thrombosis Task Force (1991) has published guidelines on testing for the lupus anticoagulant. The most important aspect of LA testing is the proper preparation of adequate platelet poor plasma (PPP) (McGlasson et al, 1989). An achievable goal is a residual platelet count of less than 10 000/µl. Failure to properly prepare PPP will compromise any test used to identify LA.

The diagnosis of LA is dependent upon three sequential steps: (1) demonstration of an abnormally prolonged phospholipid dependent test of coagulation; (2) proof the abnormal test is due to the presence of a circulating inhibitor (anticoagulant); and (3) demonstrating the inhibitor is dependent on phospholipids and is not directed against any of the specific coagulation proteins (Triplett and Brandt, 1989). Screening tests used in step 1 include the APTT, kaolin clotting time (KCT) and dilute Russell viper venom time (dRVVT) (Margolis, 1958; Thiagarajan et al, 1986; Brandt et al, 1987). Although there is a great deal of controversy, the use of a sensitive APTT test system appears to be the most sensitive screening procedure (Triplett, 1989b). Due to physiological changes noted in blood coagulation during pregnancy, the diagnosis of LA may be more difficult. Also, when there is a high index of clinical suspicion, the finding of a normal screening test does not rule out the presence of LA (Triplett and Brandt, 1989). In this circumstance, a second screening test should be performed. This approach is summarized in Figure 1.

The demonstration of an inhibitor requires mixing patient plasma and a source of normal plasma (Kaczor et al, 1991). Failure to correct is the *sine qua non* of an inhibitor/anticoagulant. The use of a thrombin time as illustrated in Figure 1 will prevent false positive results in the mixing step.

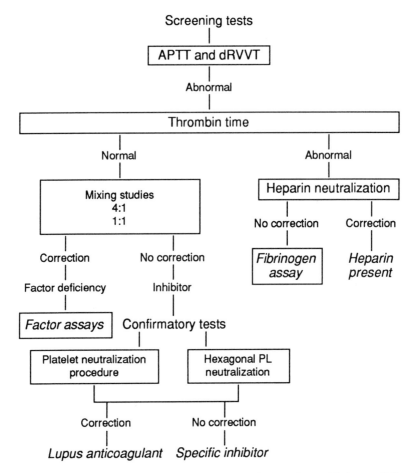

Figure 1. When the laboratory receives a request to evaluate patients with the possibility of antiphospholipid antibodies (APA), it is necessary to screen the patient sample for both lupus anticoagulants (LA) and anticardiolipin antibodies (ACA). Figure 1 illustrates a comprehensive approach to the diagnosis of LA. It is inadequate for a laboratory to merely perform an APTT as a screening test. If the APTT is found to be prolonged, then a dRVVT will not be necessary. However, if the APTT is normal, another screening test must be performed to rule out LA. The dRVVT is an excellent screening procedure to supplement the APTT. If both the APTT and dRVVT are found to be normal, no further coagulation studies are indicated. However, the laboratory should proceed with solid phase ELISA assay for ACA.

The flow diagram illustrates the subsequent approach after an abnormal APTT or dRVVT are detected in the patient's plasma. It is imperative that heparin be ruled out as an explanation for a prolonged screening study. The use of a sensitive thrombin time will effectively rule out heparin.

Assuming that the thrombin time is normal, the second step in the diagnosis is a mixing study of patient and normal plasma. The laboratory should carefully choose the source of normal plasma to ensure its relative lack of phospholipid/platelets. Many commercially available sources of lyophilized normal plasma are not acceptable for mixing studies.

If there is failure to correct upon mixing patient/normal plasma, it is necessary to proceed with the third step involving confirmation of phospholipid dependence of the inhibitor/anticoagulant. Two confirmatory tests are currently recommended: platelet neutralization

Prior to proceeding with the mixing procedure it is imperative that heparin contamination be ruled out. The thrombin time is extremely sensitive to heparin.

Confirmation of phospholipid (PL) dependence is the third step in the diagnosis of LA. Two approaches have been utilized: (1) designing a test system with decreased PL to enhance the inhibitor effect, or (2) increasing the amount or altering the configuration of the PL (Triplett and Brandt, 1988). Tests which employ decreased PL concentration include: tissue thromboplastin inhibition procedure (TTI), dilute APTT, or dRVVT (Schleider et al, 1976; Alving et al, 1985). Tests with increased or altered PL include: platelet neutralization (PNP), rabbit brain neutralization, phosphatidylserine liposomes, and hexagonal phase neutralization (Triplett et al, 1983; Rauch et al, 1989). The most reliable confirmatory procedures appear to be the PNP (Triplett et al, 1983) and the hexagonal phase neutralization (Rauch et al, 1989). Recent work suggests the epitope for LA may be the hexagonal phospholipid configuration (Rauch and Janoff, 1990). Results on the First International Workshop for Lupus Anticoagulant Identification have been recently reported (Barna and Triplett, 1991).

ACA testing has been largely converted to ELISA procedures. Various commercially available tests kits are now available. The ACA offers several distinct advantages when compared with LA testing. Serum or plasma may be used and the stringent requirements for specimen preparation and storage are not necessary. Also, it is possible to quantitate the titre of the antibodies and determine IgG, IgM, and IgA isotypes. (Harris et al (1987; Harris, 1990) have successfully conducted workshops for standardization of ACA testing. Sources of positive control are now available for all three isotypes. Utilizing these positive controls and the recommendations of the standardization workshops, laboratories can now express results in GPL, MPL, APL units. Recently, three groups have reported the need for a co-factor in the ACA ELISA assay (Galli et al, 1990; McNeil et al, 1990; Matsuura et al, 1990). This co-factor is B_2 glycoprotein I (B_2 GPI) also known as apolipoprotein H. Currently, there is some controversy regarding the epitope for ACA. Three possibilities exist: cardiolipin, a complex of cardiolipin and B_2 GPI or B_2 GPI. B_2 GPI is a physiological inhibitor of blood coagulation and an effective scavenger of negative charged substances. Therefore, the binding of APA to B_2 GPI conceivably could lead to a prothrombotic state.

---

procedure and hexagonal phospholipid neutralization. The platelet neutralization procedure relies upon an excess of disrupted platelet membranes to 'neutralize' or 'bypass' the LA. In contrast, the hexagonal phase neutralization procedure relies on the apparent specificity of LA for hexagonal configuration of phospholipids. Based on preliminary reports, the hexagonal phase neutralization procedure appears to be the most specific confirmatory procedure available.

On occasion, confirmatory tests may be discordant. With a lack of agreement, it may be necessary for the laboratory to perform factor assays to rule out other inhibitors (e.g. factor VIII inhibitors). This should, however, be a relatively rare situation. Both the platelet neutralization procedure and hexagonal phase neutralization procedure are relatively specific for LA.

MANAGEMENT OF APA-POSITIVE HIGH RISK PREGNANCIES

As previously discussed, the presence of a positive test for APA does not necessarily indicate a poor prognosis. Consequently, it is important for the physician to establish a well documented history of previous unexplained pregnancy losses or the presence of underlying autoimmune disease (SLE, APAS) prior to considering therapy.

Various different approaches have been suggested including prednisone in combination with low dose aspirin (75 mg). Lubbe et al (1983) were the first to utilize prednisone/low dose aspirin. Their reports and subsequent studies indicated a favourable response. However, Lockshin et al (1989) recently found prednisone was not effective. The maternal side-effects of prednisone are significant including: cushingoid features, diabetes, acne, hypertension and osteoporosis.

The use of low dose aspirin alone has also been suggested (Lubbe and Liggins, 1988; Lockshin et al, 1989). There is also evidence aspirin will prevent fetal growth retardation and pre-eclampsia (Wallenburg et al, 1986; Wallenburg and Rotmans, 1987).

Heparin in both low and high doses (10 000 to 36 000 IU/day) has been successfully used (Derksen et al, 1990; Rosove et al, 1990). Heparin has also been used in combination with other modalities. A disadvantage to heparin is the need for multiple subcutaneous injections and also testing to monitor the adequacy of the dose. Heparin has also been associated with osteoporosis (de Swiet et al, 1983).

Other therapeutic approaches include intravenous immunoglobulin (Carreras et al, 1988; Parke et al, 1989; Wapner et al, 1989), plasma exchange (Frampton et al, 1987; Fulcher et al, 1989) and azathioprine (Gregorini et al, 1986).

Perhaps the most important aspect in managing these patients is a well coordinated multidisciplinary support team. This team includes an obstetrician who is well versed in high risk obstetrics, a rheumatologist with an interest in APAS and a haematologist who is knowledgeable in coagulation. The patient should be carefully monitored including fetal heart rate, umbilical Doppler flow velocity waveforms, and ultrasound to monitor intrauterine fetal growth (Trudinger et al, 1988).

FUTURE POSSIBILITIES AND QUESTIONS

Although our understanding of APA has expanded significantly in the last 5 years, there are still more questions than answers. The fundamental question of whether these antibodies are pathogenic needs to be answered. If they prove to be causative, they will provide a model to approach other obstetrical and thromboembolic problems. Laboratory investigators are still attempting to identify a means of separating those antibodies which are associated with clinical complications from those with no apparent effect. These and many other questions will continue to stimulate much interest and controversy for the near future.

REFERENCES

Alarcon-Segovia D & Sanchez Guerrero J (1989) Primary antiphospholipid syndrome. *Journal of Rheumatology* **16:** 482–488.

Alving BM, Baldwin PE, Richard RL & Jackson BJ (1985) The dilute phospholipid APTT: a sensitive assay for verification of lupus anticoagulants. *Thrombosis and Haemostasis* **54:** 709–712.

Asherson RA, Khamashta MA, Ordi-Ros J et al (1989) The 'primary' antiphospholipid syndrome: major clinical and serological features. *Medicine* **68:** 366–373.

Barbui T, Cortelazzo S, Galli M et al (1987) Lupus anticoagulant and repeated abortions: a case control study. *Thrombosis and Haemostasis* **58:** 232 (abstract 856).

Barna LK & Triplett DA (1991) A report on the first international workshop for lupus anticoagulant identification. *Clinical and Experimental Rheumatology* **9:** 557–567.

Beaumont JL (1954) Syndrome hemorrhagique acquis du à un anticoagulant circulant. *Sangre* **25:** 1–15.

Berglund S & Carlsson M (1966) Clinical significance of chronic biologic false positive Wassermann reaction and 'antinuclear factors'. *Acta Medica Scandinavica* **180:** 407–412.

Blank M, Cohen J, Toder V & Shoenfeld Y (1991) Induction of anti-phospholipid syndrome in naive mice with mouse lupus monoclonal and human polyclonal anticardiolipin antibodies. *Proceedings of the National Academy of Sciences (USA)* **88:** 3069–3073.

Bowie EJW, Thompson JH, Pascuzzi CA & Owen CA (1963) Thrombosis in systemic lupus erythematosus despite circulating anticoagulants. *Journal of Clinical Investigation* **62:** 416–430.

Branch DW (1990) Antiphospholipid antibodies and pregnancy: maternal implications. *Seminars in Perinatology* **14:** 139–146.

Branch DW, Andres R, Digre KB, Rote NS & Scott JR (1989) The association of antiphospholipid antibodies with severe preeclampsia. *Obstetrics and Gynecology* **73:** 541–545.

Branch DW, Dudley DJ, Mitchell MD et al (1990) Immunoglobulin G fractions from patients with antiphospholipid antibodies cause fetal death in BALB/c mice: a model for autoimmune fetal loss. *American Journal of Obstetrics and Gynecology* **163:** 210–216.

Brandt JT, Triplett DA, Musgrave K & Orr C (1987) The sensitivity of different coagulation reagents to the presence of lupus anticoagulants. *Archives of Pathology and Laboratory Medicine* **111:** 120–124.

Brandt JT & Triplett DA (1989) The effect of phospholipid on detection of lupus anticoagulants by the dilute Russell Viper Venom Time. *Archives of Pathology and Laboratory Medicine* **113:** 1376–1378.

Cariou R, Tobelem G, Soria C & Caen J (1986) Inhibition of protein C activation by endothelial cells in the presence of lupus anticoagulant. *New England Journal of Medicine* **314:** 1193–1194.

Carreras LO, Defreyn G, Machin SJ et al (1981) Arterial thrombosis, intrauterine death and 'lupus' anticoagulant: detection of immunoglobulin interfering with prostacyclin formation. *Lancet* **i:** 244–246.

Carreras LO, Perez GN, Vega HR & Casavilla F (1988) Lupus anticoagulant and recurrent fetal loss: successful treatment with gammaglobulin. *Lancet* **ii:** 393–394.

Conley CL & Hartmann RC (1952) A hemorrhagic disorder caused by circulating anticoagulant in patients with disseminated lupus erythematosus. *Journal of Clinical Investigation* **31:** 621–622.

Cosgriff TM & Martin BA (1981) Low functional and high antigenic antithrombin III level in a patient with the lupus anticoagulant and recurrent thrombosis. *Arthritis and Rheumatism* **24:** 94–96.

Cowchock S (1991) The role of antiphospholipid antibodies in obstetric medicine. *Current Obstetrical Medicine* **1:** 229–247.

Derksen RHWM, Hasselaar P, Blokzjl L, Gmelig Meyling FHJ & DeGroot PhG (1988) Coagulation screen is more specific than the anticardiolipin antibody ELISA in defining a thrombotic subset of lupus patients. *Annals of the Rheumatic Diseases* **47:** 364–371.

Derksen RHWM, Out HJ, Bruinse HW et al (1990) Drug treatment in pregnant women with antiphospholipid antibodies. A preliminary report of a prospective study. *Clinical and Experimental Rheumatology* **8:** 219.

Derue GJ, Englert JH, Harris EN et al (1985) Fetal loss in systemic lupus erythematosus: association with anticardiolipin antibodies. *Journal of Obstetrics and Gynaecology* **5:** 207–209.

DeWolf F, Carreras LO, Moerman P, Vermylen P, VanAssche N et al (1982) Decidual vasculopathy and extensive placental infarction in a patient with repeated thromboembolic accidents, recurrent fetal loss, and a lupus anticoagulant. *American Journal of Obstetrics and Gynecology* **142:** 829–834.

Dudley DJ, Mitchell MD & Branch DW (1990) Pathophysiology of antiphospholipid antibodies: absence of prostaglandin-mediated effects on cultured endothelium. *American Journal of Obstetrics and Gynecology* **162:** 953–959.

Exner T, Triplett DA, Taberner D & Machin SJ (1991) Guidelines for testing and revised criteria for lupus anticoagulant—SSC Subcommittee for the Standardization of Lupus Anticoagulants. *Thrombosis and Haemostasis* **65:** 320–322.

Feinstein DI, Rapaport SI (1972) Acquired inhibitors of blood coagulation. In Spaet T (ed.) *Progress in Hemostasis and Thrombosis*, pp 75–95. New York: Grune and Stratton.

Frampton G, Cameron JS, Thom M, Jones S & Raftery M (1987) Successful removal of antiphospholipid antibody during pregnancy using plasma exchange and low dose prednisolone. *Lancet* **ii:** 1023–1024.

Freyssinet JM & Cazenave JP (1987) Lupus like anticoagulants modulation of the protein C pathway and thrombosis. *Thrombosis and Haemostasis* **58:** 679–681.

Fulcher D, Stewart G, Exner T, Trudinger B & Jeremy R (1989) Plasma exchange and anti-cardiolipin syndrome in pregnancy. *Lancet* **ii:** 171.

Galli M, Comfurius P, Maassen C et al (1990) Anticardiolipin antibodies (ACA) directed not to cardiolipin but to a plasma protein cofactor. *Lancet* **335:** 1544–1547.

Gleicher N, ElRoeiy A, Confino E & Friberg J (1987) Is endometriosis an autoimmune disease. *Obstetrics and Gynecology* **70:** 114–122.

Gregorini G, Setti G & Remuzzi G (1986) Recurrent abortion with lupus anticoagulant and preeclampsia: a common final pathway for two different diseases? Case Report. *British Journal of Obstetrics and Gynaecology* **93:** 194–196.

Hanly JG, Gladman DD, Rose TH, Laskin CA & Urowitz MB (1988) Lupus pregnancy, a prospective study of placental changes. *Arthritis and Rheumatism* **31:** 358–366.

Harris EN (1987) Syndrome of the black swan. *British Journal of Rheumatology* **26:** 324–326.

Harris EN (1990) The second international anticardiolipin standardization workshop/the Kingston anti-phospholipid antibody study (KAPS) group. *American Journal of Clinical Pathology* **94:** 476–484.

Harris EN & Spinnato JA (1991) Should anticardiolipin tests be performed in otherwise healthy pregnant women? *American Journal of Obstetrics and Gynecology* **165:** 1272–1277.

Harris EN, Gharavi AE, Boey ML et al (1983) Anticardiolipin antibodies; detection by radioimmunoassay and association with thrombosis in systemic lupus erythematosus. *Lancet* **ii:** 1211–1214.

Harris EN, Chan JKH, Asherson RA et al (1986) Thrombosis, recurrent fetal loss, and thrombocytopenia, predictive value of the anticardiolipin antibody test. *Archives of Internal Medicine* **146:** 2153–2156.

Harris EN, Gharavi AE, Patel SP & Hughes GRV (1987) Evaluation of the anticardiolipin antibody test: report of an international workshop held 4 April 1986. *Clinical and Experimental Immunology* **68:** 215–222.

Hasselaar P, Derksen RHWM, Blokzijl L & DeGroot PG (1988) Thrombosis associated with antiphospholipid antibodies cannot be explained by effects on endothelial and platelet prostanoid synthesis. *Thrombosis and Haemostasis* **59:** 80–85.

Hughes GVR (1983) Thrombosis, abortion, cerebral disease and the lupus anticoagulant. *British Medical Journal* **287:** 1088–1089.

Kaczor DA, Bickford NN & Triplett DA (1991) Evaluation of different mixing studies, reagents and dilution effect in lupus anticoagulant testing. *American Journal of Clinical Pathology* **95:** 408–411.

LA Working Party of the BCSH Haemostasis and Thrombosis Task Force (1991) Guidelines on testing for the lupus anticoagulant. *Journal of Clinical Pathology* **44:** 885–889.

Laurell AB & Nilsson IM (1957) Hypergamma-globulinaemia, circulating anticoagulant and biologic false positive Wassermann reaction: a study of 2 cases. *Journal of Laboratory and Clinical Medicine* **49:** 694–707.

Lockshin MD, Druzin ML, Goei S et al (1985) Antibody to cardiolipin as a predictor of fetal distress or death in pregnant patients with systemic lupus erythematosus. *New England Journal of Medicine* **313**: 152–156.

Lockshin MD, Druzin ML & Qamar T (1989) Prednisone does not prevent recurrent fetal death in women with antiphospholipid antibody. *American Journal of Obstetrics and Gynecology* **160**: 439–443.

Loizou S, McCrea JD, Rudge AC et al (1985) Measurement of anticardiolipin antibodies by an enzyme linked immunosorbent assay (ELISA): standardization and quantitation of results. *Clinical and Experimental Immunology* **62**: 738–745.

Love PE & Santoro SA (1990) Antiphospholipid antibodies: anticardiolipin and the lupus anticoagulant in systemic lupus erythematosus (SLE) and in non-SLE disorders. *Annals of Internal Medicine* **112**: 682–698.

Lubbe WF & Liggins GC (1988) Role of lupus anticoagulant and autoimmunity in recurrent pregnancy loss. *Seminars in Reproductive Endocrinology* **6**: 181–190.

Lubbe WF & Walker EB (1983) Chorea gravidarum associated with circulating lupus anticoagulant: successful outcome of pregnancy with prednisone and aspirin therapy. *British Journal of Obstetrics and Gynaecology* **90**: 487–490.

Lubbe WF, Butler WS, Palmer SJ & Liggins GC (1983) Fetal survival after prednisone suppression of maternal lupus anticoagulant. *Lancet* **i**: 1361.

McGlasson DL, Brey RL, Stickland DM & Patterson WR (1989) Differences in kaolin clotting times and platelet counts resulting from variations in specimen processing. *Clinical Laboratory Science* **2**: 109–110.

McNeil HP, Chesterman CN & Krilis SA (1989) Anticardiolipin antibodies and lupus anticoagulants comprise separate antibody subgroups with different phospholipid binding characteristics. *British Journal of Haematology* **73**: 506–513.

McNeil HP, Simpson RJ, Chesterman CN & Krilis SA (1990) Antiphospholipid antibodies are directed against a complex antigen that includes a lipid-binding inhibitor of coagulation: B$_2$ glycoprotein I (apolipoprotein H). *Proceedings of the National Academy of Sciences (USA)* **87**: 4120–4124.

Margolis J (1958) The kaolin clotting time: a rapid one stage method for diagnosis of coagulation defects. *Journal of Clinical Pathology* **11**: 406–409.

Matsuura E, Igarashi Y, Fujimoto M, Ichikawa K & Koike T (1990) Anticardiolipin cofactor(s) and differential diagnosis of autoimmune disease. *Lancet* **336**: 177–178 (letter).

Moore JE & Mohr CF (1952) Biologically false positive serologic tests for syphilis. *Journal of the American Medical Association* **150**: 467–473.

Nilsson IM, Astedt B, Hedner U & Berezin D (1975) Intrauterine death and circulating anticoagulant, 'antithromboplastin'. *Acta Medica Scandinavica* **197**: 153–159.

Out HJ, Bruinse HW & Derksen RHWM (1991a) Antiphospholipid antibodies and pregnancy loss. *Human Reproduction* **6**: 889–897.

Out HJ, Kooijman CD, Bruinse HW & Derksen RHWM (1991b) Histopathological findings in placentae from patients with intra-uterine fetal death and antiphospholipid antibodies. *European Journal of Obstetrics, Gynecology and Reproductive Biology* **41**: 179–186.

Parke A, Maier D, Wilson D, Andreoli J & Batlow M (1989) Intravenous gamma-globulin and anti-phospholipid antibodies and pregnancy. *Annals of Internal Medicine* **110**: 495–496.

Petri M, Rheinschmidt M, Whiting-O'Keefe Q et al (1987) The frequency of lupus anticoagulant in systemic lupus erythematosus. A study of sixty consecutive patients by activated partial thromboplastin time, Russell viper venom time, and anticardiolipin antibody level. *Annals of Internal Medicine* **106**: 524–531.

Rauch J & Janoff AS (1990) Phospholipid in the hexagonal II phase is immunogenic: evidence for immunorecognition of nonbilayar lipid phases in vivo. *Proceedings of the National Academy of Sciences (USA)* **87**: 4112–4114.

Rauch J, Tannenbaum M & Janoff AS (1989) Distinguishing plasma lupus anticoagulants from anti-factor antibodies using hexagonal (II) phase phospholipids. *Thrombosis and Haemostasis* **62**: 892–896.

Rosove MH, Tabsh K, Wasserstrum N et al (1990) Heparin therapy for pregnant women with lupus anticoagulant or anticardiolipin antibodies. *Obstetrics and Gynecology* **75**: 630–634.

Schleider MA, Nachman RL, Jaffe EA & Coleman M (1976) A clinical study of the lupus anticoagulant. *Blood* **48**: 499–509.

Soulier RP & Boffa MC (1980) Avortements à répétition, thromboses et anticoagulant circulant antithromboplastin. *Nouvelle Presse Médicale* **9:** 859–864.

de Swiet M, Dorrington PW, Fidler J et al (1983) Prolonged heparin therapy in pregnancy causes bone demineralization. *British Journal of Obstetrics and Gynaecology* **90:** 1129–1134.

Taylor PV, Campbell JM & Scott JS (1989) Presence of autoantibodies in women with unexplained infertility. *American Journal of Obstetrics and Gynecology* **161:** 377–379.

Thiagarajan P, Pengo V & Shapiro SS (1986) The use of the dilute Russell viper venom time for the diagnosis of lupus anticoagulants. *Blood* **68:** 869–874.

Triplett DA (1989a) Antiphospholipid antibodies and recurrent pregnancy loss. *American Journal of Reproductive Immunology* **20:** 52–67.

Triplett DA (1989b) Screening for the lupus anticoagulant. *Research in Clinic and Laboratory* **19:** 379–389.

Triplett DA & Brandt JT (1988) Lupus anticoagulant: misnomer, paradox, riddle, epiphenomenon. *Hematologic Pathology* **2:** 121–143 (review).

Triplett DA & Brandt J (1989) Laboratory identification of the lupus anticoagulant. *British Journal of Haematology* **73:** 139–142 (annotation).

Triplett DA, Brandt JT, Kaczor D & Schaeffer J (1983) Laboratory diagnosis of lupus inhibitors: a comparison of the tissue thromboplastin inhibition procedure with a new platelet neutralization procedure. *American Journal of Clinical Pathology* **79:** 678–682.

Triplett DA, Brandt JT, Musgrave KA & Orr C (1988) Relationship between lupus anticoagulants and antibodies to phospholipids. *Journal of the American Medical Association* **259:** 550–554.

Trudinger BJ, Stewart GJ, Cook CM, Connelly A & Exner T (1988) Monitoring lupus anticoagulant positive pregnancies with umbilical artery waveforms. *Obstetrics and Gynecology* **72:** 215–218.

Tsarkiris DA, Marbet GA, Maknis PE, Settas L & Duckert F (1989) Impaired fibrinolysis as an essential contribution to thrombosis in patients with lupus anticoagulant. *Thrombosis and Haemostasis* **61:** 175–177.

Wallenburg HCS & Rotmans N (1987) Prevention of recurrent idiopathic fetal growth retardation by low dose aspirin and dipyridamole. *American Journal of Obstetrics and Gynecology* **157:** 1230–1235.

Wallenburg HCS, Dekker GA, Makowitz JW & Rotmans P (1986) Low dose aspirin prevents pregnancy induced hypertension and preeclampsia in angiotensin-sensitive primigravidae. *Lancet* **i:** 1–3.

Wapner RJ, Cowchock FS & Shapiro SS (1989) Successful treatment in two women with antiphospholipid antibodies and refractory pregnancy losses with intravenous immunoglobulin infusions. *American Journal of Obstetrics and Gynecology* **161:** 1271–1272.

Wassermann A, Neisser A & Bruck C (1906) Eine serodiagnostische Reaktion bei Syphilis. *Deutsche Medizinische Wochenschrift* **32:** 745–746.

Weiner HM, Vardinon N & Yust I (1991) Platelet antibody binding and spontaneous aggregation in 21 lupus anticoagulant patients. *Vox Sanguinis* **62:** 111–121.

7

The immune system in disease: gestational trophoblastic tumours

EDWARD S. NEWLANDS
ROSEMARY A. FISHER
FRANCES SEARLE

INTRODUCTION

Gestational trophoblastic tumours (GTT) are unique in that by definition they must follow a normal or abnormal pregnancy and the tumours express paternal genes and are therefore an allograft in the maternal host.

GTT occur most commonly after the abnormal pregnancy, hydatidiform mole (HM), but can also occur after a normal pregnancy (Table 1). Trophoblast in a normal pregnancy shares some characteristics with malignancy in that the trophoblast invades the myometrium and forms intimate connections with the maternal circulation. Trophoblast from a normal pregnancy can on occasion embolize to the lungs. Sufficient trophoblast cells may be present in the circulation to allow antenatal diagnosis of genetic disorders, using the polymerase chain reaction (Mueller et al, 1990).

Table 1. Gestational trophoblastic tumours.

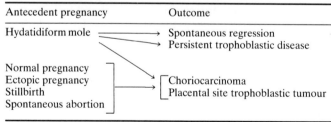

Antecedent pregnancy	Outcome
Hydatidiform mole	Spontaneous regression / Persistent trophoblastic disease
Normal pregnancy / Ectopic pregnancy / Stillbirth / Spontaneous abortion	Choriocarcinoma / Placental site trophoblastic tumour

Since GTT express not only paternal genes but paternally derived antigens, it might be anticipated that the immune system plays a major role in eliminating these diseases. However, it has been hypothesized that the process whereby the mother does not reject a normal fetus may operate in the situation where there is a trophoblastic tumour. The ABO blood group system influences the outcome of patients developing trophoblastic tumours

Baillière's Clinical Obstetrics and Gynaecology—
Vol. 6, No. 3, September 1992
ISBN 0–7020–1634–9

and patients with B or AB whose partners are either group O or A may have a worse prognosis (Bagshawe, 1976).

Lawler (1978) studied the development of anti-HLA antibodies in a large group of patients with GTT. Her results showed that (1) choriocarcinoma can follow the birth of an HLA incompatible infant but that these patients as a group had more compatible offspring than would be expected; and (2) that anti-HLA antibodies were present in a greater proportion of, and in higher titres in, pregnancies with a hydatidiform mole than in normal pregnancies. The antibodies also persisted for longer in patients with tumours than following normal pregnancies. Her conclusion was that the HLA system did not appear to exert any major influence on the chance of a woman developing a trophoblastic tumour.

All GTT synthesize varying amounts of a range of pregnancy hormones including human chorionic gonadotrophin (hCG) and its subunits and fragments (see below, Tumour markers and the role of hCG and its fragments). hCG is produced throughout a normal pregnancy and its synthesis is switched on not only in GTTs but in certain other tumours such as germ cell tumours and, less commonly, other malignancies such as bladder carcinoma. Its function both in normal pregnancy and in those tumours which produce it remains largely obscure. While hCG may stimulate the synthesis of a range of hormones and may have an immunomodulating effect, its role in malignancy is probably quite complex. On the one hand, while GTT apparently cannot grow clinically without synthesizing hCG, the same molecule can in other circumstances suppress carcinogenesis and tumour growth. This is shown in a recent study where hCG suppressed the development of carcinogen-induced mammary tumours in rats (Russo et al, 1990).

Although uncommon, GTT are important since with proper management it should now be rare for a woman to die from her tumour and in most cases fertility can be preserved. The main reasons for this success are threefold: (1) for reasons that are not clearly understood, GTT are highly sensitive to a range of currently available therapeutic agents; (2) the universal production of a serological tumour marker, hCG, makes possible a sensitivity and accuracy of screening, monitoring, management and follow-up of patients which is unique in clinical cancer; (3) detailed analysis of large groups of patients with these rare diseases has allowed the recognition of a range of prognostic factors, permitting the adjustment of intensity of treatment so that each patient only receives the minimum treatment necessary to eliminate her disease.

PATHOLOGY

The terminology in GTT and gestational trophoblastic disease (GTD) remains confusing partly due to the interchangeable use of histopathological and clinical terms. Since the management of patients at risk of developing a GTT is focused on the behaviour of the serum concentration of hCG, the curability of most of these patients means that frequently clinical decisions are made without further pathological specimens being obtained.

Hydatidiform moles (HM)

HM are premalignant conditions and in most cases remit spontaneously once the HM has been evacuated from the uterus. Molar pregnancies are now clearly distinguished both on morphological and cytogenetic grounds into complete and partial HM (Szulman and Surti, 1978a,b).

Complete hydatidiform mole

A complete HM forms a multivesicular mass composed of grossly distended chorionic villi without a gestational sac or fetus. Hydropic change usually affects all the villi and trophoblastic hyperplasia is present to a variable extent.

Partial hydatidiform mole

A partial HM is one in which only a proportion of the chorionic villi are affected by vesicular change, the abnormal villi being admixed with normal villi. The vesicular villi tend to be smaller than those in the complete HM, frequently showing a deeply indented outline. The presence of a fetus may be recognized either macroscopically or by the presence of nucleated red cells. It is likely that many partial HM are classified as 'products of conception' at uterine evacuation for a 'miscarriage'. Without genetic analysis to confirm that a specimen is a partial HM, underdiagnosis will continue.

The natural history of partial HM has recently been better defined. While the malignant sequelae following partial HM is much less than after complete HM, a small number (approximately 1 in 200) of patients with partial HM require chemotherapy for a GTT and therefore all patients need to be registered and followed up in the same way as for complete HM (Bagshawe et al, 1990).

Invasive hydatidiform mole

This term is applied when a HM (complete or partial) invades into the myometrium. Since this is part of the normal behaviour of molar tropho-blast, this is common, as is confirmed both on ultrasound examination of the uterus and by the hCG profile following evacuation of the uterine cavity. Pathologically this condition can only be confirmed by either having curettings containing a significant amount of myometrium or in the occasional case where a hysterectomy is performed rather than evacuation of the uterine cavity for a molar pregnancy.

Choriocarcinoma

Choriocarcinoma is composed of both cyto- and syncytiotrophoblastic cells, characteristically surrounded by necrosis and haemorrhage. Choriocarcinoma is unusual in stimulating virtually no connective tissue support for the tumour and this is reflected by its clinical behaviour in its rapid haematogenous spread and haemorrhagic complications at sites where the tumour is growing. In the past choriocarcinoma was a rapidly lethal neoplasm but with proper management and modern chemotherapy, most patients should achieve complete remission.

Placental site trophoblastic tumour

This rare tumour is composed mainly of cytotrophoblast with very little syncytiotrophoblast. It can occur after both normal and molar pregnancies (Fisher et al, 1992b). The tumour tends to grow locally with a lower metastatic potential than choriocarcinoma. In most cases described so far its spread is mainly by local infiltration rather than widespread dissemination. The management of these tumours is different from other GTT in that they are less chemosensitive and if localized to the uterus the treatment of choice is surgery. Occasional long-term remissions have been obtained with intensive chemotherapy (Dessau et al, 1990).

EPIDEMIOLOGY

The epidemiology of GTT is still poorly understood although major progress in this area is likely to come from modern molecular genetics. The identification of the abnormal gene expression associated with the different clinical and pathological syndromes is fundamental to further progress in our understanding of these conditions. Many reports in the past, before the recognition by Szulman and Surti (1978a,b) that there are two different pathological syndromes of complete and partial HM, contain patients with both conditions and makes the earlier published data difficult to interpret. However, there is considerable evidence in the literature that the incidence of HM in different parts of the world varies considerably. In a number of countries including Japan and the Far East the incidence would appear to be much higher than it is in Europe and North America. Matsuura et al (1984) analysed the incidence of HM in Hawaii between 1968 and 1981. In 278 cases, 69.4% were complete HM, 24.5% were partial HM and 6.1% were non-molar pregnancies. This is a complete:partial HM ratio of 2.9:1. The population studied was of particular interest since several different racial groups live in Hawaii and have more or less equal access to hospital facilities. In Table 2 the incidence in the different racial groups in Hawaii are shown. This study confirms that molar pregnancies are more common in Filipino, Japanese and Oriental groups. The fact that the incidence is similar in Caucasians and native Hawaiians suggests that an environmental cause does not explain this difference in incidence between racial groups.

　　Molar pregnancies are more common at the extremes of the reproductive age range. In a study of over 8000 cases of HM registered in England and Wales between 1973 and 1983 the relative risk of a HM in patients under 15 years was 6 and in patients over 50 years was 411 (when compared with the incidence in patients aged between 25 and 29 years) (Bagshawe et al, 1986).

Table 2. Incidence of complete hydatidiform moles by maternal race in Hawaii (1968–1981).

	Rate/10 000	Incidence
White	8.0	1:1256
Filipino	17.5	1:571
Japanese	16.5	1:607
Hawaiian	7.7	1:1304
Orientals (Chinese, Koreans)	17.5	1:571
All	12.1	1:825

Modified with permission from Matsuura et al, 1984.

Analysis of this large group of patients confirmed the increased risk of a second HM with an incidence of 1 in 76 and of a third HM of 1 in 6.5. **This increased risk of further GTT following subsequent pregnancies is an important feature in their follow-up in that they need confirmation that the hCG returns to normal following each subsequent pregnancy.**

GTT occur after approximately 1 in 50 000 full-term pregnancies. Where histology is available, these tumours are choriocarcinoma or occasionally placental site trophoblastic tumours. In Charing Cross Hospital, London, a referral centre for trophoblastic tumours, this pattern of disease accounted for 137 (12.9%) of 1058 patients treated between 1968 and 1985. GTT following a full-term pregnancy behave aggressively and form that subgroup described in the older literature of women presenting with fulminating disease and dying within a matter of weeks.

The clinical pattern in the patients presenting with choriocarcinoma following a full-term pregnancy is intriguing. In all the patients in the Charing Cross series the pregnancy reached term normally and no abnormality was noted in any placenta, yet the patient frequently presented with widespread disease within a matter of weeks of delivery. This raises the possibility that the presence of the fetus may suppress the malignant trophoblast until after delivery. We have attempted to identify an inhibitory factor in cord serum from pregnancies using normal adult serum as a control. No inhibitory factor has been identified in vitro or in vivo with choriocarcinoma xenografts. However, in a recent review of the literature Flam et al (1989) identified nine cases in which both mother and infant have had tumour invasion with choriocarcinoma.

The influence of exogenous hormones on the behaviour of molar trophoblast is an area of considerable interest. Stone and Bagshawe (1976) suggested that patients who were exposed to oestrogen and/or progesterone had an increased incidence of malignant sequelae following a molar pregnancy. We have recently analysed the patients registered between 1973 and 1989 (Table 3). These data indicate that there is probably very little effect of exogenous hormones in patients whose hCG has already returned to normal, indicating minimal or no residual abnormal trophoblast. However, in patients given exogenous hormones while their hCG is still raised, the proportion requiring chemotherapy is 30.7%, compared with 8–9% in the overall population (Bagshawe et al, 1986). This subgroup of patients should not, therefore, receive oral contraceptives owing to the

Table 3. Effects of taking oral contraceptives within 6 months of evacuation of a hydatidiform mole, Charing Cross Hospital (1973–1989).

Total number of patients	8882
Total number of patients requiring chemotherapy	663 (7.5%)
Numbers who received oral contraceptive	1384 (15.6%)
A. Patients with normal hCG prior to oral contraceptive	1049
Number requiring chemotherapy (0.0047%)	5*
B. Patients with raised hCG given oral contraceptives	335
Number requiring chemotherapy	103 (30.7%)
A versus B, $P < 0.001$	

* 3 patients required chemotherapy after a subsequent pregnancy; 1 patient required chemotherapy after a subsequent hydatidiform mole; 1 patient required chemotherapy after 18 months post hydatidiform mole.

stimulatory effect of oestrogen and progesterone on the persisting abnormal trophoblast.

GENETICS

Hydatidiform mole

The first suggestion that HM were in any way unusual genetically came from the observations of Barr bodies in these tissues which showed that the majority of HM were female (Park, 1957). This was confirmed by early karyotype studies which showed 46XX to be the commonest karyotype amongst HM. A small number of triploid HM were also described and further genetic studies of HM which were carefully characterized pathologically showed that it was the complete HM which was diploid while partial HM were triploid (Szulman and Surti, 1978a). This clearly defined partial HM as a separate genetic entity and not a transitional stage between normal placenta and complete HM.

Using cytogenetic polymorphisms as a means of identifying whether particular chromosomes were maternally or paternally derived, two groups of workers made the surprising observation that all 46 chromosomes in the complete HM were paternally derived (Kajii and Ohama, 1977; Wake et al, 1978) and that the conceptus was thus androgenetic in origin. It is now known that, although indistinguishable pathologically (Kajii et al, 1984), complete HM may be genetically homozygous if they arise by fertilization of an anucleate egg by a single haploid sperm which then duplicates (Lawler et al, 1979, 1982b; Jacobs et al, 1980), or heterozygous if they arise by dispermy (Ohama et al, 1981). The former have a 46XX karyotype, homozygosity for the Y chromosome being non-viable: the latter may be 46XX or 46XY. About 25% of complete HM are heterozygous (Fisher et al, 1989) but the majority are homozygous which explains the female nature of most complete HM. Despite the androgenetic nature of the nuclear genome the mitochondrial DNA of complete HM is maternally derived, as in a normal conceptus (Wallace et al, 1982; Edwards et al, 1984).

Studies of the parental origin of triploid partial HM show that it is the paternal nuclear genome which is important in molar development. Partial HM are different to complete HM in having a maternal contribution to the genome, but have been shown, like complete HM, to have two paternal sets of chromosomes (Jacobs et al, 1982; Lawler et al, 1982a). Where the origin of partial HM has been examined they have generally been shown to arise by dispermy (Jacobs et al, 1982; Lawler et al, 1982a). Digynic triploids with two maternal contributions to the nuclear genome are generally associated with non-molar placenta (Jacobs et al, 1982) and thus in most partial HM, as in complete HM, the characteristic abnormal pathology is associated with the presence of two paternal genomes.

Occasional tetraploid partial HM (Sheppard et al, 1982; Surti et al, 1986; Vejerslev et al, 1987) have been observed but, like triploid partial HM, they have an excess of paternal genomes, their most likely origin being fertilization of an egg by three sperm or two sperm, one of which was diploid. The origin of two unusual cases of triploid complete HM were consistent with androgenesis (Verjerslev et al, 1987). HM thus appear to be an example of genomic imprinting, a phenomenon whereby genes function differently depending on their parental origin. Where only paternal chromosomes are present a complete HM develops while the presence of a maternal genome in partial HM is associated with some fetal development.

The unusual genetic constitution of HM has implications for the immune response elicited by a pregnancy with HM. In a normal pregnancy the fetus represents a partial allograft having both a maternal and paternal contribution to the nuclear genome. The androgenetic nature of complete HM results in their having greater potential to be antigenically different from the maternal host than a normal conceptus. Either an increase in the number of antigenic differences between the molar pregnancy and the mother or an increase in the dose of antigenic products produced by the HM could result in a greater immune response in the mother.

Gestational trophoblastic tumours

That genomic imprinting also plays a role in tumorigenesis is suggested by the very high incidence of GTT which occurs after the androgenetic complete HM compared with normal term pregnancy or other types of abnormal conceptuses. A pregnancy with HM is approximately a thousand times more likely to progress to choriocarcinoma than a normal term pregnancy (Bagshawe and Lawler, 1982). Since the evidence suggests that there is no difference between the frequency with which homozygous and heterozygous complete HM progress to GTT (Lawler et al, 1991) or that heterozygous complete HM may in fact have a more malignant potential than homozygous complete HM (Wake et al, 1987), it would appear that it is the paternal nature of the genome rather than homozygosity for specific genes which is the important factor in tumorigenesis.

Genetic studies of choriocarcinomas have shown that they generally have grossly abnormal karyotypes with a wide range of ploidies and a number of chromosomal rearrangements (Wake et al, 1981; Sasaki et al, 1982;

Sheppard et al, 1985; Lawler and Fisher, 1986). However, no specific chromosome abnormalities have yet been found to be associated with this group of tumours. Studies of the origin of GTT have confirmed that choriocarcinoma may arise from a normal term pregnancy (Wake et al, 1981; Chaganti et al, 1990; Osada et al, 1991; Fisher et al, 1992a) from a homozygous complete HM or from a heterozygous complete HM (Fisher et al, 1988, 1992a). One of these reports also confirmed an earlier suggestion from the results of studies of antibodies to major histocompatibility antigens (Lawler et al, 1976) that the antecedent pregnancy is not always the causative pregnancy in cases of GTT. A patient with a history of HM 4 years previously was shown, following a subsequent term pregnancy, to have a tumour which was clearly molar in origin (Fisher et al, 1992a).

Few cases of placental site trophoblastic tumour have been examined genetically. Two cases have been reported to be diploid (Eckstein et al, 1985; Lathrop et al, 1988) in contrast to the more aneuploid karyotypes of most choriocarcinomas. Although placental site trophoblastic tumours are less often associated with an antecedent molar pregnancy, they have been shown by genetic studies to originate both from normal conceptuses and in HM (Fisher et al, 1992b).

The very nature of a GTT makes it unlike any other type of tumour since it arises not from the patient's own tissue but from an allograft. GTT thus have a unique potential to be antigenically different from the host in which they develop, differences which may again vary according to the type of pregnancy in which the tumour arose.

TUMOUR MARKERS AND THE ROLE OF HUMAN CHORIONIC GONADOTROPHIN (hCG) AND ITS FRAGMENTS

The measurement of hCG by antisera directed to the immunologically distinct part of the molecule, the β-hCG, is fundamental to the management of patients with GTT. However, the role of intact hCG in normal pregnancy is imperfectly understood and the situation in patients with GTT and other tumours producing either hCG or its fragments is even more complex. The fact that GTT never grows clinically without hCG production implies a very fundamental role for this molecule. It is possible that hCG and its fragments may have a growth regulatory role for the placenta in a normal pregnancy, in GTT and other tumours producing them.

Nicked and fragmented β-subunits of hCG

There is considerable homology between the β-subunits of the four glyco-protein hormones FSH, hCG, LH and TSH. hCG can be converted into a follitropin merely by substituting hFSH-β residues 88–108 in place of the carboxyl terminus (CTP) of hCG-β, i.e. residues 94–145 (Campbell et al, 1991). Determinant loop sequences β 38–57 and β 93–100 have been implicated in distinguishing the biological activity of hCG (Keutmann et al, 1987, 1989). Alterations in the β-subunit of hCG, whether by 'nicking' of bonds between amino acids or by loss of peptide sequences, will affect the biological potency of the β-subunit and could remove distinctive epitopes which might render discrepant the levels of apparent β-subunit (measured in serum or urine samples) in different types of assay even though standard preparations are consistent (Kardana et al, 1991).

The 'nicked' β-subunit, generated from intact β-hCG by human leukocyte elastase, or prepared directly from urine samples, is cleaved between amino acids 47 and 48 or, to a lesser extent, 44 and 45. It binds with diminished affinity to receptors in luteinized rat ovary homogenates and steroidogenesis declines linearly with increase in the percentage of nicked material (Cole et al, 1991). Nicked β-subunits of hCG have been demonstrated in urines in early pregnancy and from patients with HM or choriocarcinoma (Kardana and Cole, 1991). Conclusions drawn from ratios of β-subunit to intact hCG in these diseases depend to some extent on the capacity of an assay to measure both complete and nicked β-subunit. In particular, assays which depend on the captive antibody IE5 in a sandwich format respond to a much smaller extent to the presence of nicked β-hCG than do assays utilizing antibodies of the characteristics of FBT 11 and B 204 (Kardana and Cole, 1991).

The β core fragment of hCG (BCF) consists of disulphide-linked amino acid sequences β 6–40 and β 55–92. The CTP is missing and with it the O-linked oligosaccharide chains (Cole et al, 1989). The N-linked oligosaccharide chains, in preparations from urine, lack sialic acid and much of the galactose (Birken et al, 1988) which implies a possible alternative glycosylation pathway. BCF will not combine with α-subunit, a characteristic probably attributable to the loss of residues 41–50 (Birken et al, 1988).

Ectopic production of hCG and/or β-subunit, as defined by β-directed antisera, has been identified as a fairly wide-ranging occurrence in patients with non-trophoblastic tumours (Braunstein, 1983) with the highest incidence reported for 48.5% of patients with breast cancer (Tormey et al, 1977).

Ectopic production of BCF seems to be even more widespread. A monoclonal antibody, 2C2, raised in the Department of Medical Oncology at Charing Cross Hospital, London, bound to 93% of tumours, examined by immunohistochemistry, including those of breast, lung, colon, stomach, pancreas and ovary (Kardana et al, 1988).

BCF has been detected in 66% of urines from women with active gynaecological malignancies (Cole and Birken, 1988). Large series in other malignancies have yet to be measured but the preliminary indications all suggest that BCF is found in more tumours than intact ectopic hCG. Also, cross-reactivity between β-hCG and BCF has not necessarily been excluded from early surveys with β-directed antisera.

The presence of BCF in urine was attributed at first to renal breakdown of either hCG or β-subunit (Wehmann and Nisula, 1980). Recent evidence suggests that BCF circulates in serum though its definitive epitope is masked in a larger protein complex (Kardana and Cole, 1990). The evidence from immunohistochemistry suggests that BCF is produced in or near malignant cells.

A single α-subunit gene is transcribed to make the α-subunit mRNA for all four glycoprotein hormones (Fiddes and Goodman, 1981). The genes for β-hCG and β-LH have been mapped to a complex cluster of inverted and tandem genes on chromosome 19, of which six are for β-hCG and the terminal seventh for β-LH (Boorstein et al, 1982; Policastro et al, 1986; Graham et al, 1987). Only genes 5 and 3 of the available cluster in placenta and choriocarcinoma cells appear to give rise to mRNA (Jameson et al, 1987). It is not known yet which genes are activated in non-gestational tumours but it is believed that ectopic expression of β-hCG by bladder tumours is the result of altered gene regulation rather than amplification of the gene cluster (Iles et al, 1989).

If BCF has its own role, it is not yet defined. Assertions of its occurrence based on antibodies to one epitope must be treated with caution until all cross-reactions with allied truncated glycoproteins have been completely excluded. However, the changing levels of intact hCG, β-hCG, nicked β-hCG, BCF and free α-subunit in pregnancy argue a regulatory pattern for these molecules which may not be restricted to the primary role of hCG in sustaining the steroid hormone secretory capacity of the corpus luteum.

CLINICAL PRESENTATION

The most common prodrome to a GTT is a patient presenting with a HM. Clinically these patients usually present towards the end of the first trimester as a threatened abortion with vaginal bleeding. The uterus may be 'large for dates' and they may suffer from rather more nausea and vomiting than would be expected with a normal pregnancy.

Since the quantity of hCG produced in a normal pregnancy varies considerably, the serum hCG concentration is rarely diagnostic of a molar pregnancy although it is commonly greater than 1×10^6 IU/litre before evacuation of a HM. The main investigation in these patients is pelvic ultrasound imaging to confirm the presence of a molar pregnancy and the absence of a fetus. Initial clinical management is evacuation of the uterine cavity. The method of evacuation which gives the lowest incidence of sequelae is suction evacuation (Bagshawe et al, 1986). Since the molar trophoblast usually invades the myometrium, it is relatively easy to perforate the uterus if a metal curette is used.

It has been common practice in the United Kingdom for gynaecologists to perform a second evacuation of the uterine cavity in patients with molar pregnancies. We have analysed our data between 1973 and 1986 and the results are shown in Table 4. This shows that where the clinical indications have resulted in only a single evacuation of the uterus, the complication rate in terms of requiring chemotherapy is low but rises to 18% in those patients in whom it is thought a second evacuation is necessary. However, it is clear that a third and fourth evacuation of the uterus is contraindicated since most of these patients require chemotherapy. Therefore our current recommendation is the initial evacuation of the uterine cavity to confirm the diagnosis, and if there are clinical indications such as bleeding or if repeat

Table 4. Hydatidiform moles and number of uterine evacuations, Charing Cross Hospital (1973–1986).

Number of evacuations	Patients not treated	Patients treated	% Patients treated
1	4481	109	2.4
2	1495	267	18
3	106	106	50
4	5	22	81
5	3	0	0

ultrasound shows a considerable amount of molar trophoblast still within the uterine cavity, a second evacuation of the uterus is probably justified.

GTT can present after any form of pregnancy without an initial history of a HM. In these cases diagnosis may be very difficult. **It is important to bear in mind the possibility of a GTT in a young woman presenting with evidence of a malignancy elsewhere** (particularly in the lungs and brain). The probable presence of a trophoblastic tumour can be confirmed by performing a pregnancy test or a quantitative hCG assay. However, since other tumours can produce hCG (the most common being germ cell tumours) followed by bladder and gastrointestinal tract tumours, a raised serum hCG is not in itself diagnostic of a GTT.

The pattern of spread in those patients with metastatic GTT has recently been reviewed by Hunter et al (1990). Where there were metastases, these involved lungs (93%), vagina (16%), pelvis (7%), central nervous system (7%), liver (4%), bowel (2%), and other sites were only occasionally involved by metastases.

GTT can occasionally present as multiple pulmonary emboli. This is important to recognize because the pathology is unusual in that the tumour grows in the pulmonary artery and the presence of a GTT can be confirmed by the significantly raised hCG which is present in these cases (Seckl et al, 1991).

REGISTRATION AND FOLLOW-UP

Because all GTT synthesize hCG, a national follow-up service has been instituted in the United Kingdom since 1973 based on three laboratories for hCG estimation in Dundee, Sheffield and London. The success of this screening service has been reported in detail (Bagshawe et al, 1986). After registration the patient's details and pathology and blood and urine samples are sent through the post to one of the reference laboratories for serial hCG estimations. Table 5 summarizes the operation of this service. Following a complete HM between 7% and 8% of patients require chemotherapy.

Since a molar pregnancy is a premalignant condition, in the majority of cases the molar tissue dies out spontaneously. This is reflected in the return to normal of the hCG concentration. Once the hCG has reached normal, our recommendation is that the patient should not start a further pregnancy until the hCG has been normal for 6 months. In the review by Bagshawe et al

Table 5. UK hydatidiform mole follow-up service.

Year	London	Sheffield	Dundee	Total
	Number of patients registered 1981–1990			
1981	548	289	59	896
1982	644	*	66	*
1983	679	327	76	1082
1984	566	374	83	1023
1985	625	358	98	1081
1986	676	356	90	1122
1987	663	390	78	1131
1988	634	413	82	1129
1989	582	358	75	1015
1990	684	377	89	1150

* Number unavailable.

(1986), in those patients whose hCG fell to normal within 8 weeks of evacuation follow-up could be safely reduced to 6 months. In those patients where the hCG is still elevated beyond 8 weeks from the date of evacuation, the follow-up is continued for a total of 2 years. Since patients who have had a previous GTT are more at risk of having a second, all patients should have further estimation of hCG at 6 and 10 weeks following the completion of each subsequent pregnancy.

The indications for intervention with chemotherapy in patients who have had a HM are shown in Table 6.

Table 6. Indications for chemotherapy.

Serum hCG above 20 000 IU/litre more than 4 weeks after evacuation, because of the risk of uterine perforation
Histological evidence of choriocarcinoma
Evidence of metastases in brain, liver or gastrointestinal tract, or radiological opacities greater than 2 cm on chest X-ray
Long-lasting uterine haemorrhage
Rising hCG values
hCG in body fluids 4–6 months after evacuation

PROGNOSTIC FACTORS AND STAGING

GTT form a wide spectrum of disease from those which can be eliminated with minimally toxic chemotherapy to highly aggressive disease where the initial extent of disease at the time of presentation or the late development of drug resistance remain problems. The main prognostic variables which have been identified in GTT are summarized in Table 7, which is a minor modification of the scoring system proposed by Bagshawe (1976). The most important prognostic variables in this table which also carry the highest score are as follows: (1) the duration of the disease because drug resistance of GTT varies inversely with time from the original antecedent pregnancy; (2) the concentration of hCG in the serum which is a semiquantitative

Table 7. Scoring system for gestational trophoblastic tumours (1.8.83).

	0	1	2	6
Age (years)	<39	>39		
Antecedent pregnancy (AP)	Mole	Abortion or unknown	Term	
Interval (end of AP to chemo at CXH in months)	<4	4–7	7–12	>12
hCG (IU/litre)	10^3–10^4	$<10^3$	10^4–10^5	$>10^5$
ABO (woman × partner)		A × O O × A O or A × unknown	B × A or O AB × A or O	
No. of metastases	Nil	1–4	4–8	>8
Site of metastases	Not detected Lungs Vagina	Spleen Kidney	GI tract Liver	Brain
Largest tumour mass	<3 cm	3–5 cm	>5 cm	
Previous chemotherapy	Nil		Single drug	2 or more drugs

Low risk, 0–5; medium risk, 6–9; high risk, >9; CXH, Charing Cross Hospital, London.

assessment of the volume of viable tumour in the body; (3) failure of previous chemotherapy to eliminate the GTT.

A purely anatomical staging system is included in the World Health Organisation report (WHO, 1983) but, although the above scoring system appears complex, a detailed comparison (Smith et al, 1992) has confirmed that it can identify a small subgroup of patients who would be either under- or overtreated if their treatment was based solely on anatomical staging. This scoring system can also be applied in centres without high technology equipment since the important variables include only the history, examination, chest X-ray and a quantitative hCG estimation.

TREATMENT

At the Charing Cross Hospital, London we have used the prognostic scoring system in Table 7 and have subdivided the patients into low, medium and high risk categories. We have retained the medium risk category of patients since this allows the assessment of a new anticancer agent in a patient population where the survival is already 100%, but without compromising their subsequent treatment (for discussion, see Newlands et al, 1986). However, for many centres it is probably simpler to have two risk categories, low and high risk, since the toxicity with our current high risk schedule (the EMA/CO regimen; see below) is only moderately more than our medium risk schedule and may induce complete remission more rapidly.

Our management of these three risk categories has each been reviewed recently: the results with the low risk patients in Bagshawe et al (1989), the medium risk patients in Newlands et al (1986) and the high risk patients in Newlands et al (1991). These results are summarized briefly here.

Low risk patients

Since 1964 these patients have been treated with a simple schedule of methotrexate 50 mg i.m. given on days 1, 3, 5 and 7, and folinic acid 6 mg i.m. on days 2, 4, 6 and 8, with a 6-day interval between courses. This schedule is, in general, well tolerated although 5% of patients need to change treatment because of toxicity (usually severe pleuritic chest pain or drug-induced hepatitis). However, even in correctly stratified patients 20% will need to change because of the development of drug resistance. This means that methotrexate is not a simple 'wonder drug' for this group of patients since a total of 25% will need to change treatment because of either drug resistance or toxicity. Therefore these patients need to be carefully monitored to ensure that they achieve complete remission.

The survival in these patients is excellent even though they may need to change treatment and the only deaths in patients treated with this schedule

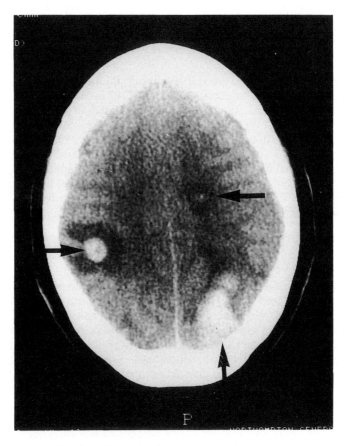

Figure 1. Patient presenting several months after a normal pregnancy with symptoms of a subarachnoid haemorrhage and a hemianopia. CT scan confirmed three cerebral metastases (arrowed).

following the introduction of the prognostic scoring system were one from concurrent but not therapy-induced non-Hodgkin's lymphoma and one from hepatitis (Bagshawe et al, 1989).

Medium risk patients

These patients need to be treated with chemotherapy either using drugs in sequence or in combination. Between 1974 and 1979 2 patients out of 75 (3%) in this category died from their tumours despite intensive treatment. Following the introduction of etoposide (Newlands and Bagshawe, 1980), there have been no further deaths in this subgroup of patients.

High risk patients

Since 1979 we have used a weekly chemotherapy schedule, trying to

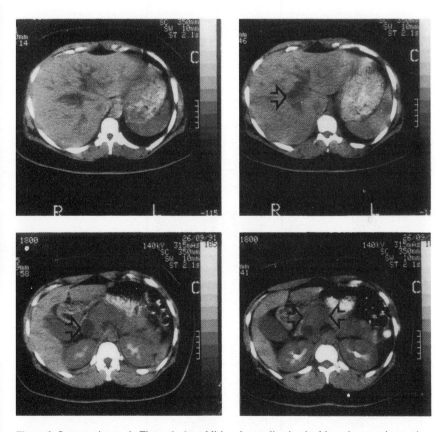

Figure 2. Same patient as in Figure 1. An additional complication in this patient was increasing obstructive jaundice due to a pancreatic mass of tumour obstructing the common bile duct (CT showing dilated bile ducts and pancreatic mass, arrowed). This required stenting so that intensive chemotherapy with EMA/CO was not delayed by the impaired liver function.

Table 8. Follow-up for gestational trophoblastic tumour patients who have received chemotherapy.

Low risk		Medium risk		High risk	
Score value 0–5		Score value 6–9		Score value >9	
Urine	Blood	Urine	Blood	Urine	Blood
Fortnightly ×10	Fortnightly ×5	As for low risk	Fortnightly ×5	Fortnightly ×20	Fortnightly ×20
Monthly ×10	Monthly ×5		Monthly ×10	Monthly ×20	Monthly ×10
2-Monthly ×10	Then only if necessary		Then only if necessary	2-Monthly ×20	2-Monthly ×10
3-Monthly ×10				3-Monthly ×20	Then only if necessary
Then every 6 months				Then every 6 months	

maximize dose intensity in order to minimize the development of drug resistance. The EMA/CO schedule contains etoposide, methotrexate and actinomycin D, cyclophosphamide and vincristine (Oncovin). In our recent analysis (Newlands et al, 1991) of 148 patients receiving this schedule, the overall survival was 85%. There were two subgroups of patients: 76 who had received no prior chemotherapy and whose survival was 82%. Ten of the 14 patients who died in this group died early from the following causes: respiratory failure (five), cerebral metastases (three), hepatic failure (one), pulmonary embolism (one). Some of the clinical problems presented by this variant of GTT are illustrated in Figures 1 and 2. In none of these cases was the antecedent pregnancy a HM (they were: livebirth, six; stillbirth, one; spontaneous abortion, three). It will be difficult to improve the survival in this particular subgroup of patients since there was no immediate antecedent pregnancy to allow them to be entered into a screening programme such as that for patients who have had a HM. The ready awareness that widespread malignancy in a young woman may possibly be choriocarcinoma which can be confirmed by a very high hCG will minimize the number of patients presenting with this disease extent and consequent mortality.

The second group of high risk patients are those relapsing after previous chemotherapy, either our own treatment failures or those referred from centres abroad. The survival in these 72 patients was 89%. These patients were all on follow-up and therefore their disease extent was less than in the previous group. The cause of death in these patients was usually the development of drug-resistant disease and these patients could not be saved either by extensive surgery or by the addition of cis-platinum (cisplatin) to the chemotherapy (Newlands et al, 1991).

POST-TREATMENT FOLLOW-UP AND FERTILITY

Following completion of their chemotherapy, patients need to be followed up regularly with hCG estimations to confirm that their disease is in remission. Initially the follow-up is with serum and urine samples (Table 8). In due course the follow-up is only on urine samples. In the UK this is computerized and automatic reminders are sent to patients so that they do not get lost to follow-up. Patients are advised to avoid a subsequent pregnancy until 12 months after completing their chemotherapy, in order to minimize the potential teratogenicity of the treatment.

Even in the high risk patients receiving intensive chemotherapy, patients return to normal activity within a few months and most side-effects of the treatment are reversible. Chemotherapy-induced alopecia is always reversible. To date, late sequelae from chemotherapy have been remarkably rare. Two patients receiving extensive treatment (lasting more than 6 months) developed acute myeloid leukaemia which was probably therapy-induced. This emphasizes the importance of achieving complete remission as rapidly as possible to minimize this recognized complication of intensive chemotherapy. In the population analysed between 1968 and 1978 there was no increase in second tumours in 457 long-term survivors (Rustin et al, 1983).

The outcome of subsequent pregnancies following chemotherapy is usually successful. In an analysis of 445 long-term survivors treated at the Charing Cross Hospital, London, 90% of those who wished to become pregnant succeeded and 86% of these had at least one livebirth (Rustin et al, 1984). However, there was a tendency for patients who had received three or more drugs to be less likely to have a livebirth than those who had received only one or two drugs. There was no increase in the incidence of congenital malformation compared with the normal population.

SUMMARY

Trophoblastic tumours form a spectrum of disease from the borderline malignancy of HM to highly aggressive choriocarcinoma. Their management requires the integration of the information derived from serial hCG estimations, the clinical history and pattern of spread of the disease, so that our understanding of the prognostic variables can be applied appropriately. This maximizes the patient's chances of complete remission from her disease with the minimum of toxicity. Given our knowledge of this group of diseases and an integrated approach to management, it should be uncommon for any woman to die from her trophoblastic tumour.

REFERENCES

Bagshawe KD (1976) Risk and prognostic factors in trophoblastic neoplasia. *Cancer* **38:** 1373–1385.

Bagshawe KD & Lawler SD (1982) Choriocarcinoma. In Schottenfeld D & Fraumeni JF (eds) *Cancer Epidemiology and Prevention*, pp 909–924. Philadelphia: Saunders.

Bagshawe KD, Dent J & Webb J (1986) Occasional survey: hydatidiform mole in England and Wales 1973–83. Lancet **ii:** 673–677.

Bagshawe KD, Dent J, Newlands ES et al (1989) The role of low dose methotrexate and folinic acid in gestational trophoblastic tumours (GTT). *British Journal of Obstetrics and Gynaecology* **96:** 795–802.

Bagshawe KD, Lawler SD, Paradinas FJ et al (1990) Gestational trophoblastic tumours following initial diagnosis of partial hydatidiform mole. *Lancet* **335:** 1074–1076.

Birken S, Armstrong EG, Kolks MAG et al (1988) Structure of the human chorionic gonadotrophin beta subunit fragment from pregnancy urine. *Endocrinology* **123(1):** 572–583.

Boorstein WR, Vamkakopoulos NC & Fiddes JC (1982) Human chorionic gonadotrophin beta subunit is encoded by at least eight genes arranged in tandem and inverted pairs. *Nature* **300:** 419–422.

Braunstein GD (1983) HCG expression in trophoblastic and non-trophoblastic tumours. In Braunstein GD (ed.) *Oncodevelopmental Markers. Biologic, Diagnostic and Monitoring Aspects*, pp 351–357. New York: Academic Press.

Campbell RK, Dean-Emig DM & Moyle WR (1991) Conversion of human chorionic gonadotrophin into a follitropin by protein engineering. *Proceedings of the National Academy of Sciences (USA)* **88:** 760–764.

Chaganti RSK, Kodura PRK, Chakraborty R et al (1990) Genetic origin of a trophoblastic choriocarcinoma. *Cancer Research* **50:** 6330–6333.

Cole LA & Birken S (1988) Origin and occurrence of human chorionic gonadotrophin beta subunit core fragment. *Molecular Endocrinology* **2:** 825–830.

Cole LA, Kardana A & Birken S (1989) The isomers, subunits and fragments of hCG. *Serono Symposia Publications* **65:** 59–78.

Cole LA, Kardana A, Andradegordon P et al (1991) The heterogeneity of human chorionic gonadotrophin (hCG). 3. The occurrence and biological and immunological activities of nicked hCG. *Endocrinology* **129(3):** 1559–1568.

Dessau R, Rustin GJS, Dent J et al (1990) Surgery and chemotherapy in the management of placental site tumor. *Gynecologic Oncology* **39:** 56–59.

Eckstein RP, Russell P, Friedlander ML et al (1985) Metastasizing placental site trophoblastic tumor: a case study. *Human Pathology* **16:** 632–636.

Edwards YH, Jeremiah SJ, McMillan S et al (1984) Complete hydatidiform moles combine maternal mitochondria with a paternal nuclear genome. *Annals of Human Genetics* **48:** 119–127.

Fiddes JC & Goodman HM (1981) The gene encoding the common beta-subunit of the four human glycoprotein hormones. *Journal of Molecular and Applied Genetics* **1:** 13–18.

Fisher RA, Lawler SD, Povey S & Bagshawe KD (1988) Genetically homozygous choriocarcinoma following pregnancy with hydatidiform mole. *British Journal of Cancer* **58:** 788–892.

Fisher RA, Povey S, Jeffreys AJ et al (1989) Frequency of heterozygous complete hydatidiform moles, estimated by locus-specific minisatellite and Y chromosome-specific probes. *Human Genetics* **82:** 259–263.

Fisher RA, Newlands ES, Jeffreys AJ et al (1992a) Gestational and non-gestational trophoblastic tumours distinguished by DNA analysis. *Cancer* **69:** 839–845.

Fisher RA, Paradinas FJ, Newlands ES & Boxer GM (1992b) Genetic evidence of placental site trophoblastic tumours originating from hydatidiform mole or a normal conceptus. *British Journal of Cancer* **65:** 355–358.

Flam F, Lundstrom V & Silfversward C (1989) Choriocarcinoma in mother and child. Case report. *British Journal of Obstetrics and Gynaecology* **96:** 241–244.

Graham MY, Otani T, Boime I et al (1987) Cosmid mapping of hCG beta subunit genes by field inversion gel electrophoresis. *Nucleic Acids Research* **15:** 4437–4448.

Hunter V, Raymond E, Christensen C et al (1990) Efficacy of the metastatic survey in the staging of gestational trophoblastic disease. *Cancer* **65:** 1647–1650.

Iles RK, Czepulkowski BH, Young BD et al (1989) Amplification or rearrangement of the beta-hCG-human LH cluster is not responsible for the ectopic production of beta-hCG by bladder tumour cells. *Journal of Molecular Endocrinology* **2:** 113–117.

Jacobs RA, Wilson CM, Sprenkle JA et al (1980) Mechanisms of origin of complete hydatidiform moles. *Nature* **286:** 714–716.

Jacobs PA, Szulman AE, Funkhouser J et al (1982) Human triploidy: relationship between parental origin of the additional haploid complement and development of partial hydatidiform mole. *Annals of Human Genetics* **46:** 223–231.

Jameson JL, Lindell CM & Habener JF (1987) Gonadotrophin and thyrotrophin and subunit gene expression in normal and neoplastic tissues characterized by using specific mRNA hybridization probes. *Journal of Clinical Endocrinology and Metabolism* **64:** 319–326.

Kajii T & Omaha K (1977) Androgenetic origin of hydatidiform mole. *Nature* **268:** 633–634.

Kajii T, Kurashige H, Ohama K & Uchino F (1984) XY and XX complete moles. Clinical and morphologic correlations. *American Journal of Obstetrics and Gynecology* **150:** 57–64.

Kardana A & Cole LA (1990) Serum hCG beta core fragment is masked by associated macromolecules. *Journal of Clinical Endocrinology and Metabolism* **71(5):** 1393–1395.

Kardana A & Cole LA (1991) Polypeptide nicks cause erroneous results in assays of human chorionic gonadotrophin free beta subunit. *Clinical Chemistry* **38:** 26–33.

Kardana A, Taylor M, Southall P et al (1988) Urinary gonadotrophin peptide: isolation and purification and its histochemical distribution in normal and neoplastic tissues. *British Journal of Cancer* **58:** 281–286.

Kardana A, Elliott MM, Gawinowicz MA et al (1991) The heterogeneity of human chorionic gonadotrophin (hCG). 1. Characterization of peptide heterogeneity in 13 individual preparations of hCG. *Endocrinology* **129(3):** 1541–1551.

Keutmann HT, Charlesworth MC, Mason KA et al (1987) A receptor-binding region in human gonadotrophin/lutropin beta subunit. *Proceedings of the National Academy of Sciences (USA)* **84:** 2038–2042.

Keutmann HT, Mason KA, Kitzmann K et al (1989) Role of the 93–100 determinant loop sequence in receptor binding and biological activity of human luteinizing hormone and chorionic gonadotrophin. *Molecular Endocrinology* **3:** 526–531.

Lathrop JC, Lauchlan S, Nayak R & Ambler M (1988) Clinical characteristics of placental site trophoblastic tumor (PSST). *Gynecologic Oncology* **31:** 32–42.

Lawler SD (1978) HLA and trophoblastic tumours. *British Medical Bulletin* **34(3):** 305–308.

Lawler S & Fisher RA (1986) Genetic aspects of gestational trophoblastic tumours. In Ichinoe K (ed.) *Trophoblastic Diseases*, pp 23–33. Tokyo, New York: Igaku-Shoin.

Lawler SD, Klouda PT & Bagshawe KD (1976) The relationship between HLA antibodies and the causal pregnancy in choriocarcinoma. *British Journal of Obstetrics and Gynaecology* **83:** 651–655.

Lawler SD, Pickthall VJ, Fisher RA et al (1979) Genetic studies of complete and partial hydatidiform moles. *Lancet* **ii:** 58.

Lawler SD, Fisher RA, Pickthall VJ et al (1982a) Genetic studies on hydatidiform moles. I. The origin of partial moles. *Cancer Genetics and Cytogenetics* **5:** 309–320.

Lawler SD, Povey S, Fisher RA & Pickthall VJ (1982b) Genetic studies on hydatidiform moles. II. The origin of complete moles. *Annals of Human Genetics* **46:** 209–222.

Lawler SD, Fisher RA & Dent J (1991) A prospective study of hydatidiform mole. *American Journal of Obstetrics and Gynecology* **164:** 1270–1277.

Matsuura J, Chiu D, Jacobs P et al (1984) Complete hydatidiform mole in Hawaii: an epidemiological study. *Genetic Epidemiology* **1:** 271–284.

Mueller UW, Hawes CS, Wright AE et al (1990) Isolation of fetal trophoblast cells from peripheral blood of pregnant women. *Lancet* **336:** 197–200.

Newlands ES & Bagshawe KD (1980) Antitumour activity of the epipodophyllin derivative VP16-213 (etoposide: NSC-141540) in gestational choriocarcinoma. *European Journal of Cancer* **16:** 401–405.

Newlands ES, Bagshawe KD, Begent RHJ et al (1986) Developments in chemotherapy for medium and high risk patients with gestational trophoblastic tumours (1979–1984). *British Journal of Obstetrics and Gynaecology* **93:** 63–69.

Newlands ES, Bagshawe KD, Begent RHJ et al (1991) Results with the EMA/CO (etoposide, methotrexate, actinomycin D, cyclophosphamide, vincristine) regimen in high risk gestational trophoblastic tumours, 1979 to 1989. *British Journal of Obstetrics and Gynaecology* **98:** 550–557.

Ohama K, Kajii T, Okamoto E et al (1981) Dispermic origin of XY hydatidiform moles. *Nature* **292:** 551–552.

Osada H, Kawata M, Yamada M, Okumura K & Takamizawa H (1991) Genetic identification of pregnancies responsible for choriocarcinomas after multiple pregnancies by restriction fragment length polymorphism analysis. *American Journal of Obstetrics and Gynecology* **165:** 682–688.

Park WW (1957) The occurrence of sex chromatin in chorionepitheliomas and hydatidiform moles. *Journal of Pathology and Bacteriology* **74:** 197–206.

Policastro PF, Daniels-McQueen S, Carle G et al (1986) A map of the hCG beta-LH beta gene cluster. *Journal of Biological Chemistry* **261:** 5907–5916.

Russo IH, Koszalka M & Russo J (1990) Human chorionic gonadotrophin and rat mammary cancer prevention. *Journal of the National Cancer Institute* **82:** 1286–1289.

Rustin GJS, Rustin F, Dent J et al (1983) No increase in second tumours after cytotoxic chemotherapy for gestational trophoblastic tumours. *New England Journal of Medicine* **308:** 473–476.

Rustin GJS, Booth M, Dent J et al (1984) Pregnancy after cytotoxic chemotherapy for gestational trophoblastic tumours. *British Medical Journal* **288:** 103–106.

Sasaki S, Katayama PK, Roesler M et al (1982) Cytogenetic analysis of choriocarcinoma cell lines. *Acta Obstetrica et Gynecologica Japonica* **34:** 2253–2256.

Seckl MJ, Rustin GJS, Newlands ES et al (1991) Pulmonary embolism, pulmonary hypertension, and choriocarcinoma. *Lancet* **338:** 1313–1315.

Sheppard DM, Fisher RA, Lawler SD & Povey S (1982) Tetraploid conceptus with three paternal contributions. *Human Genetics* **62:** 371–374.

Sheppard DM, Fisher RA & Lawler SD (1985) Karyotypic analysis and chromosome polymorphisms in four choriocarcinoma cell lines. *Cancer Genetics and Cytogenetics* **16:** 251–259.

Smith DB, Holden L, Newlands ES & Bagshawe KD (1992) Correlation between clinical staging (FIGO) and prognostic groups in gestational trophoblastic disease. Submitted to *British Journal of Obstetrics and Gynaecology*.

Stone M, Dent J, Kardana A et al (1976) Relationship of oral contraception to development of trophoblastic tumour after evacuation of a hydatidiform mole. *British Journal of Obstetrics and Gynaecology* **83:** 913–916.

Surti U, Szulman AE, Wagner K et al (1986) Tetraploid partial hydatidiform moles: two cases with a triple paternal contribution and a 92,XXXY karyotype. *Human Genetics* **72:** 15–21.

Szulman A & Surti U (1978a) The syndromes of hydatidiform mole. I. Cytogenetic and morphologic correlations. *American Journal of Obstetrics and Gynecology* **131:** 665–671.

Szulman A & Surti U (1978b) The syndromes of hydatidiform mole. II. Morphologic evidence of the complete and partial mole. *American Journal of Obstetrics and Gynecology* **132:** 20–27.

Tormey DC, Waalkes PT & Simon RM (1977) Biological markers in breast carcinoma. *Cancer* **39:** 2391–2396.

Vejerslev LO, Fisher RA, Surti U & Wake N (1987) Hydatidiform mole: cytogenetically unusual cases and their implications for the present classification. *American Journal of Obstetrics and Gynecology* **157:** 180–184.

Wake N & Sasaki M (1978) Androgenesis as a cause of hydatidiform mole. *Journal of the National Cancer Institute* **60:** 51–57.

Wake N, Tanaka K-I, Chapman V, Matsui S & Sandberg AA (1981) Chromosomes and cellular origin of choriocarcinoma. *Cancer Research* **41:** 3137–3143.

Wake N, Fujino T, Hoshi S et al (1987) The propensity to malignancy of dispermic heterozygous moles. *Placenta* **8:** 319–326.

Wallace DC, Surti U, Adams CW & Szulman AE (1982) Complete moles have paternal chromosomes but maternal mitochondrial DNA. *Human Genetics* **61:** 145–147.

Wehmann RE & Nisula BC (1980) Characterization of a discrete degradation product of hCG beta subunit in humans. *Journal of Clinical Endocrinology and Metabolism* **51:** 101–107.

World Health Organisation (1983) Gestational trophoblastic diseases. Report of a WHO scientific group. *Technical Report Series* 692. Geneva: WHO.

8

Alloimmune conditions and pregnancy

G. MARC JACKSON
JAMES R. SCOTT

Many studies in maternal–fetal immunology have already contributed important findings that are relevant to reproductive biology, organ transplantation, and tumour immunology. Rh immunization first demonstrated that the transplacental passage of cells is not of mere academic interest, and other alloimmune diseases have now become extremely relevant to the practice of modern obstetrics. It is beyond the scope to this chapter to review all aspects of these disorders. Rather, we have chosen to discuss new developments in three specific alloimmune pregnancy disorders (Rh immunization, alloimmune thrombocytopenia, and graft-versus-host disease) which are of practical importance to the obstetrician. The emphasis is on modern management to decrease fetal morbidity and mortality.

RED BLOOD CELL ANTIGEN SENSITIZATION

Immunology and pathophysiology of Rh isoimmunization

Although erythrocytes contain multiple surface antigens, antigens of the Rh blood group have the most clinical importance in obstetrics. The Rh antigens are a family of small integral proteins associated with the lipid component of the red blood cell membrane which are scattered across the cell surface in an ordered manner (James and James, 1978; Brown et al, 1983). The Rh antigens are designated C, c, E, e, and D. As no antibody to a d antigen has been identified, the designation d actually describes the absence of the D antigen. Additionally, a large number of variants including C^w and D^u have been identified. Although sensitization to the C, E, D, and e antigens can cause fetal anaemia, sensitization to D is by far the most common and clinically important.

When an Rh-negative individual is first exposed to an adequate volume of Rh-positive red blood cells, a primary immune response is mounted following a latent period of several weeks. IgM is the primary immunoglobulin produced, increasing in exponential fashion to a plateau, then decreasing over a period of months. Because IgM antibodies are unable to cross the placenta, there is no fetal effect of a primary response. However, IgM (and, if present, IgG) can be detected on screening of the mother's blood, identifying her as having been sensitized. The primary response also involves expansion of a population of memory B cells with high affinity for binding the Rh antigen, primed to produce IgG antibody earlier and in much greater quantity on subsequent exposure to antigen.

With later exposure to Rh-positive red blood cells, a secondary response occurs. Immunoglobulin G is the main antibody produced, with a much smaller antigenic requirement, a shorter lag phase, a much longer plateau, and a titre of perhaps ten times that of the primary response. Immunoglobulin G actively crosses the placenta by Fc binding to specific receptors on trophoblastic cells and produces the clinical effects of Rh isoimmunization: fetal anaemia and hydrops fetalis.

In the case of sensitization to the D antigen, fetal erythrocytes are covered with D antigen sites and maternally derived IgG specifically attaches to antigen. Fetal haemolysis then occurs through a mechanism which does not appear to involve complement activation and intravascular cellular lysis; rather, intravascular opsonization, phagocytosis, and intracellular cytolysis occur. Fetal red blood cells coated with anti-D IgG are bound via the Fc receptor of the IgG by macrophages and monocytes in the fetal reticulo-endothelial system, especially within the fetal spleen. Macrophages produce defects in the red cell membrane, resulting in alterations in cell wall deformability and a predisposition to haemolysis (LoBuglio, 1967).

In addition, antibody-dependent cell-mediated cytotoxicity may play a role in fetal red cell destruction. In vitro, phagocytic mononuclear cells and cytotoxic killer T cells can bind to the Fc receptor of IgG adherent to fetal erythrocytes, and cause rupture of the red cell without phagocytosis or complement activation. The extent of in vivo haemolysis due to this mechanism remains to be clearly defined (Rote, 1982; Jones and Need, 1988).

Progressive fetal anaemia results in tissue hypoxia and stimulation of erythropoietin production which in turn incites medullary, then extra-medullary, erythropoiesis. Hepatic erythropoiesis leads to hepatomegaly, portal and umbilical venous obstruction, and hypertension. The impaired liver function results in decreased albumin production, eventually contributing to ascites, generalized oedema, and, often, pleural effusion. Placental hypertrophy secondary to erythropoiesis is common. The spleen, kidneys, and adrenal glands also contribute to extramedullary red cell production, with various derangements in organ function. Although high-output heart failure may be present in severely affected fetuses, it is now thought to be a late finding and not part of the causative mechanism of hydrops (Rote, 1982; Bowman, 1989).

MANAGEMENT STRATEGIES IN Rh IMMUNIZED PREGNANCIES

Because there are clinical variations between patients with Rh-immunized pregnancies, protocols for fetal assessment and treatment must be individualized. The severity of previously affected pregnancies, the possibility of an Rh-negative fetus, and the results of testing in the current pregnancy are important factors in formulating a management plan for fetal evaluation, treatment, and delivery. Because the interpretation of data and timing of interventions are based on gestational age, an ultrasound examination should be obtained in the late first or early second trimester of all immunized pregnancies.

ASSESSMENT OF THE Rh IMMUNIZED PREGNANCY

Maternal history and anti-D titres

In a first sensitized gestation, there is a very low risk of fetal involvement. Thus, women in their first immunized pregnancy and those without a history of a moderate to severely affected fetus should be evaluated with monthly anti-D titres and serial ultrasound examinations. So long as the titre remains low, there is little risk of significant fetal anaemia and the pregnancy can usually be allowed to continue to term without other testing or intervention. However, after the first affected pregnancy, maternal anti-D titres are poorly predictive of fetal status and closer evaluation is required. Although each laboratory has its own 'critical titre', anti-D titres of 1 : 16 or greater in most centres justify amniocentesis and analysis of amniotic fluid bilirubin concentration.

Unlike first immunized pregnancies where the incidence of significant fetal anaemia and hydrops is less than 10%, the pattern of fetal involvement in successive pregnancies is generally one of equal or progressive severity at the same or earlier gestational age. If hydrops occurred in one pregnancy, the next Rh-incompatible fetus has an 80–90% chance of becoming hydropic. When previous fetuses have been moderately to severely affected, amniotic fluid analysis is begun as early as 18–22 weeks' gestation.

Amniotic fluid bilirubin analysis

Assessment of amniotic fluid in Rh immunization is based on the original observations of Bevis (1956) that spectrophotometric determinations of amniotic fluid bilirubin correlated with the severity of fetal haemolysis. Using a semilogarithmic plot, the curve of optical density of normal amniotic fluid is approximately linear between wavelengths of 525 and 375 nm. Bilirubin causes a shift in the spectrophotometric density with a peak at a wavelength of 450 nm. The amount of shift in optical density from linearity at 450 nm (the ΔOD 450) is used to estimate the degree of fetal red cell haemolysis.

Liley (1961) provided a framework for the management of immunized pregnancies based on ΔOD 450 values across gestational ages. Retrospectively, he correlated amniotic fluid ΔOD 450 values with newborn outcome by dividing the graph of gestational age versus ΔOD 450 into three zones. Fetuses unaffected or with mild anaemia had ΔOD 450 values in zone I (the lowest zone), fetuses severely affected had ΔOD 450 values in zone III (the highest zone), and fetuses with zone II values (the middle zone) had

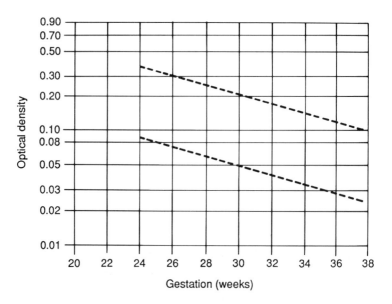

Figure 1. Modification of the Liley curve currently used at the University of Utah. Amniotic fluid ΔOD 450 values are plotted against gestational age after 24 weeks, and clinical management is based on the zone and trend of values.

disease ranging from mild to severe (Figure 1). Management prior to this time consisted primarily of early induced delivery, but Liley's method identified pregnancies that could be safely allowed to continue without great risk of hydrops and stillbirth. In this way, iatrogenic prematurity was avoided in many cases, with a significant reduction in neonatal morbidity and mortality.

It became clear with further study that a single measurement of ΔOD 450 was poorly predictive of fetal condition unless it was very high or very low (Liley, 1963). Thus, management now includes serial amniocenteses to determine the trend of ΔOD 450 values over time (Queenan, 1982; Bowman, 1989). Timing of repeat amniocenteses is determined by the level or trend of ΔOD 450 values: upper zone II values, whether trending horizontally or upward require weekly sampling, and downward trends in the lower half of zone II or zone I are repeated every 2–3 weeks.

Umbilical cord blood sampling

Three decades of clinical use has confirmed the reliability of third-trimester amniotic fluid analysis of ΔOD 450 to assess the fetus in Rh immunization. Because of recent advances in ultrasound technology and intrauterine transfusion techniques, fetal assessment and treatment are now being undertaken as early as 18 weeks' gestation. However, data for ΔOD 450 analysis were originally obtained from third-trimester pregnancies, and interpretation of amniotic fluid bilirubin values prior to 27 weeks is controversial. Several investigators have arbitrarily extrapolated the Liley graph backward and interpreted the results as for third-trimester fetuses (Berkowitz and Hobbins, 1981).

However, Nicolaides and colleagues (1986a) have questioned this approach. They obtained amniotic fluid and umbilical cord blood samples from 59 fetuses with Rh immunization between 18 and 25 weeks' gestation and correlated ΔOD 450 values with fetal haemoglobin; in 25 amniotic fluid was also obtained by amniocentesis between 6 and 16 days before fetoscopy. While the ΔOD 450 correlated with the degree of fetal anaemia, the ΔOD 450 values were widely scattered and did not accurately predict the haematocrit in an individual fetus. The authors concluded that second-trimester amniotic fluid bilirubin analysis is unreliable and that umbilical cord blood sampling is the only accurate method of assessing fetal anaemia (Figure 2).

These results have been widely accepted, and standard recommendations for second-trimester fetal assessment have been modified to include fetal blood sampling instead of amniocentesis (ACOG, 1990). Nevertheless, others have found amniotic fluid bilirubin analysis to be valuable. Ananth and Queenan (1989) studied ΔOD 450 values and trends in 32 Rh-immunized pregnancies between 16 and 20 weeks' gestation. They found that ΔOD 450 values greater than or trending above 0.15 predicted severe

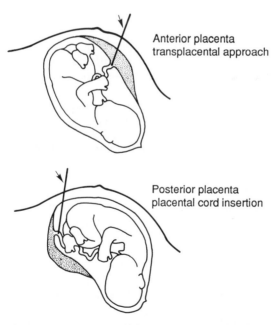

Anterior placenta
transplacental approach

Posterior placenta
placental cord insertion

Figure 2. Needle placement for umbilical cord blood sampling and intravascular fetal transfusion. For needle insertion at the placental insertion site, an anterior placenta must by necessity be traversed. With a posterior placentation, the needle must pass through the amniotic cavity.

isoimmunization, while ΔOD 450 values below 0.09 indicated mild or absent disease. They concluded that umbilical blood sampling is necessary only in pregnancies with ΔOD 450 values greater than 0.15; fetuses with ΔOD 450 values below 0.15 can be managed with serial amniocenteses to determine whether the trend indicates severe disease.

Spinnato and co-workers (1991) suggested that the ΔOD 450 results of Nicolaides et al (1986a) were misleading because no correction for amniotic fluid contamination was utilized. They found that chloroform extraction of amniotic fluid in Rh-immunized pregnancies (to recover bilirubin and remove contaminants such as blood and meconium) resulted in a decrease in ΔOD 450 values in 90% of samples by a mean of 20% and allowed accurate clinical categorization of each patient tested. Nicolaides' group also included hydropic fetuses in their analysis, perhaps underutilized trend analysis, and did not address the risk/benefit ratio for routine umbilical cord blood sampling. Spinnato et al (1991) concluded that second-trimester chloroform-extracted amniotic fluid bilirubin analysis permits accurate fetal assessment and avoids umbilical cord blood sampling in all but 15% of patients.

Adoption of umbilical cord blood sampling has not been universal because of concern for potential fetal and maternal morbidity. The procedure is successful in greater than 95% of cases, but fetal mortality rates of up to 2% have been reported even by experienced investigators (Daffos et al, 1985). In approximately 7% of patients complications such as acute refractory fetal distress, umbilical cord haematoma, amnionitis with maternal adult respiratory distress syndrome, and placental abruption have been described (Pielet et al, 1988; Wilkins et al, 1989; Feinkind et al, 1990). Moreover, there is a significant risk of fetal–maternal bleeding with umbilical cord blood sampling and the potential for worsened maternal sensitization and fetal involvement (Bowell et al, 1988; Nicolini et al, 1988a). Because of the technical difficulty and increased hazard associated with the procedure, umbilical cord blood sampling should be performed only by properly trained personnel in a tertiary referral centre.

Despite the increased hazard of umbilical cord blood sampling over amniocentesis, some groups advocate its use in virtually all Rh-immunized pregnancies. One such protocol calls for cord blood sampling at 18–20 weeks for all patients with a maternal anti-D titre above a critical level and an Rh-positive paternal blood type (or doubtful paternity) (Reece et al, 1988). Rh-negative fetuses require no further testing, and Rh-positive fetuses with low haematocrits at the time of initial sampling have treatment begun immediately. Unfortunately, a number of disadvantages are inherent in this scheme: (1) only a minority of fetuses thus tested will be Rh negative; (2) most fetuses will require continued testing; (3) no data have been presented to indicate the number of fetuses with anaemia severe enough to require transfusion at 20 weeks; and (4) there are a number of procedure-related risks associated with umbilical cord blood sampling. This protocol is of greater value in the management of isoimmunization with the minor antigens such as Kell because with rare antigens a high proportion of fetuses are antigen negative and require no further surveillance.

Ultrasound

Because of the invasive nature of amniocentesis, ultrasound has been studied to identify factors that might predict the severity of erythroblastosis fetalis. Polyhydramnios, placental thickness greater than 4 cm, pericardial effusion, dilatation of the cardiac chambers (especially the right atrium), chronic enlargement of the spleen and liver, visualization of both sides of the fetal bowel wall, and dilation of the umbilical vein have all been proposed as indicators of significant prehydropic fetal anaemia (DeVore et al, 1981; Benacerraf and Frigoletto, 1985; Frigoletto et al, 1986).

In an effort to determine which, if any, ultrasound parameters are most predictive, Chitkara et al (1988) reviewed the ultrasound findings just prior to umbilical cord blood sampling on 35 occasions between 21 and 33.5 weeks' gestation in 15 severely sensitized pregnancies. The relationship of sonographic findings of polyhydramnios, increased placental thickness, increased umbilical vein diameter, and hydrops to fetal haematocrit was studied. All fetuses with hydrops had a haematocrit < 15%, but two of eight fetuses with a haematocrit < 15% had a normal ultrasound and another had only moderate polyhydramnios. Of fetuses with a haematocrit between 16% and 29%, 11 of 19 (58%) had a normal ultrasound; 8 of the 19 (42%) had mild to moderate polyhydramnios, and 3 had placental thickening. Poly-hydramnios was the first and only sonographic sign before fetal anaemia (haematocrit < 26%) in 6 of 10 patients studied serially. Although poly-hydramnios may be an early indication of significant haemolysis and fetal anaemia, the absence of this sonographic finding did not preclude significant anaemia; 13 of 27 (48%) fetuses with normal ultrasound examinations had haematocrits < 30%. It is important to note that there was no normal control group for comparison, and many sonograms were performed when fetuses had already undergone at least one transfusion.

Nicolaides et al (1988) measured fetal head circumference, abdominal circumference, head:abdomen ratio, estimated intraperitoneal volume, placental thickness, and extrahepatic and intrahepatic umbilical vein diameters in 50 patients prior to umbilical cord blood sampling for severe Rh disease. No fetus had been transfused, and the measurements were compared with those from 410 healthy women with normal singleton pregnancies. The presence of hydrops predicted a fetal haemoglobin < 5 g/dl in all 12 cases so affected. In the absence of hydropic changes on ultrasound, none of the parameters differentiated mild from severe anaemia: 4 of 8 fetuses with a haemoglobin < 5 g/dl had no sonographic abnormality, and no consistent pattern was apparent in the 4 with abnormal ultrasound findings. Of the 19 fetuses with a haemoglobin level of 5–10 g/dl, 13 (68%) had a normal ultrasound examination. Nicolaides et al (1988) concluded that the role of ultrasound in the monitoring of fetuses with severe Rh immunization is limited to the search for hydropic changes.

Doppler flow–velocity analysis

Doppler flow–velocity waveforms have also been investigated as non-invasive predictors of fetal anaemia. In a retrospective study of 21 Rh-immunized fetuses about to undergo fetoscopic blood sampling, Rightmire et al (1986) found that the mean blood velocity in the descending aorta and the ratio of systolic to diastolic velocity in the umbilical artery were inversely proportional to fetal haematocrit. Additionally, the mean velocity in the descending aorta was significantly higher in affected fetuses than in normal controls. Unfortunately, a great deal of overlap in velocities between anaemic fetuses and normal controls limited the usefulness of these findings. Also, inclusion of data from hydropic fetuses in the study group may not have been appropriate. The hydropic fetuses identified clinically as needing transfusion had the highest aortic flow velocities, which exaggerated the difference between affected and normal fetuses.

Nicolaides et al (1990) also used retrospective and cross-sectional data to compare fetal aorta Doppler blood velocities in 68 severely immunized fetuses and 218 normal controls. Overall, there was a positive correlation between degree of anaemia and deviation in mean aortic velocity. Considering non-hydropic and hydropic fetuses separately, they found a linear positive correlation and a linear negative correlation, respectively. In the non-hydropic fetus, an aortic mean velocity above the normal range suggested fetal anaemia and a normal mean velocity made significant anaemia unlikely. However, they concluded that Doppler measurements of the aortic blood flow cannot accurately predict the degree of fetal anaemia because of the great overlap in values.

In a similar retrospective study, Copel et al (1988) found that a calculation based on the peak velocity in the descending aorta was predictive of a fetal haematocrit above or below 25% with a high degree of sensitivity. However, their formula and its modifications was not useful in predicting the haematocrit after fetal transfusion. Most importantly, this group was unable to predict the degree of fetal anaemia in a prospective evaluation of their method (Copel et al, 1989).

Doppler indices are currently of limited clinical usefulness for identifying those fetuses that require transfusion, and properly designed prospective studies of Doppler blood flow analysis are necessary before it can be utilized in the obstetric management of isoimmunization.

Assessment: conclusions

Our usual approach to assess the non-hydropic fetus is to follow the trend of ΔOD 450 values in the second and third trimesters. Umbilical cord blood sampling is performed if the initial ΔOD 450 value is near or in zone III, and when the ΔOD 450 trend is upward into the middle or upper zone II. Fetal cord blood is analysed for haemoglobin and haematocrit, and for Rh-antigen status if no anaemia is present. If hydrops is evident by ultrasound, umbilical blood sampling is performed regardless of ΔOD 450 values. However, patient assessment is individualized, and those with a history of severe second-trimester disease or previous severe disease with misleading ΔOD 450 values are also considered for umbilical cord blood sampling as their primary mode of fetal evaluation.

MANAGEMENT OF THE SEVERELY AFFECTED FETUS

Before the introduction of amniotic fluid analysis and in utero transfusion, the management of Rh isoimmunization was limited to induced preterm delivery. With the introduction of ΔOD 450 analysis, fetuses specifically at risk for death in utero could be targeted for early delivery, reducing unnecessary prematurity. The direct treatment of fetal anaemia by intrauterine transfusion of red blood cells now allows even later delivery of healthier infants.

Intrauterine intraperitoneal transfusion

Placement of erythrocytes in the fetal peritoneal cavity reverses fetal anaemia by uptake of red blood cells into the fetal circulatory system via the subdiaphragmatic lymphatics. Perinatal survival following intraperitoneal transfusion is related to gestational age at delivery and the severity of fetal disease, particularly with regard to whether hydrops develops. When transfusions were performed with X-ray guidance, overall neonatal survival was approximately 60%, survival of non-hydropic infants was near 70%, and less than 40% of those developing hydrops survived (Bowman, 1978). The routine use of ultrasound for transfusion and monitoring, improvements in transfusion technique, and advances in neonatal care have now resulted in more favourable outcomes (Table 1).

Table 1. Neonatal survival of fetuses with severe Rh immunization treated with red blood cell transfusion in the time since introduction of ultrasound guidance.

	Non-hydropic	Hydropic	Overall
Intraperitoneal transfusion: neonatal survival			
Bowman & Manning (1983)	16/16 (100%)	6/8 (75%)	22/24 (92%)
Scott et al (1984)	12/14 (86%)	4/6 (67%)	16/20 (80%)
Watts et al (1988)	26/26 (100%)	4/9 (44%)	30/35 (86%)
Harman et al (1990)	19/23 (83%)	10/21 (48%)	29/44 (66%)
Total	73/79 (92%)	24/44 (55%)	97/123 (79%)
Intravascular transfusion: neonatal survival			
Nicolaides et al (1986b)	8/8 (100%)	9/10 (90%)	17/18 (94%)
Berkowitz et al (1988)	13/16 (81%)	0/1 (0%)	13/17 (76%)
Grannum et al (1988)	5/6 (83%)	16/20 (80%)	21/26 (81%)
Poissonnier et al (1989)	55/60 (92%)	29/47 (62%)	84/107 (79%)
Harman et al (1990)	22/23 (96%)	18/21 (86%)	40/44 (91%)
Weiner et al (1991)	35/35 (100%)	11/13 (85%)	46/48 (92%)
Total	138/148 (93%)	83/112 (74%)	221/260 (85%)

Ultrasound has dramatically reduced the procedure-related morbidity and mortality associated with intraperitoneal transfusion. Confirmation of appropriate needle placement is usually straightforward, but inadvertent transfusion into the bowel, liver, abdominal wall, and retroperitoneum still occur. Infection, premature rupture of the membranes, refractory preterm labour, and fetal distress necessitating immediate delivery continue to pose a hazard. Bowman and Manning (1983) reported 5 traumatic deaths in 53 transfusions (9.4%) during the 2 years prior to instituting ultrasound guidance; there were no deaths in the 64 transfusions immediately afterward. In a similar analysis, Scott et al (1984) observed a reduction in traumatic death rate from 8.0% to 2.3% per transfusion. Most recently, Harman et al (1990) have reported a traumatic death rate of 7.6% per procedure; nearly 75% of the fetal and neonatal deaths in this series were due to trauma or complications of prematurity and not to Rh disease. Thus, while intraperitoneal transfusion has evolved into a relatively safe procedure, it is not without risk for fetal loss.

Intrauterine intravascular transfusion

First described by Rodeck et al (1981) using fetoscopy, intravascular fetal transfusion has been widely adopted in modified form using ultrasound to guide placement of a needle into the umbilical vein. Direct access to the fetal circulation for transfusion offers a number of advantages over the intraperitoneal approach: (1) fetal haematocrit can be measured, allowing a more precise calculation of the volume of blood required for transfusion; (2) in some cases, fetuses will have a higher haematocrit than expected and transfusion can be delayed; (3) at times, the fetus will be found to be Rh negative. A post-transfusion haematocrit can be used to determine whether the transfusion was adequate and when the next one should be scheduled. Transfusion into the fetal vascular system ensures complete uptake of the intended red blood cell mass with a more rapid correction of fetal anaemia. This is especially important in hydropic fetuses who often do not adequately absorb intraperitoneally transfused erythrocytes. Potential disadvantages of intravascular fetal transfusion include: (1) the rare possibility of volume overload in the compromised fetus; (2) procedure-related complications; and (3) the risk of increasing the severity of maternal sensitization due to fetal–maternal haemorrhage.

Despite the recent popularity of intravascular transfusion, perinatal survival in pregnancies managed with intravascular transfusion is convincingly improved over that with intraperitoneal transfusion only for hydropic fetuses. Overall survival rates are 76–94% (Table 1). The perinatal survival of non-hydropic fetuses exceeds 90%, and among fetuses with hydrops, 75% survive with intravascular transfusion.

Morbidity and mortality related to the technique of vascular access and transfusion are similar to those with intraperitoneal transfusion. Nicolaides et al (1986b), in a large experience with intravascular transfusion, reported fetal bradycardia in 12.5% of procedures and one fetal death in a hydropic fetus (1%) occurring 4 days after transfusion. Pielet et al (1988) had a complication rate of 9.4% and a mortality rate of 4.7% per transfusion in a series of 64 procedures, and Poissonnier et al (1989) had five procedure-related fetal deaths in 200 transfusions (2.5%). Harman et al (1990) reported a procedural complication rate of 9.8% and a traumatic death rate of 0.6% per transfusion ($n = 173$). Weiner et al (1991), in a review of 142 intravascular transfusions, noted an incidence of fetal bradycardia of 8%

(requiring immediate delivery in only one instance), a single case of intra-amniotic infection, three cases of premature rupture of membranes, and two fetal losses. Overall, intravascular transfusion in experienced hands seems to have a procedure-related complication rate of 5–10%, and a mortality rate of between 1 and 4%.

However, concern about the intravascular route has been raised because of the possibility of increasing maternal sensitization with worsened disease in subsequent pregnancies. Bowell et al (1988) measured anti-D levels before and 2 weeks after amniocentesis, umbilical cord blood sampling, and transfusion with an ultrasound-guided needle. Five of 18 (28%) umbilical cord blood samplings were followed by an anti-D titre rise of greater than 50%, as compared with 31% (11 of 36) following amniocentesis. Seven pregnancies with multiple sampling showed a rise in anti-D, and five (71%) of these were after the first procedure. No information is available on placental location, but the data suggest that boosted maternal anti-D levels may increase the severity of fetal anaemia and worsen the prognosis in subsequent pregnancies. Nicolini et al (1988a), using maternal serum α-fetoprotein as a marker for fetomaternal haemorrhage, reported similar results with 68 intravascular transfusions. When an anterior placenta was traversed, 66% of patients had a significant increase in maternal serum α-fetoprotein, as compared with 17% of those with a posterior placenta. The estimated volume of fetal–maternal bleeding correlated with increases in the maternal anti-D titre. Weiner et al (1989) reported a rise in maternal serum α-fetoprotein in 44% of patients undergoing umbilical cord blood sampling and intravascular fetal transfusion with an anterior placenta and an increase in only 4% of those with a posterior placenta. There was no difference between patients undergoing blood sampling and transfusion, and avoidance of an anterior placenta when performing diagnostic or therapeutic umbilical cord procedures was recommended.

These studies indicate that umbilical cord blood sampling and intravascular transfusion can be associated with significant fetal–maternal bleeding and a heightened maternal immune response, but actual clinical data from subsequent pregnancies do not yet exist. Additionally, comparative data from intraperitoneal procedures are not available, and it is not certain whether increases in α-fetoprotein and anti-D are worse following intravascular transfusion than following intraperitoneal transfusion.

Treatment options

Intraperitoneal versus intravascular transfusion

Analysis of the collective experience of the last decade with intrauterine treatment of the hydropic fetus definitely shows an improved survival rate using intravascular transfusion when compared with treatment with intraperitoneal transfusion. However, the difference in outcome between the two techniques is much less clear in non-hydropic fetuses. Survival rates of 80–100% have been documented for both methods, with near-identical rates of survival when the published series are combined (Table 1). Unfortunately, a prospective, randomized clinical trial designed to determine the superior technique in the non-hydropic fetus has not been performed.

In an attempt to compare the two methods, Harman et al (1990) analysed their results in patients who underwent intravascular and intraperitoneal transfusions for severe fetal anaemia. Forty-four patients undergoing 173 intravascular transfusions were compared retrospectively with 44 fetuses treated with 104 intraperitoneal transfusions in the same institution and matched for severity of disease, placental location, and gestational age. The authors concluded that intravascular transfusion was superior, based on a higher survival rate, a greater gestational age at delivery, and significant reductions in Apgar scores <7, caesarean section rate, the need for and number of neonatal exchange transfusions, and intensive care nursery admissions and duration of stay. Additionally, the intraperitoneal group had higher procedure-related mortality (7.7% versus 0.6% per transfusion) and overall rate of maternal complication (12.5% versus 3%). However, the survival of non-hydropic fetuses was not significantly different between the two treatment groups, and the morbidity data were not analysed separately for hydropic and non-hydropic fetuses. Acknowledging that the difference in survival for non-hydropic fetuses was statistically unconvincing, the authors argued that the lower procedure-related loss rate with intravascular treatment was clinically significant and that intraperitoneal transfusion should be reserved for those situations where intravascular transfusion is impossible due to position of the fetus and cord.

Combined intravascular/intraperitoneal transfusion

In an effort to reduce the number of transfusions necessary during treatment of a severely involved pregnancy, Nicolini et al (1989) have combined intravascular and intraperitoneal transfusions. After an intravascular transfusion to a fetal haematocrit of approximately 40%, enough blood to raise the intravascular haematocrit to 60% was then transfused intraperitoneally. Although cases were not randomized, comparison of 32 patients who had combined procedures to 17 who received only intravascular transfusions revealed a significantly increased interval between transfusions (24.2 ± 4.1 versus 21.6 ± 3.6 days, $P < 0.05$) and a higher fetal haematocrit at the time of the subsequent procedure (27.0 ± 5.8 versus 23.2 ± 5.7, $P < 0.05$). Careful examination of these data suggests that the clinical benefit of a combined procedure would be minimal, but some authors (Lenke et al, 1990) have advocated routinely combining intravascular with intraperitoneal transfusions.

Management: conclusions

It is clear that intravascular transfusion is more effective than intraperitoneal transfusion in treating hydropic fetuses and is life saving in many cases. However, it is not clear whether the intravascular route is superior for the fetus who is not hydropic or for the fetus who has resolved hydrops and is receiving subsequent transfusions. Recent series indicate that fetal survival rates are excellent and comparable by either technique. It is possible that indications for combining intraperitoneal and intravascular transfusions will eventually be better defined and this may become the optimum treatment in the future.

Based on the available data, we currently treat all Rh-immunized pregnancies with evidence of hydrops fetalis by intravascular transfusion, reserving intraperitoneal transfusion for situations where the intravascular route is not technically feasible. Because even hydropic fetuses can usually tolerate bolus transfusion, and because the technique is easier and less time-consuming than exchange transfusion, we perform simple transfusions. While there is still a role for intraperitoneal transfusion in the non-hydropic fetus, we use intravascular transfusion when the umbilical vein is accessible, because a relatively precise estimate of the required volume of blood is possible, complete uptake of erythrocytes is assured, and a post-transfusion haematocrit can be obtained which allows an estimate of the timing of the next transfusion. Intraperitoneal transfusion is routinely used in cases where the umbilical cord is not easily accessible and the fetus is not hydropic.

Increased maternal sensitization after intravascular transfusion is likely to be due to the transplacental approach rather than intravascular access. If an anterior placenta must be traversed to gain access to the fetal peritoneal cavity, intravascular transfusion is preferred because access to the target vessel is easier with no difference in risk of increasing sensitization. Intraperitoneal transfusion can be considered for patients who have a non-hydropic fetus in good position, particularly those who expect to have additional pregnancies.

MINOR ANTIGEN SENSITIZATION

In addition to the D antigen, there are other distinct antigens found on the red blood cell surface. Known as minor or atypical antigens, their frequency varies between populations. Because of the reduction in Rh immunization brought about by Rh immune globulin prophylaxis, minor antigen sensitization has become relatively more frequent in pregnancy. Blood banks do not routinely assess donor–recipient compatibility for antigens other than ABO and Rh, and transfusion is a major cause of sensitization to the non-Rh antigens. A partial listing of atypical red blood cell antigens is found in Table 2.

A number of the minor antigens can result in fetal anaemia and hydrops as reviewed by Weinstein (1982), and the pathogenesis of fetal anaemia is similar for the minor antigens as for Rh disease. Thus, management of the pregnant patient with antibody to one of the significant minor antigens is much the same as for Rh immunization, with frequent measurement of maternal antibody titres, serial amniocenteses after a critical titre is reached, and transfusion or delivery based on the ΔOD 450 values and trends (Weinstein, 1982; Bowman, 1989). However, few centres have a significant number of pregnancies affected by minor antigen sensitization, so establishment of a critical maternal titre is difficult. Also, the reliability of maternal antibody titre or ΔOD 450 analysis to assess fetal status is more controversial.

Kell is the most frequent irregular antigen to cause haemolytic disease of the newborn. More than 90% of the general population is Kell negative, and over 90% of cases of Kell immunization are the result of transfusion of

Table 2. Atypical or minor red blood cell antigens.

Blood group system	Antigens related to haemolytic disease	Severity of haemolytic disease
CDE	C	Mild to moderate
	c	Mild to severe
	D	Mild to severe
	E	Mild to severe
	e	Mild to moderate
Lewis		Not a proved cause of haemolytic disease of the newborn
Kell	K	Mild to severe with hydrops fetalis
Kidd	Jk^a	Mild to severe
	Jk^b	Mild to severe
Duffy	Fy^a	Mild to severe with hydrops fetalis
	Fy^b	Not a cause of haemolytic disease of newborn
I		Not a proved cause of haemolytic disease of the newborn
Lutheran	Lu^a	Mild
	Lu^b	Mild
Diego	Di^a	Mild to severe
	Di^b	Mild to severe
MNSs	M	Mild to severe
	N	Mild
	S	Mild to severe
	s	Mild to severe
P	PP, P^k (T^{ja})	Mild to severe
Public	Co^a	Severe
	En^a	Moderate
	Jr^a	Mild
	Lan	Mild
	Y^{ta}	Moderate to severe
	Y^{tb}	Mild
Private antigens	Co^{a-b}	Mild
	Becker	Mild
	Berrens	Mild
	Good	Severe
	Heilbel	Moderate
	Hunt	Mild
	Radin	Moderate
	Wright^a	Severe
	Wright^b	Mild
	Zd	Moderate

Patients sensitized to antigens that cause only mild fetal anaemia can be followed expectantly, with no need for amniocentesis or fetal blood sampling. Patients sensitized to antigens that can cause moderate or severe haemolytic disease require serial fetal assessment with analysis of amniotic fluid ΔOD 450 or fetal haematocrit (modified from Weinstein, 1982).

incompatible blood. Fetal involvement in cases of Kell sensitization may be qualitatively different from in Rh disease. For example, Berkowitz et al (1982) reported a case of fetal hydrops and death due to Kell sensitization despite amniotic fluid ΔOD 450 values trending downward in the lower third of the Liley midzone. Similarly, Copel et al (1986) reported one case of fetal hydrops with a maternal anti-Kell titre of 1:4 and another patient with an anti-Kell titre rise from 1:32 to 1:2048 while carrying a Kell-negative fetus.

Caine and Mueller-Huebach (1986) described their 16-year experience with Kell-sensitized pregnancies. In 127 pregnancies, 13 (10.2%) had an affected Kell-positive fetus, and 5 of these 13 (38%) had severe disease. Only 2.6% of pregnancies with a maternal titre ≤1:16 had a Kell-positive fetus, as compared with 28.5% of those with a titre >1:16. No patients with a titre ≤1:16 had a fetal death, and all patients with a poor perinatal outcome had a titre ≥1:128 at delivery. No patient with a poor outcome had an amniotic fluid ΔOD 450 value in the highest Liley zone, suggesting that serious haemolytic disease develops at lower ΔOD 450 values than with Rh sensitization.

Leggat and co-workers (1991) described 194 pregnancies over 25 years in which anti-Kell was the only antibody identified. Of the 178 unaffected babies, 106 (60%) had maternal titres ≥1:16. There were 16 affected infants (9% of the total), ten with mild disease and six with moderate or severe anaemia. Of the six mothers who delivered affected infants, four had titres ≥1:16 while two had titres ≤1:8. Amniotic fluid analysis was also performed in pregnancies which resulted in 16 unaffected and 5 affected newborns; fetuses with disease of moderate or greater severity had ΔOD 450 values trending upward or in the upper part of the Liley midzone, but four unaffected fetuses had ΔOD 450 values associated with moderate to severe haemolysis in Rh disease. The authors concluded that neither maternal antibody titres nor amniotic fluid analysis are satisfactory predictors of fetal status.

Based on these data, Kell sensitization may justify a modification of the obstetric management scheme used for Rh disease. Determination of paternal antigen status is important, as less than 10% of the population are Kell positive and less than 3% of those are homozygous positive. Because 60–70% of fetuses of mothers with elevated anti-Kell titres are actually Kell negative and fetal condition may not be accurately reflected by amniotic fluid analysis, a more liberal use of umbilical cord blood sampling is suggested for pregnant patients with anti-Kell antibody and a Kell-positive partner. However, the value of serial umbilical cord samplings is yet to be determined, and it has not been proven to significantly improve the perinatal outcome of affected pregnancies.

ALLOIMMUNE THROMBOCYTOPENIA

Like erythrocytes, platelets contain specific surface antigens, and maternal sensitization to platelet antigens may occur when there is an incompatibility between fetus and mother. In a situation analogous to Rh isoimmunization, alloimmune thrombocytopenia is the result of maternal sensitization to incompatible fetal platelets and transfer of immunoglobulin to the fetus with subsequent destruction of platelets. Although a number of antigens can produce isoimmune thrombocytopenia (including those of the HLA system), sensitization to the Pl^{A1} antigen is the cause in the majority of cases. Approximately 3% of the population is negative for Pl^{A1}, and alloimmune thrombocytopenia occurs in about 1:2000 births (Burrows and Kelton, 1988; Mueller-Eckhardt et al, 1989).

For reasons that are unclear, alloimmune thrombocytopenia can result in maternal IgG production in the first pregnancy. Primigravidae account for approximately half of identified cases, and mothers at risk are usually identified only after the birth of an affected newborn. There are several reasons why all pregnant women are not screened for the presence of antiplatelet antibodies: approximately a third of cases of isoimmune neonatal thrombocytopenia are not due to the Pl^{A1} antigen; the maternal immune response seems to be influenced by other factors such as HLA type and only a minority of fetuses of mothers negative for the Pl^{A1} antigen will develop significant thrombocytopenia; and, there is no relationship between the level of antibody to Pl^{A1} and the degree of fetal thrombocytopenia (Shulman and Jordan, 1987).

Following delivery of an affected newborn, the incidence of recurrent fetal thrombocytopenia of equal or greater severity is up to 95% in the next pregnancy (Shulman and Jordan, 1987). Approximately 90% of affected newborns will have diffuse petechiae, but central nervous system bleeding accounts for the most serious sequelae. Postnatal mortality is about 5%, and of the 9–12% of newborns who suffer an intracerebral haemorrhage, about 45% occur before birth (Shulman and Jordan, 1987; Mueller-Eckhardt et al, 1989).

Before the availability of umbilical cord blood sampling, the management of pregnancies at risk for alloimmune thrombocytopenia was based on the avoidance of fetal trauma with bed rest during the pregnancy and caesarean delivery before labour (Mennuti et al, 1974; Sitarz et al, 1976). However, since approximately half of fetuses who suffer intracranial bleeding do so before labour, avoidance of labour and vaginal delivery only partially reduces the associated morbidity and mortality. Maternal platelet count is normal, and maternal antibody levels are not predictive of fetal platelet count (Kaplan et al, 1988). Umbilical cord blood sampling and direct measurement of fetal platelet count is currently the only method to assess fetal status.

Several strategies have been proposed for the management of pregnancies at risk for alloimmune thrombocytopenia. Bussel and co-workers (1988) serially measured fetal platelet counts and administered intravenous immunoglobulin to seven mothers on a weekly basis until delivery. They found a mean increase in fetal platelet count of 72.5×10^9 per litre, and all neonates had platelet counts $\geq 30 \times 10^9$ at birth. No infant in the series had an intracranial haemorrhage compared with three of seven previously affected siblings. They recommended that pregnant patients with a previously affected infant undergo umbilical blood sampling at 20–22 weeks' gestation, and that mothers whose fetuses had a platelet count $< 100 \times 10^9$ per litre should receive weekly infusions of immunoglobulin. However, others have been unable to show a benefit of maternal immunoglobulin infusion, even with a documented increase in fetal immunoglobulin levels (Kaplan et al, 1988; Nicolini et al, 1990).

Kaplan et al (1988) have advocated umbilical cord blood sampling at 21 weeks' gestation for analysis of fetal platelet count and Pl^{A1} antigen typing. If the diagnosis of alloimmune thrombocytopenia is made, they recommended strict bed rest until 37 weeks to avoid fetal bleeding from maternal trauma. At that time, umbilical cord blood sampling is repeated, and if the fetal platelet count is normal, labour can be induced safely; if the platelet count is less than 50×10^9 per litre, maternal platelets are transfused into the fetal circulation to allow induction of labour and vaginal delivery. This approach still fails to address the problem of intracranial haemorrhage before labour.

In an effort to prevent antepartum intracranial bleeding, Nicolini et al (1988b) used serial platelet transfusions throughout the third trimester. Their patient had a previous infant with Pl^{A1} antigen alloimmune thrombocytopenia leading to severe intracranial haemorrhage with neurological sequelae. Fetal thrombocytopenia was documented and weekly platelet transfusions were begun at 26 weeks. The pregnancy was carried to 32 weeks and delivered by caesarean section. Neonatal platelet counts were greater than 44×10^9 per litre, and the infant had no evidence of intracranial bleeding. However, further data are needed to confirm the efficacy of this approach because of the risk of procedure-related complications and the difficulty of obtaining sufficient Pl^{A1}-negative platelets. The need for frequent transfusions makes it difficult to use only maternal platelets, and donor platelets carry a small but real risk of infections such as cytomegalovirus, hepatitis, and HIV.

The best prenatal management of alloimmune thrombocytopenia has not been established despite the availability of fetal blood sampling. However, there have been few reported cases of intracranial haemorrhage before 30 weeks' gestation, and the outcome of the first affected pregnancy is somewhat predictive of the prognosis for subsequent affected siblings (Mueller-Eckhardt et al, 1989). We advocate serial sonograms in all pregnancies during the third trimester to detect intracranial bleeding. If there is a history of a previous fetus with intracranial haemorrhage, maternal administration of intravenous immune globulin 1.0 g/kg of body weight, although expensive, is one option. In these cases, we sample umbilical cord blood for a platelet count at 30–34 weeks' gestation and begin maternal platelet transfusions in the markedly thrombocytopenic fetus. In patients at lower risk, the first fetal platelet count is obtained at 35–37 weeks' gestation. All thrombocytopenic infants are delivered by caesarean when mature, but preparations are made for emergency caesarean at the time of umbilical cord blood sampling should that become necessary. This regimen avoids serial invasive procedures in an immature fetus when the risk of intracranial bleeding is lower and when an umbilical cord accident would be fatal.

GRAFT-VERSUS-HOST DISEASE

Although the obstetrician is very familiar with fetal diseases caused by maternal alloantibodies, much less is known about the maternal cellular immune system and its relationship to potential fetal disorders. In the conventional graft-to-host relationship, transplantation of an allograft to an immunologically mature individual normally results in destruction of the entire alien cell population. Since peripheral blood contains circulating stem cells, engraftment and subsequent development of immunocompetent donor lymphocytes can occur if the recipient is immunologically immature or profoundly immunosuppressed. When HLA-foreign stem cells are not destroyed, graft-versus-host disease can develop in the recipient, character-ized by a rash, mucositis, diarrhoea, hepatic dysfunction, failure to thrive, and death. Graft-versus-host disease or the 'runting syndrome' has been extensively studied in animals (Figure 3), and there is now increasing

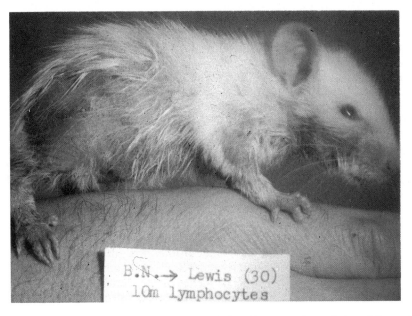

Figure 3. White rat with graft-versus-host disease induced by neonatal transfusion of allogeneic lymphocytes.

experience with acute and chronic forms of the disease in the human because of congenital and acquired immunodeficiency disorders and as the result of bone marrow transplantation.

Fetal immunological responses to antigenic challenge develop at various specific stages in utero, and a spectrum ranging from complete tolerance to sensitization may be elicited depending upon such variables as the strength, dose, physical form, route of administration, and age and species of the fetus at the time of antigen exposure. Fetal lambs respond immunologically to inoculation with bacteriophage virus as early as 41 days post-conception and reject skin and kidney allografts at mid-gestation. Fetal rats and mice are immunologically less mature and primates more mature, at the same relative stages of gestation. During the second and third weeks of gestation in the human fetus, pluripotential yolk sac stem cells form the precursors of all the blood cell series. The thymus develops at about 6 weeks' gestation, and lymphocyte differentiation proceeds in the complete absence of foreign antigens. Small lymphocytes appear in the peripheral blood at about 7 weeks and in connective tissue around lymphocyte plexuses by 8 weeks. Primary lymph node development and lymphopoiesis begins at 12 weeks' gestation, T cells capable of responding to mitogens and recognizing histocompatible cells appear at 13 weeks, and lymphocyte aggregates form in the fetal spleen by 14 weeks' gestation. Thus, by 20–22 weeks' gestation the human fetus is relatively immunologically mature as evidenced by response to congenital infections with the production of antibody and phytohaemagglutinin stimulation of fetal lymphocytes (Scott, 1990).

It is possible that if sufficient numbers of maternal small lymphocytes gained access to an immunogenetically appropriate fetus and were not promptly rejected, graft-versus-host disease could occur. Indeed, there have been sporadic reports during the past 25 years of infants who develop a clinical picture resembling the disease with persistent circulating maternal white blood cells. These have usually occurred in immunodeficiency states (Kodawaki et al, 1965; Lischner et al, 1967; Pollack et al, 1982) and in infants who have received intrauterine transfusions (Turner et al, 1966; Naiman et al, 1969). Fortunately, intrauterine transfusions are normally begun after mid-gestation, and graft-versus-host disease can be prevented by irradiating all blood products prior to transfusion. However, in utero haematopoietic stem cells transplanted into fetal rhesus monkeys at 60 days' gestation survive in the neonate (Crombleholme et al, 1991), and permanent chimerism has been shown in twins which shared placental circulation (Owen, 1945). Little is known in the human about exactly when in gestation and by what mechanism tolerance and the risk for graft-versus-host disease is lost, but rhesus monkey experiments suggest it is not before 16.5 weeks' gestation. Accurate information about this would be clinically useful because fetal graft-versus-host disease could then perhaps be prevented. On the other hand, if tolerance could be safely produced, each child born could have a potential donor organ allograft (without the need for immuno-suppressive drugs) should one become necessary later in life.

In summary, placental haemodynamics favour the passage of cells from the fetus to the mother. Although the nature and extent of transfer in the opposite direction is unknown, the relative difficulty with which maternal white cells cross the placenta probably accounts for the fact that colonization of the fetus is distinctly uncommon. Nevertheless, obstetricians and neo-natologists should be aware of this possibility in infants who are immuno-deficient or who display signs and symptoms suggestive of graft-versus-host disease.

SUMMARY

Transfer of fetal red blood cells and platelets to the maternal circulation can stimulate an immune response with production of immunoglobulin that can cross the placenta. Similarly, passage of maternal stem cells to an immunologically incompetent fetus can theoretically produce graft-versus-host disease.

Maternal sensitization to red blood cell antigens such as D and Kell can result in anaemia, hydrops, and death in an incompatible fetus. Current assessment of these pregnancies involves serial analysis of amniotic fluid bilirubin concentration, with umbilical cord blood sampling reserved for special circumstances; neither ultrasound or Doppler blood flow analysis are accurate in the prediction of fetal haematocrit. Intravascular transfusion is the treatment of choice for hydropic fetuses. Perinatal survival in non-hydropic fetuses is similar with either intravascular or intraperitoneal transfusion, and the choice of procedures is individualized.

Isoimmune fetal thrombocytopenia is usually the result of maternal sensitization to the Pl^{A1} antigen. There is significant risk of intracranial haemorrhage, both antepartum and during labour and delivery. Umbilical cord blood sampling at term can determine fetal platelet count and the need for platelet transfusion, and can aid in deciding the appropriate route of delivery.

REFERENCES

ACOG (1990) Management of D isoimmunization in pregnancy. *ACOG Technical Bulletin 148*. Washington DC: American College of Obstetricians and Gynecologists.

Ananth U & Queenan JT (1989) Does midtrimester ΔOD 450 of amniotic fluid reflect severity of Rh disease? *American Journal of Obstetrics and Gynecology* **161**: 47–49.

Benacerraf BR & Frigoletto FD (1985) Sonographic sign for the detection of early ascites in the management of severe isoimmune disease without intrauterine transfusion. *American Journal of Obstetrics and Gynecology* **152**: 1039–1041.

Berkowitz RL & Hobbins JC (1981) Intrauterine transfusion utilizing ultrasound. *Obstetrics and Gynecology* **57**: 33–36.

Berkowitz RL, Beyth Y & Sadovsky E (1982) Death in utero due to Kell sensitization without elevation of the ΔOD 450 value in amniotic fluid. *Obstetrics and Gynecology* **60**: 746–749.

Berkowitz RL, Chitkara U, Wilkins IA et al (1988) Intravascular monitoring and management of erythroblastosis fetalis. *American Journal of Obstetrics and Gynecology* **158**: 783–795.

Bevis DCA (1956) Blood pigments in haemolytic disease of the newborn. *Journal of Obstetrics and Gynaecology of the British Commonwealth* **63**: 68–75.

Bowell PJ, Selinger M, Ferguson J, Giles J & MacKenzie IZ (1988) Antenatal fetal blood sampling for the management of alloimmunized pregnancies: effect upon maternal anti-D potency levels. *British Journal of Obstetrics and Gynaecology* **95**: 759–764.

Bowman JM (1978) The management of Rh isoimmunization. *Obstetrics and Gynecology* **52**: 1–16.

Bowman JM (1989) Hemolytic disease (erythroblastosis fetalis). In Creasy RK & Resnik R (eds) *Maternal–Fetal Medicine: Principles and Practice*, 2nd edn, pp 613–655. Philadelphia: W. B. Saunders Company.

Bowman JM & Manning FA (1983) Intrauterine fetal transfusions: Winnipeg 1982. *Obstetrics and Gynecology* **61**: 203–209.

Brown PJ, Evans JP, Sinor LT et al (1983) The rhesus antigen: a dicyclohexylcarbodiimide-binding proteolipid. *American Journal of Pathology* 110: 127–134.

Burrows RF & Kelton JG (1988) Incidentally detected thrombocytopenia in healthy mothers and their infants. *New England Journal of Medicine* 319: 142–145.

Bussel JB, Berkowitz RL, McFarland JG, Lynch L & Chitkara U (1988) Antenatal treatment of neonatal alloimmune thrombocytopenia. *New England Journal of Medicine* 319: 1374–1378.

Caine ME & Mueller-Huebach E (1986) Kell sensitization in pregnancy. *American Journal of Obstetrics and Gynecology* 154: 85–90.

Chitkara U, Wilkins I, Lynch L, Mehalek K & Berkowitz RL (1988) The role of sonography in assessing severity of fetal anemia in Rh- and Kell immunized pregnancies. *Obstetrics and Gynecology* 71: 393–398.

Copel JA, Scioscia A, Grannum PA et al (1986) Percutaneous umbilical blood sampling in the management of Kell isoimmunization. *Obstetrics and Gynecology* 67: 288–290.

Copel JA, Grannum PA, Belanger K, Green J & Hobbins JC (1988) Pulsed Doppler flow–velocity waveforms before and after intrauterine intravascular transfusion for severe erythroblastosis fetalis. *American Journal of Obstetrics and Gynecology* 158: 768–774.

Copel JA, Grannum PA, Green JJ, Belanger K & Hobbins JC (1989) Pulsed Doppler flow–velocity waveforms in the prediction of fetal hematocrit of the severely immunized pregnancy. *American Journal of Obstetrics and Gynecology* 161: 341–344.

Crombleholme TM, Langer JC, Harrison MR & Zanjani ED (1991) Transplantation of fetal cells. *American Journal of Obstetrics and Gynecology* 164: 218–230.

Daffos F, Capella-Pavlovsky M & Forestier F (1985) Fetal blood sampling during pregnancy with use of a needle guided by ultrasound: A study of 606 consecutive cases. *American Journal of Obstetrics and Gynaecology* 153: 655–660.

DeVore GR, Mayden K, Tortora M, Berkowitz RL & Hobbins JC (1981) Dilation of the fetal umbilical vein in rhesus hemolytic anemia: a predictor of severe disease. *American Journal of Obstetrics and Gynecology* 141: 464–466.

Feinkind L, Nanda D, Delke I & Minkoff H (1990) Abruptio placentae after percutaneous umbilical cord sampling: a case report. *American Journal of Obstetrics and Gynecology* 162: 1203–1204.

Frigoletto FD, Greene MF, Benacerraf BR, Barss VA & Saltzman DH (1986) Ultrasonographic fetal surveillance in the management of the immunized pregnancy. *New England Journal of Medicine* 315: 430–432.

Grannum PAT, Copel JA, Moya FR et al (1988) The reversal of hydrops fetalis by intravascular intrauterine transfusion in severe isoimmune fetal anemia. *American Journal of Obstetrics and Gynecology* 158: 914–919.

Harman CR, Bowman JM, Manning FA & Menticoglou SM (1990) Intrauterine transfusion-intraperitoneal versus intravascular approach: A case-control comparison. *American Journal of Obstetrics and Gynecology* 162: 1053–1059.

James NT & James V (1978) Nearest neighbor analysis on the distribution of Rh antigens on erythrocyte membranes. *British Journal of Haematology* 40: 657–659.

Jones WR & Need JA (1988) Maternal–fetal cell surface antigen incompatibilities. *Clinical Immunology and Allergy* 2: 577–605.

Kaplan C, Daffos F, Forestier F et al (1988) Management of alloimmune thrombocytopenia: antenatal diagnosis and in utero transfusion of maternal platelets. *Blood* 72: 340–343.

Kodawaki J, Thompson RI, Zuelzer WW et al (1965) XX/YY lymphoid chimerism in congenital deficiency syndrome with thymic alymphoplasia. *Lancet* ii: 1152–1156.

Leggat HM, Gibson JM, Barron SL & Reid MM (1991) Anti-Kell in pregnancy. *British Journal of Obstetrics and Gynaecology* 98: 162–165.

Lenke RR, Persutte WH & Nemes JM (1990) Combined intravascular and intraperitoneal transfusions for erythroblastosis fetalis. A report of two cases. *Journal of Reproductive Medicine* 35: 425–428.

Liley AW (1961) Liquor amnii in the management of the pregnancy complicated by rhesus sensitization. *American Journal of Obstetrics and Gynecology* 82: 1359–1370.

Liley AW (1963) Errors in assessment of hemolytic disease from amniotic fluid. *American Journal of Obstetrics and Gynecology* 86: 485–494.

Lischner HW, Punnett HH & diGeorge AM (1967) Lymphocytes in congenital absence of the thymus. *Nature* 214: 580–582.

LoBuglio AFL (1967) Red cells coated with immunoglobulin G: binding and sphering by mononuclear cells in man. *Science* 158: 1582–1585.

Mennuti M, Schwarz RH & Gill F (1974) Obstetric management of isoimmune thrombocytopenia. *American Journal of Obstetrics and Gynecology* 118: 565–566.

Mueller-Eckhardt C, Grubert A, Weisheit M et al (1989) 348 cases of suspected neonatal alloimmune thrombocytopenia. *Lancet* i: 363–366.

Naiman JL, Punnett HH, Lischner HW, Destine ML & Arey JB (1969) Possible graft-versus-host reaction after intrauterine transfusion for Rh erythroblastosis fetalis. *New England Journal of Medicine* 281: 697–701.

Nicolaides KH, Rodeck CH, Mibashan RS & Kemp JR (1986a) Have Liley charts outlived their usefulness? *American Journal of Obstetrics and Gynecology* 155: 90–94.

Nicolaides KH, Soothill PW, Rodeck CH et al (1986b) Rh disease: intravascular blood transfusion by cordocentesis. *Fetal Therapy* 1: 185–192.

Nicolaides KH, Fontanarosa M, Gabbe SL & Rodeck CH (1988) Failure of ultrasonographic parameters to predict the severity of fetal anemia in rhesus isoimmunization. *American Journal of Obstetrics and Gynecology* 158: 920–926.

Nicolaides KH, Bilardo CM & Campbell S (1990) Prediction of fetal anemia by measurement of the mean blood velocity in the fetal aorta. *American Journal of Obstetrics and Gynecology* 162: 209–212.

Nicolini U, Kochenour NK, Greco P et al (1988a) Consequences of fetomaternal haemorrhage after intrauterine transfusion. *British Medical Journal* 297: 1379–1381.

Nicolini U, Rodeck CH, Kochenour NK et al (1988b) In-utero platelet transfusion for alloimmune thrombocytopenia. *Lancet* ii: 506.

Nicolini U, Kochenour NK, Greco P, Letsky E & Rodeck CH (1989) When to perform the next intra-uterine transfusion in patients with Rh allo-immunization: combined intravascular and intraperitoneal transfusion allows longer intervals. *Fetal Therapy* 4: 14–20.

Nicolini U, Tannirandorn Y, Gonzalez P et al (1990) Continuing controversy in alloimmune thrombocytopenia: fetal hyperimmunoglobulinemia fails to prevent thrombocytopenia. *American Journal of Obstetrics and Gynecology* 163: 1144–1146.

Owen RD (1945) Immunogenetic consequences of vascular anastomoses between bovine twins. *Science* 102: 400–401.

Pielet BW, Socol ML, MacGregor SN, Ney JA & Dooley SL (1988) Cordocentesis: an appraisal of risks. *American Journal of Obstetrics and Gynecology* 159: 1497–1500.

Poissonnier M-H, Brossard Y, Demedeiros N et al (1989) Two hundred intrauterine exchange transfusions in severe blood incompatibilities. *American Journal of Obstetrics and Gynecology* 161: 709–713.

Pollack MS, Kirkpatrick D, Kapoor N, Dupont B & O'Reilly RJ (1982) Identification by HLA typing of intrauterine-derived maternal T cells in four patients with severe combined immunodeficiency. *New England Journal of Medicine* 307: 662–666.

Queenan JT (1982) Current management of the Rh-sensitized patient. *Clinical Obstetrics and Gynecology* 25: 293–301.

Reece EA, Copel JA, Scioscia AL et al (1988) Diagnostic fetal umbilical blood sampling in the management of isoimmunization. *American Journal of Obstetrics and Gynecology* 159: 1057–1062.

Rightmire DA, Nicolaides KH, Rodeck CH & Campbell S (1986) Fetal blood velocities in Rh isoimmunization: relationship to gestational age and to fetal hematocrit. *Obstetrics and Gynecology* 68: 233–236.

Rodeck CH, Holman CA, Karnicki J et al (1981) Direct intravascular fetal blood transfusion by fetoscopy in severe rhesus isoimmunization. *Lancet* i: 625–627.

Rote NS (1982) Pathophysiology of Rh isoimmunization. *Clinical Obstetrics and Gynecology* 25: 243–253.

Scott JR (1990) Immunologic disorders in pregnancy. In Scott JR, DiSia PJ, Hammond CB & Spellacy WN (eds) *Danforth's Obstetrics and Gynecology*, 6th edn, pp 461–493. Philadelphia: J.B. Lippincott Company.

Scott JR, Kochenour NK, Larkin RL & Scott MJ (1984) Changes in the management of severely Rh-immunized patients. *American Journal of Obstetrics and Gynecology* 149: 336–340.

Shulman NR & Jordan Jr JV (1987) Platelet immunology. In Colman RW, Hirsh J, Marder VJ & Salzman EW (eds) *Hemostasis and Thrombosis*, 2nd edn, pp 452–529. Philadelphia: J.B. Lippincott Company.

Sitarz AL, Driscoll Jr JM & Wolff JA (1976) Management of isoimmune neonatal thrombocytopenia. *American Journal of Obstetrics and Gynecology* **124:** 39–42.

Spinnato JA, Ralston KK, Greenwell ER et al (1991) Amniotic fluid bilirubin and fetal hemolytic disease. *American Journal of Obstetrics and Gynecology* **165:** 1030–1035.

Turner JH, Wald N & Wuinlivan WLG (1966) Cytogenetic evidence concerning possible transplacental transfer of leukocytes in pregnant women. *American Journal of Obstetrics and Gynecology* **95:** 831–833.

Watts DH, Luthy DA, Benedetti TJ et al (1988) Intraperitoneal fetal transfusion under direct ultrasound guidance. *Obstetrics and Gynecology* **71:** 84–88.

Weiner C, Grant S, Hudson J et al (1989) Effect of diagnostic and therapeutic cordocentesis on maternal serum α-fetoprotein concentration. *American Journal of Obstetrics and Gynaecology* **161:** 706–708.

Weiner CP, Williamson RA, Wenstrom KD et al (1991) Management of fetal hemolytic disease by cordocentesis. II. Outcome of treatment. *American Journal of Obstetrics and Gynecology* **165:** 1302–1307.

Weinstein L (1982) Irregular antibodies causing hemolytic disease of the newborn: a continuing problem. *Clinical Obstetrics and Gynecology* **25:** 321–332.

Wilkins I, Mezrow G, Lynch L et al (1989) Amnionitis and life-threatening respiratory distress after percutaneous umbilical blood sampling. *American Journal of Obstetrics and Gynecology* **160:** 427–428.

9

Autoimmune disease in pregnancy

ROBERT M. SILVER
D. WARE BRANCH

Autoimmune diseases encompass a variety of disorders characterized by humoral or cellular immune damage to various tissues. This represents a failure of self-tolerance and can lead to severe and debilitating illness. The pathophysiology of most autoimmune diseases is unknown, although genetic, immunological, infectious, environmental, and hormonal factors have been implicated. These disorders occur primarily in women of reproductive age, and simultaneous pregnancies are common; this is particularly true for MHC class II associated diseases (Talal, 1989).

Sex hormones have been proposed as a reason for the preponderance of females affected by autoimmune disorders. In the B/W mouse model of systemic lupus erythematosus (SLE) (Talal, 1989) females develop auto-antibodies, clinical disease, and eventual death more rapidly than males (Steinberg et al, 1979), the onset of SLE is accelerated by oestrogen (Metz et al, 1980), and both the onset and course of disease are retarded by testosterone (Roubinian et al, 1978; Metz et al, 1980). Androgens also reduce lacrimal and submandibular inflammation in the Sjögren's syndrome mouse model (Ariga et al, 1989). SLE exacerbations in women taking oestrogens (Jungers et al, 1982a), decreased testosterone levels in males with SLE (Mackworth-Young et al, 1983), and the occurrence of SLE in males with Klinefelter's syndrome (Stern et al, 1977) all implicate increased oestrogen:testosterone ratios as a risk factor. Oestradiol metabolism in both males and females with SLE is abnormal, with increased oestrogen activity (Lahita et al, 1979, 1982).

Because of markedly increased oestrogen production in pregnancy, there is logical concern over its potential to exacerbate or accelerate auto-immunity. This concern is amplified by evidence that immune function as measured by several parameters is increased in women compared with men (Purtilo and Sullivan, 1979). Conversely, there is evidence that oestrogen depresses cell-mediated immunity (Luster et al, 1984) and pregnancy has long been considered a state of relative immunosuppression (Billingham and Beer, 1984). These latter observations suggest that autoimmune diseases may actually improve during pregnancy. In light of these conflicting theoretical influences of pregnancy on the course of autoimmune disease, it is not surprising that there are divergent clinical data on the impact that SLE has on pregnancy. Other autoimmune diseases are consistently improved (rheumatoid arthritis) or worsened (polyarteritis nodosa) by pregnancy.

There are other challenges to the physician caring for pregnant women with autoimmune disorders. Since these diseases may influence the course of pregnancy, consideration of both the mother and fetus is necessary with all therapeutic and medical intervention. Finally, there are special circumstances in which the fetus can be directly affected by maternal autoimmunity. Though rare, these conditions may provide insight into the overall pathogenesis of autoimmunity.

This chapter will focus primarily on SLE, considered to be the prototypical autoimmune disease. Other topics to be covered include autoimmune thrombocytopenic purpura (ATP), myasthenia gravis (MG), autoimmune thyroid disorders, and rheumatoid arthritis (RA).

SYSTEMIC LUPUS ERYTHEMATOSUS

Systemic lupus erythematosus (SLE) is a complex, systemic, and chronic inflammatory disease. It can affect any organ, but most commonly involves the musculoskeletal, cutaneous, renal, central nervous, cardiac, and pulmonary systems. Specific clinical and serological criteria for the diagnosis of SLE have been published by the American Rheumatic Association (Tan et al, 1982) (Table 1). Additionally, many patients have several features of a lupus-like illness without fulfilling criteria for the diagnosis. These patients, while not having SLE by accepted criteria, require special care during pregnancy.

Table 1. 1982 Revised criteria for the classification of SLE.*

Molar rash
Discoid rash
Photosensitivity
Oral ulcers
Arthritis
Serositis (pleuritis and/or pericarditis)
Renal disorder (proteinuria > 0.5 g/day or cellular casts)
Neurological disorder (psychosis and/or seizures)
Haematological disorder (haemolytic anaemia or
    thrombocytopenia or leukopenia or lymphopenia)
Immunological disorder (anti-DNA or anti-Sm or LE cell
    or false-positive STS)
Antinuclear antibody

* American Rheumatic Association (Tan et al, 1982). Four or more of the 11 criteria must be present serially or simultaneously, for a patient to be considered to have SLE.

The intensity of the disease fluctuates over time. Periods of active disease are often termed flares, while symptom-free intervals are termed remissions. Flares are often difficult to define, especially during pregnancy. Common symptoms include rash, joint pain, alopecia, fatigue, fever, anorexia, malaise, and lymphadenopathy, but many of these symptoms can also be seen in normal pregnant women.

SLE, like many autoimmune diseases, is characterized by autoantibody production. Antinuclear antibodies (ANA) are the most common. Of these, antibodies to double-stranded DNA are the most specific for SLE. A variety of other autoantibodies may be found, including antibodies against nucleic acids, nucleoproteins, and phospholipids (Hardin, 1986). These antibodies may play a role in the pathogenesis of SLE, perhaps via deposition of immune complexes in the basement membranes of systemic organs and tissues. Other laboratory abnormalities include thrombocytopenia, leukopenia, and hypocomplementaemia. Several relatively common problems that require special consideration in pregnancy include renal disease, anti-Ro (SSA) antibodies, and antiphospholipid antibodies (APA).

The influence of pregnancy on SLE

Most older reports suggest that pregnancy exacerbates SLE, with the incidence of flares ranging from 6 to 55% (Garenstein et al, 1962; Mund et al, 1963; Devoe and Taylor, 1979; Zulman et al, 1979; Gimovsky et al, 1984) while several recent studies have shown no increase in exacerbations in pregnant patients compared with non-pregnant controls (Lockshin et al, 1984; Mintz et al, 1986; Meehan and Dorsey, 1987; Lockshin, 1989). This disparity may reflect improved care for these patients as well as the discontinuance of an earlier practice of withholding medications from pregnant patients for fear of untoward fetal effects. Moreover, older studies were hampered by a lack of appropriate control groups, poorly defined definitions of lupus flares, and a lack of differentiation between pregnancy complications and true lupus flares (Lockshin, 1989). In a well controlled prospective study of 80 women with SLE during pregnancy, fewer than 25% had exacerbations. If pregnancy abnormalities were excluded, less than 13% had demonstrably worse SLE during pregnancy (Lockshin, 1989). However, three very recent studies revealed exacerbation rates of 58% (Wong et al, 1991), 74% (Nossent and Swaak, 1990), and 60% (Petri et al, 1991) during pregnancy; these series had much less stringent criteria for defining flares and most cases were mild-to-moderate. Table 2 summarizes the results of several controlled trials which examined the influence of pregnancy on SLE. Older publications also suggested that SLE worsened in the postpartum period (Garenstein et al, 1962; Mund et al, 1963; Devoe and Taylor, 1979; Zulman et al, 1979); the occurrence of several maternal deaths labelled the postpartum period as a time of extreme risk (Zulman et al, 1979; Imbasciati et al, 1984). Again, most recent studies have shown a low risk of flare in the postpartum period (Gimovsky et al, 1984; Lockshin et al, 1984; Meehan and Dorsey, 1987) including a study by Petri et al in which an increased rate of antepartum flares was found (Petri et al, 1991). There is no evidence that termination of pregnancy improves maternal outcome or alters the risk of exacerbation. Therefore, termination should not be performed with the expectation of improving the symptoms of SLE.

Some authors believe that this decrease in postpartum exacerbations is

Table 2. Frequency of lupus flares: controlled studies during pregnancy.

Authors	Study group			Control group		
	Patients	Pregnancies	Flares	Patient type	Patients	Flares
Zulman et al, 1979	23	24	13 (55%)	Same patients in 6 months prior to pregnancy	23	1 (4%)
Lockshin et al, 1984[a]	28	33	7 (21%)	Matched non-pregnant	33	6 (18%)
Meehan & Dorsey, 1987	18	22	10 (45%)	Matched non-pregnant	22	12 (54%)
Petri et al, 1991[c]	36	39	23 (59%) 1.6337 ± 0.3008[b]	Matched non-pregnant	185	N/A 0.6518 ± 0.0539[b]
				Same patients after delivery	29	N/A 0.6392 ± 0.1507[b]

[a] Flares defined as a requirement for increased medical therapy. There was also no difference in flares defined by a flare scoring system.
[b] Mean $\pm$ SEM—flare rates per person-years.
[c] Two control groups used.

due to the use of steroids (McGee and Makowski, 1970; Bobrie et al, 1987). In fact, many advocate their use prophylactically in the postpartum period (Mund et al, 1963; McGee and Makowski, 1970), and throughout gestation as well (Mintz et al, 1986; Wong et al, 1991). Others do not (Lockshin, 1989) and there are no well designed prospective studies that can yield definitive conclusions. There is general agreement, however, that steroid use should not be modified in pregnancy (Fine et al, 1981; Varner et al, 1983). In the study by Varner et al, 7/10 (70%) patients who had their prednisone dosages decreased during pregnancy experienced flares, and this has been demonstrated by others as well (Zurier et al, 1978; Fine et al, 1981).

Active disease at the time of conception may also increase the risk of exacerbation during pregnancy in patients with SLE (Devoe and Taylor, 1979; Varner et al, 1983; Ramsey-Goldman, 1988). In addition, the rate of exacerbation may be even greater in patients with active renal disease at conception, with some studies suggesting flares in 50% or more (Hayslett and Lynn, 1980; Houser et al, 1980; Jungers et al, 1982b; Bobrie et al, 1987). Not all studies, however, have found that active SLE at the time of conception bodes a particularly ominous course in gestation (Nossent and Swaak, 1990; Wong et al, 1991). A separate, important question is whether underlying lupus nephropathy worsens in pregnancy. In an excellent summary of lupus nephritis cases reported prior to 1980, Burkett noted a high rate of progression of renal disease in pregnancy with frequent maternal deaths (Burkett, 1985). The same author (Burkett, 1985) summarized the pregnancy experience in several large recent series (Hayslett and Lynn, 1980; Houser et al, 1980; Fine et al, 1981; Jungers et al, 1982b; Gimovsky et al, 1984; Imbasciati et al, 1984). In 242 pregnancies in 156 women with lupus nephritis, there was no change in 142 women (59%), a transient renal impairment occurred in 73 (30.2%), and 17 (7.1%) developed permanent renal insufficiency. A recent large series had similar findings: a 34% exacerbation rate (18/53) with 7.5% (4/53) of patients progressing to end stage renal failure (Bobrie et al, 1987). Serum creatinine levels greater than 1.5 mg/dl have been associated with an increased risk of deterioration during pregnancy (Bear, 1976; Jungers et al, 1982b; Burkett, 1985; Katz and Lindheimer, 1985). Despite these trends however, several patients with serum creatinine levels greater than 2.0 mg/dl have had uncomplicated pregnancies (Hayslett and Lynn, 1980; Katz and Lindheimer, 1985). Renal histology also has not been a consistent predictor of pregnancy outcome (Fine et al, 1981; Imbasciati et al, 1984).

The initial presentation of SLE during pregnancy or the postpartum state often heralds a particularly severe course (Friedman and Rutherford, 1956; Zurier et al, 1978; Jungers et al, 1982b; Varner et al, 1983; Imbasciati et al, 1984). The reasons for this are unknown, but may be due to delay in diagnosis and treatment. Furthermore, the initial presentation of SLE is often one of the most severe, especially in patients with renal disease (Fries and Holman, 1975).

Influence of SLE on pregnancy

Pregnancy loss

Fetal outcome is probably adversely affected by SLE. Most authors have reported an increased risk of spontaneous abortions, fetal deaths, pre-term deliveries, and small-for-gestation fetuses in infants born to mothers with lupus (Garenstein et al, 1962; McGee and Makowski, 1970; Fraga et al, 1974; Zurier et al, 1978; Zulman et al, 1979; Hayslett and Lynn, 1980; Jungers et al, 1982b; Imbasciati et al, 1984; Mintz et al, 1986). Table 3 lists fetal outcome in several large recent series. Overall, fetal loss rates range from 10 to 46%. The same risk factors that appear to increase the chance of SLE flare also appear to worsen the prognosis for the fetus. These include renal disease (Hayslett and Lynn, 1980; Fine et al, 1981; Gimovsky et al, 1984; Imbasciati et al, 1984), active disease at conception (Hayslett and Lynn, 1980), and first presentation during pregnancy or the postpartum period (Varner et al, 1983). Many studies need to be interpreted cautiously when evaluating fetal loss. Often, basic information regarding prior obstetric history and evaluation for non-lupus causes of pregnancy loss is unavailable. Overall, in patients in remission and without other risk factors (renal disease, hypertension, antiphospholipid syndrome), fetal mortality is probably no higher, or only marginally higher than in the general population.

Table 3. Pregnancy loss in patients with SLE.[a]

Authors	Number of patients	Number of pregnancies	Spontaneous abortions[b]	Fetal death[c]	Total losses
Fraga et al, 1974	20	42	N/A	N/A	17 (40%)
Zurier et al, 1978	13	25	7 (28%)	2 (8%)	9 (36%)
Zulman et al, 1979	23	24	0	3 (12%)	3 (12%)
Hayslett and Lynn, 1980	N/A	46	6 (13%)	4 (9%)	10 (22%)
Fine et al, 1981	44	45	3 (7%)	10 (22%)	13 (29%)
Jungers et al, 1982a	N/A	23	3 (13%)	0	3 (13%)
Varner et al, 1983	31	34	3 (9%)	2 (6%)	5 (15%)
Gimovsky et al, 1984	39	65	23 (35%)	7 (11%)	30 (46%)
Imbasciati et al, 1984	19	24	1 (4%)	7 (29%)	8 (33%)
Lockshin et al, 1984	28	32	3 (9%)	7 (22%)	10 (31%)
Nossent and Swaak, 1990	18	24	3 (13%)[d]	2 (8%)[d]	5 (21%)
Mintz et al, 1986	75	92	16 (17%)[d]	4 (4%)[d]	20 (22%)
Wong et al, 1991	17	19	2 (10%)	0	2 (10%)
Petri et al, 1991	37	40	5 (13%)	1 (3%)[e]	6 (15%)
Medians			13%	8%	22%

[a] Includes only those pregnancies in patients with an antenatal diagnosis of SLE. Elective terminations are not included. Distinctions are not made (or unavailable) in patients with renal disease, antiphospholipid antibodies, or in remission at the time of conception.
[b] Losses prior to 13 weeks' gestation.
[c] Losses after 13 weeks' gestation.
[d] In these studies, spontaneous abortions included all losses < 21 weeks' gestation. Fetal deaths included those after 21 weeks.
[e] Neonatal death after pre-term birth due to lupus flare.

The 10–30% of SLE patients with antiphospholipid antibodies (APA) are at increased risk for fetal loss, especially second- and third-trimester fetal death (Branch et al, 1985; Lockshin et al, 1987b; Derue et al, 1985). It appears that APAs are the most predictive risk factor for fetal death in lupus pregnancy. In one series, 10 of 11 fetal deaths in 42 lupus pregnancies were predicted by the presence of anticardiolipin (ACA), lupus anticoagulant (LA), or both (Lockshin et al, 1987b). Moreover, among patients with APA, pregnancies proceeding to livebirth are often complicated by pre-eclampsia and small-for-gestation fetuses (Branch and Scott, 1991). The APAs that have most consistently been associated with fetal loss are the LA and IgG ACA. The lupus anticoagulant interferes with phospholipid-dependent coagulation, thus prolonging the activated partial thromboplastin time, or other phospholipid-dependent coagulation assays. The prolongation of clotting is not corrected by the addition of normal plasma. The detection of ACA is done by immunoassay, usually an ELISA, using standard sera available from the Antiphospholipid Standardization Laboratory in Louisville, Kentucky (Harris et al, 1992) and the Department of Immunology, Royal Hallamshire Hospital, Sheffield (Standard 90/656). Although patients with these antibodies *and* a well documented history of recurrent pregnancy loss or fetal death have a marked risk of fetal wastage (Derksen et al, 1986), the presence of these antibodies in asymptomatic patients may not be associated with pregnancy loss (Harris and Spinnato, 1991; Infante-Rivard et al, 1991). Several studies have reported improved fetal outcome after treatment with low dose aspirin (LDA) and prednisone (Lubbe et al, 1983; Reece et al, 1984; Branch et al, 1985) or LDA and heparin (Rosove et al, 1990; Cowchock et al, 1992). Others have not found prednisone to be helpful (Lockshin et al, 1989). In one small randomized trial, treatment with heparin and LDA was found to be as efficacious as treatment with prednisone and LDA (Cowchock et al, 1992). In addition to fetal losses, symptomatic patients with these antibodies may have thrombocytopenia, haemolytic anaemia, and both arterial and venous thromboses. This has been termed the antiphospholipid syndrome (Harris, 1990).

The cause of fetal loss in patients with SLE and/or APA is unclear. Proposed aetiologies have been decidual vasculopathy (Abramowsky et al, 1980), immune complex deposition in the placenta (Grennan et al, 1978; Guzman et al, 1987), and lymphocytotoxic antibodies against trophoblast (Bresnihan et al, 1977; Lom-Orta et al, 1979). Findings of decreased placental weight, placental infarcts, and intraplacental haematoma all point to abnormal placentation as a cause of fetal loss (Branch et al, 1985; Hanly et al, 1988). Conversely, fetal outcome has not consistently correlated with either serological abnormalities or placental changes (Hanly et al, 1988). Other factors may be involved such as hypertension (Tervila et al, 1973) and renal disease (Hou, 1985) which have been associated with increased fetal loss.

Pregnancy-induced hypertension (pre-eclampsia)

Overall, 20–30% of SLE pregnancies are complicated by pre-eclampsia (Lockshin et al, 1987a). The influence of underlying renal disease is unmistakable. In one series, pre-eclampsia occurred in 8 of 11 (72%) pregnancies in women with SLE and nephropathy, but in only 12 of 53 (22%) pregnant women with SLE alone (Lockshin et al, 1987a). The reason for the relatively high rate of pre-eclampsia among women with SLE is unknown, but probably is due to underlying renal disease, which may occur in many patients with SLE (Schur, 1989).

Distinguishing an exacerbation of SLE involving active nephritis from pre-eclampsia presents a clinical dilemma. Symptoms and signs are similar, including proteinuria, hypertension, and multiorgan dysfunction. The distinction may be useful in deciding the timing of delivery. Some investigators have advocated using complement levels or activation products (Buyon et al, 1986), antithrombin III levels (Weiner et al, 1985), cellular fibrinectin (Ballegeer et al, 1989; Lockwood and Peters, 1990), or hypocalciuria (Taufield et al, 1987) to distinguish pre-eclampsia from other conditions. With the possible exception of renal biopsy proving lupus nephritis, no single test is likely unequivocally to distinguish SLE flare from pre-eclampsia and sound clinical judgement is always required. Table 4 lists some parameters which may be helpful in making this distinction.

Table 4. Laboratory parameters that may be useful in distinguishing SLE from pre-eclampsia.

Test	Pre-eclampsia	SLE
Serological		
Decreased complement	±	+++
Antithrombin III deficiency	++	±
Elevated ANA (most specifically anti-DNA)	±	+++
Haematological		
Thrombocytopenia	++	++
Leukopenia	−	++
Coombs' positive haemolytic anaemia	−	++
Microangiopathic haemolytic anaemia	++	−
Liver		
Serum transaminases	++	±
Renal		
Haematuria	+	+++
Cellular casts	−	+++
Elevated serum creatinine	±	++
Elevated ratio of serum blood urea nitrogen/creatinine	++	±

Pre-term delivery

Pre-term delivery is fairly common among women with SLE, occurring in about 30% of cases (Varner et al, 1983; Lockshin et al, 1985; Mintz et al, 1986; Wong et al, 1991). Pre-term delivery is most often iatrogenic due to pre-eclampsia (Varner et al, 1983; Gimovsky et al, 1984), abnormal fetal surveillance (Druzin et al, 1987), or lupus flare (Mintz et al, 1986). Pre-term labour is probably not more common among women with SLE (Lockshin et al, 1987a).

Small-for-gestational-age (SGA) infants

SGA infants are probably more prevalent among women with SLE than among normal patients; however, supporting data are sparse. In one large prospective series, 23% of infants were SGA (Mintz et al, 1986). Other smaller series also suggest a high rate of SGA infants (Fine et al, 1981; Varner et al, 1983; Nossent and Swaak, 1990; Wong et al, 1991). One important risk factor for SGA infants may be APA (Branch and Scott, 1991).

Neonatal lupus (NLE)

NLE is an uncommon syndrome of the fetus/neonate characterized by dermatological, cardiac, or haematological abnormalities. Typical skin lesions are similar to those of adult subacute cutaneous lupus and usually appear after birth (Watson et al, 1984). The hallmark cardiac lesion is congenital complete heart block (CHB), but widespread endomyocardial involvement may also occur. Haematological lesions include haemolytic anaemia and thrombocytopenia (Watson et al, 1984; Olson and Lindsley, 1987).

NLE is attributed to immune damage mediated by maternal autoantibodies which cross the placenta. The most strongly associated is antibody to SSA (Ro), a cytoplasmic ribonucleoprotein (Hardin, 1986). Anti-SSA (Ro) has been found in 83 (JS Scott et al, 1983) to 100% (Watson et al, 1984) of mothers of affected infants and in the serum of most infants with NLE (JS Scott et al, 1983; Watson et al, 1984). Fifty to 70% of these mothers also have anti-SSB (La) (Watson et al, 1984). In some cases, anti-SSB (La) alone is present (Buyon et al, 1987) and rarely, an antibody to ribonucleoprotein is the only autoantibody found in the serum of these patients (Provost et al, 1987).

The cutaneous and haematological symptoms, as well as these antibodies, disappear after 6 months, suggesting that the disease is antibody mediated (Watson et al, 1984). Other evidence for this includes the demonstration of antibodies against myocardial tissue in the sera of affected fetuses and their mothers (Taylor et al, 1986) as well as the demonstration of Ro antigen (Deng et al, 1987) and IgG deposition in affected fetal hearts (Lee et al, 1987). CHB is thought to be mediated by inflammation and fibrosis of the conduction system (Chameides et al, 1977) (Figure 1), although this process occurs throughout the myocardium (Chameides et al, 1977).

The risk to a patient with SLE for delivering an infant with NLE is unknown but can be estimated. In women with SLE and anti-SSA, the risk of NLE is reported to range from 5 to 10% (Ramsey-Goldman et al, 1986; Lockshin et al, 1988). As anti-SSA occurs in approximately 30% of patients with SLE (Scopelitis et al, 1980), the risk in all SLE patients can be estimated at 1–2% (Ramsey-Goldman, 1988). It is clear that factors other than the presence of antibody are required for disease to occur. The risk of recurrence of NLE in infants born to mothers with previous affected infants was 25% (3/12) in one series (McCune et al, 1987). Twins are frequently discordant for the development of NLE (Lockshin et al, 1988) and HLA

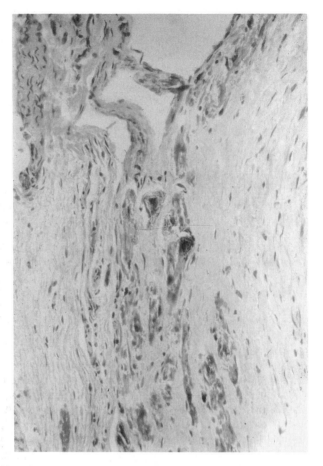

Figure 1. Photomicrograph of a histological section of heart in an infant affected by congenital heart block and neonatal lupus erythematosus. The conduction system is interrupted by calcifications and inflammation.

type may be important (Lee et al, 1983; Watson et al, 1984; Buyon et al, 1987). A large proportion of affected infants will be born to asymptomatic mothers (McCune et al, 1987; Lockshin et al, 1988), although in one series a majority of these women (8/11) subsequently developed connective tissue disease (McCune et al, 1987).

Cutaneous and haematological manifestations do not pose long-term risks to the infant. These signs usually appear soon after birth and resolve by 6 months without treatment (Lockshin, 1990). Conversely, CHB can appear in utero and can be fatal (Watson et al, 1984; Buyon et al, 1987) (Figure 2). There is no proven therapy for in utero treatment although steroids and plasmapheresis have been used (Buyon et al, 1987; Bierman et al, 1988; Richards et al, 1990). Most infants who survive the neonatal period do well,

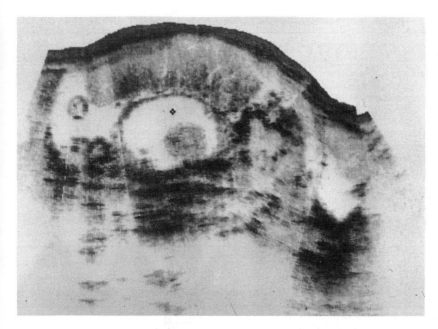

Figure 2. Ultrasound of a hydropic fetus in utero with congenital heart block due to neonatal lupus erythematosus. The cursor is on ascitic fluid.

although many require permanent pacemakers (McCune et al, 1987). Long-term follow-up is unavailable on most infants with NLE, but a handful have developed connective tissue disease early in life (Jackson and Gulliver, 1979; Lanham et al, 1983).

Management of SLE pregnancy

Ideally, care of the pregnant patient with SLE should be provided by a team of obstetricians and rheumatologists (Varner et al, 1983; Mintz et al, 1986). Recommended care beyond the usual obstetric evaluation is summarized in Table 5. This includes an initial evaluation of renal function and platelets as well as screening for APA and anti-Ro/La. Although findings in asymptomatic patients may not change their management in all cases, these tests are of useful prognostic value. Some investigators have advocated serial testing for serum ANA titres (Mintz et al, 1986) and complement levels (Devoe and Taylor, 1979; Devoe and Loy, 1984). This has not been found to be useful in more recent investigations (Varner et al, 1983; Wong et al, 1991). Increased maternal surveillance for the development of flares and pre-eclampsia as well as fetal surveillance for growth and well-being are also recommended. Druzin and Lockshin have noted spontaneous decelerations in the second trimester in several fetuses who subsequently died in utero (Druzin et al, 1987). The authors have also noted a significant rate of abnormal fetal heart rate tracings and impaired fetal growth in patients with SLE and APA;

Table 5. Care of the pregnant patient with SLE.[a]

	Initial visit	Second trimester	Third trimester
Laboratory evaluation			
Complete blood count and platelets	×	×	×
Activated partial thromboplastin time[b]	×		
Anticardiolipin antibodies	×		
Anti-Ro and anti-La antibodies	×		
Microscopic urinalysis	×		
Creatinine clearance and total protein (24-hour urine collection)	×	×	×
Clinical evaluation			
Office visits[c]	Biweekly	Biweekly	Weekly
Obstetrical ultrasound	×	Monthly/ bimonthly	Monthly
Non-stress testing			Weekly
Other fetal surveillance[d]		×	×

[a] Guidelines for care. Each case should be individualized.
[b] Any sensitive test for the 'lupus anticoagulant' may be used.
[c] Visits should be tailored to individual patients; and may need to be more frequent.
[d] Other adjunctive forms of fetal surveillance may be helpful. These include doppler velocimetry, biophysical profiles, and amniotic fluid volume assessment. Their efficacy in these patients is unproven.

intervention with preterm delivery may improve fetal outcome in severe cases (Druzin et al, 1987; Branch and Scott, 1991). Caesarean section should only be performed for the usual obstetric indications. As stated earlier, the use of prednisone in pregnant patients with SLE should be similar to that in non-pregnant patients. Prednisone or hydrocortisone are preferred corticosteroids because the placenta oxidizes these steroids to a relatively inactive 11-keto form (Blanford and Murphy, 1977). Two large summaries of corticosteroid use in pregnancy found no evidence of increased malformations or untoward effects on the fetus (Burkett, 1985; Crowley et al, 1990). It is important to screen for glucose intolerance and hypertension as these patients are at increased risk. It is crucial to use stress doses of steroids at the time of delivery in patients on chronically administered steroids as Addisonian crisis and death have been reported (Devoe and Taylor, 1979). Steroids should be continued in the postpartum period but their initiation prophylactically is controversial.

There is less information available about other drugs commonly used to treat SLE. Antimalarials have been reported to cause loss of vision and ototoxicity (Hart and Naughton, 1964; Carr et al, 1968) and are avoided by most authors (Lockshin, 1990) although some feel that the benefits outweigh the risks (Parke, 1988). Cyclophosphamide and chlorambucil are contraindicated in the first trimester (Lockshin, 1985) and should be used only in extreme circumstances thereafter. Azathioprine has been associated with SGA infants (Scott, 1977) and neonatal immune suppression (Cote et al, 1974) and should be used when the potential benefits clearly outweigh these risks. Non-steroidal anti-inflammatory drugs (NSAIDs) are best avoided due to concerns about premature closure of the ductus (Moise et al, 1988b; Besinger et al, 1991) and fetal renal effects (Vanhaesebrouck et al, 1988). Aspirin in full dosage taken late in pregnancy may prolong labour and cause neonatal bleeding (Stuart et al, 1982).

Several well designed studies indicate that prophylactically administered low dose aspirin (LDA) prevents or ameliorates pre-eclampsia in patients at risk for this disease (Imperiale, 1991). In addition, LDA is thought to be safe in pregnancy (Imperiale and Petrulis, 1991). Since patients with SLE are at substantial risk for pre-eclampsia, LDA should be considered, especially in patients with underlying renal disease.

The management of patients at risk of delivering an infant with NLE is controversial. CHB is the only life-threatening manifestation. The prospective risk of CHB in patients with SLE or SLE with anti-SSA is so low that prophylactic measures are not warranted (Lockshin et al, 1988). Some authors have suggested prophylactic treatment of mothers who have previously delivered infants with CHB using glucocorticoids and/or plasmapheresis (Buyon et al, 1987), but the efficacy of this approach is unproven. In mothers with a history of affected infants, more frequent assessment of the fetal heart rate and serial ultrasounds for development of fetal hydrops are reasonable precautions. In newly discovered cases of CHB in utero, evaluation should include sonographic evaluation of the fetal heart and determination of maternal anti-SSA and anti-SSB status.

AUTOIMMUNE THROMBOCYTOPENIA

Autoimmune thrombocytopenic purpura (ATP) is a syndrome of immunologically mediated thrombocytopenia in which autoantibodies to platelets lead to increased platelet destruction by the reticuloendothelial system (Karpatkin, 1980; McMillan, 1981). In adults, ATP is usually chronic and has a female to male prevalence of $3:1$.

ATP is a diagnosis of exclusion. Evaluation of thrombocytopenic patients should include an evaluation for concurrent disease (especially SLE, antiphospholipid syndrome, bone marrow suppression, infection, and pre-eclampsia), drug exposure, or chemical exposure. Bone marrow aspiration may be required to clarify the diagnosis. Symptoms of ATP include minor bleeding and easy bruising when the platelet count is less than $70\,000/mm^3$ and can include life-threatening spontaneous bleeding when platelets are less than $20\,000/m^3$.

Pregnancy and ATP

Maternal considerations

The incidence of true ATP in pregnancy is uncertain since most studies consist of numerator data from tertiary care centres. Moreover, the criteria used to establish the diagnosis of ATP vary from study to study, with few studies using the presence of a normal or megakaryocytic bone marrow as diagnostic criteria in all patients. The recently introduced concept of essential thrombocytopenia of pregnancy further compounds the problem of diagnosis. It is possible, and probably likely, that many patients considered to have ATP in past studies actually had essential thrombocytopenia of pregnancy. Burrows and Kelton recently reported thrombocytopenia (platelet count less than 150 000/mm³) in 513 of 6715 consecutive deliveries; (7.6%) (Burrows and Kelton, 1990b). Of these, over three quarters had essential thrombocytopenia.

Beyond delivery issues, care for these patients should include periodic determination of the maternal platelet count. In non-pregnant patients, the treatment of thrombocytopenia is usually reserved for patients with bleeding or an extremely low platelet count (i.e. < 20 000/mm³). Bleeding is also an indication for treatment in the pregnant patient. However, it is controversial as to whether a certain platelet count (e.g. < 50 000/mm³ or < 30 000/mm³) is sufficient indication for prophylactic therapy in the pregnant patient. The first line of treatment is prednisone, usually started in doses of 60–80 mg per day. After a response is noted, the dose is tapered to the lowest that will maintain the maternal platelet count in an acceptable range. Cases refractory to glucocorticoids are treated with splenectomy or intravenous γ-globulin. In acute situations, platelet transfusions may be used to temporize. Splenectomy during pregnancy should be reserved for extreme cases and the risks of surgery and fetal loss must be considered (Martin et al, 1984). Intravenous γ-globulin is efficacious but very expensive (Gounder et al, 1986), while platelet transfusions are a temporary measure best reserved for haemorrhage or surgery in the markedly thrombocytopenic patient (McMillan, 1981). Vinca alkaloids, colchicine, other immunosuppressive agents, and danazol are best avoided in pregnancy because of the potential for adverse fetal effects. Patients with ATP should be instructed to avoid NSAIDs and trauma, and special attention must be given to infections in splenectomized patients (McMillan, 1981). Although not always predictive of fetal platelet count, antiplatelet antibody determination may be helpful in distinguishing ATP from essential thrombocytopenia.

Fetal considerations

Antiplatelet IgG molecules can cross the placenta placing the fetus at risk for developing thrombocytopenia. This can lead to serious bleeding problems and is a crucial issue to the obstetric care of women with ATP. Most cases of intracranial haemorrhage (ICH) have been reported in infants born vaginally (Jones et al, 1977; Samuels et al, 1990), but it is not clear that vaginal delivery *per se* was a causative factor. Most cases of ICH have occurred in fetuses with platelet counts below 50 000/mm³ (Scott et al, 1980). Based on these inconclusive data, it has been recommended that caesarean section be performed in cases of fetal platelet count less than 50 000/mm³ (Scott et al, 1980).

Although potentially serious, the rate of fetal bleeding due to ATP is quite low. Table 6 lists the incidence of severe fetal thrombocytopenia and bleeding complications in a representative sample of recent series. The median

Table 6. Fetal platelet counts and bleeding complications in women with thrombocytopenia.

| Authors | Pregnancies | Fetal platelets <50 000/mm³ | Serious haemorrhage | |
			ICH[a]	Total
Cook et al, 1991	32	2 (6%)	0	1 (3%)
Kaplan et al, 1990[b]	33	4 (12%)	0	0
Moise et al, 1988[a]	22	1 (4.5%)	0	0
Burrows and Kelton, 1990[a]	61	3 (4.9%)	0	0
Scioscia et al, 1988	19	1 (5.2%)	0	0
Samuels et al, 1990[b]	88	18 (20%)	2[c] (2%)	5 (6%)
Jones et al, 1977	20	6 (30%)	1 (5%)	1 (5%)
Scott JR et al, 1983	25	5 (20%)	0	0

[a] Intracranial haemorrhage.
[b] In these studies, ATP was differentiated from essential thrombocytopenia. Only ATP cases are included.
[c] In one neonate ICH occurred with a neonatal platelet count of 78 000/mm³.

proportion of infants with platelet counts below 50 000/mm³ born to mothers with thrombocytopenia was 7.8%; but not all series strictly selected patients with ATP. In two large series, none of 334 (Burrows and Kelton, 1990a,b) and none of 74 (Samuels et al, 1990) infants born to mothers with asymptomatic thrombocytopenia had platelet counts below 50 000/mm³. ICH occurred in 0 (Burrows and Kelton, 1990b) and 5% (Samuels et al, 1990) of cases. One of the cases of ICH was diagnosed by screening sonography in an asymptomatic infant with a neonatal platelet count of 78 000/m³ (Samuels et al, 1990), suggesting that a 'cut-off' platelet count of 50 000/mm³ does not identify all cases at risk.

Current investigations have focused on a method for predicting infants who are at risk for ICH (i.e. platelet count less than 50 000/mm³). Ideally, this test would be non-invasive, reproducible, and sensitive in identifying patients at risk. Unfortunately, no such test is presently available. It appears that one of the best predictors of low fetal risk is the absence of maternal symptoms or history of ATP (Burrows and Kelton, 1990b; Samuels et al, 1990). Samuels and colleagues noted fetal thrombocytopenia in 18 of 88 (20%) mothers in whom a diagnosis of ATP antedated pregnancy compared with 0 of 74 mothers with asymptomatic thrombocytopenia diagnosed for the first time in pregnancy (Samuels et al, 1990). However, several cases of patients with no history of ATP who delivered thrombocytopenic infants have been reported (Rauch et al, 1990). Samuels et al also advocated the measurement of circulating antiplatelet antibodies (indirect test) to predict patients at risk (Samuels et al, 1990). Of his patients with clinical ATP, 18 of 70 (26%) women with circulating antiplatelet antibodies delivered thrombocytopenic infants (platelet count below 50 000/mm³) versus 0 of 18 women with negative circulating antiplatelet antibodies. Unfortunately the assay is considered difficult to perform and is not readily available in most centres. Moreover, exceptional cases have been reported (Rauch et al, 1990). Other initially promising signs and tests that have since been shown to correlate poorly with fetal platelets are a maternal history of splenectomy, low maternal platelet count, and detectable direct antiplatelet antibodies (JR Scott et al, 1983).

When formulating a strategy to avoid fetal thrombocytopenia and haemorrhage, three observations require consideration (McMillan, 1981); no test or clinical feature predicts the presence or absence of feto/neonatal risk in all cases (Burrows and Kelton, 1990a), caesarean section is not proven to prevent feto/neonatal haemorrhage in thrombocytopenic infants, and (Samuels et al, 1990) the apparent risk of serious feto/neonatal haemorrhage in ATP is quite low. Clinicians have developed three strategies for deciding the mode of delivery for patients with ATP. None is clearly superior and all have favourable and unfavourable aspects. First, several authors have advocated the use of fetal scalp sampling (FSS) in labour to determine fetal platelet count (Ayromlooi, 1978; Scott et al, 1980). If the platelet count is greater than $50\,000/mm^3$, vaginal delivery is attempted; if it is less than $50\,000/mm^3$, caesarean section is performed. This strategy has the advantage of being low risk to mother and fetus and uses an assay (platelet count) that is widely available and inexpensive. The major drawback is an incidence of falsely low platelet counts resulting in unnecessary caesarean birth (Christiaens and Helmerhorst, 1987). Also, the FSS cannot always be easily accomplished and there is a theoretical risk of ICH during the labour required to reach a cervical dilatation permissible for the procedure.

Secondly, some groups are performing cordocentesis prior to the onset of labour to determine the fetal platelet count (Moise et al, 1988a; Scioscia et al, 1988; Kaplan et al, 1990). The procedure is usually deferred until fetal maturity is secure (36–38 weeks' gestation). Management based on fetal platelet count is similar to that for FSS. If attempted vaginal delivery is deemed safe (i.e. fetal platelet count $>50\,000/mm^3$), induction is often initiated within an arbitrary time period. This method avoids some of the pitfalls of FSS. The fetal platelet count is accurate and falsely low determinations have not been reported. Also, the platelet count is known prior to labour. However, cordocentesis is not always easily accomplished (Moise et al, 1988a) and the skills required are more sophisticated than those needed for FSS.

The worst potential complication of cordocentesis is haemorrhage from the cord puncture site or cord spasm with fetal bradycardia. Overall mortality rates for cordocentesis are 1–2% in groups skilled at the procedure (Daffos et al, 1985), but the risk is probably lower in otherwise healthy term neonates. Procedure-related complications were seen in 3 of 105 (2.8%) ATP cases reported in three recent series of cordocentesis (Moise et al, 1988a; Scioscia et al, 1988; Kaplan et al, 1990). All of the complications occurred in one series (Moise et al, 1988a), and included haemorrhage at the cord puncture site in two cases. Two of the three patients required urgent delivery by caesarean section. *It is important to note that the risk of cordocentesis in fetuses proven to have thrombocytopenia is unknown.* In fact, only five cases of successful cordocenteses in fetuses with platelet counts below $50\,000/mm^3$ due to ATP have been reported in the English-language literature (Moise et al, 1988; Scioscia et al, 1988; Kaplan et al, 1990). There were no complications in these five cases, but there have been two cases of exsanguination associated with cordocentesis performed in infants with Glanzmann's thrombasthenia (Daffos et al, 1988). It is possible that the risks of serious haemorrhage due to cordocentesis in thrombocytopenic fetuses is greater than the risk of serious haemorrhage associated with vaginal delivery!

The third approach to delivery in cases of maternal ATP is that of expectant management, with caesarean section only for the usual obstetric reasons. This approach is based (McMillan, 1981) on the absence of the clear superiority of the above two approaches, and (Burrows and Kelton, 1990a) the apparently low risk of an adverse fetal outcome (Aster, 1990). This may be the best course of action in the absence of a history of ATP, although an unaffected infant is not guaranteed. Patients should be informed about all of these options with their attendant risks and benefits. Neonatologists should be alerted to a maternal history of ATP. Neonatal platelet counts may not reach a nadir for 2–4 days and these infants require surveillance and occasional treatment (Pearson and McIntosh, 1978).

Although advocated by some (Karpatkin et al, 1981), maternal treatment to increase fetal platelet count is not proven. Dexamethasone did not prevent neonatal thrombocytopenia in one case reported by Yin et al (Yin, 1985). Furthermore, Kaplan found no effect on fetal platelets from maternal administration of prednisone or intravenous γ-globulin in a small number of patients (Kaplan et al, 1990).

MYASTHENIA GRAVIS

Myasthenia gravis (MG) is an autoimmune disorder characterized by skeletal muscle weakness and excessive fatiguability. Common signs and symptoms include difficulty in speaking, swallowing, and clearing secretions, diplopia, and ptosis. The disease is classified based on clinical severity, ranging from ophthalmic symptoms alone to severe involvement of respiratory muscles. Thymus abnormalities including thymoma (10%) and hyperplasia are frequent (Grouse and Young, 1983). The elicitation of a characteristic decrease in muscle strength with repetitive use and the dramatic, transient restoration of strength with anticholinesterase drugs is the traditional approach to the diagnosis (Grouse and Young, 1983). More sophisticated tests are now available, including single fibre electromyography and repetitive nerve stimulation studies.

MG is thought to be mediated by autoantibodies against acetylcholine receptors (AChR), probably with complement-dependent destruction of the postsynaptic portion of the neuromuscular junction (Plauche, 1983). These antibodies have been detected in 80–90% of patients with MG (Lindstrom et al, 1976; Soliven et al, 1988), and can induce MG in experimental animal models (Engel et al, 1979). MG occurs in twice as many females as males with an estimated prevalence of 1 in 20000 (Chambers et al, 1967; Fenichel, 1978; Grouse and Young, 1983).

The influence of pregnancy on MG

The effect of pregnancy on the natural history of MG is uncertain, and there are no large series from which to draw conclusions. The best available data come from a summary of retrospectively collected cases and small series (Plauche, 1983). This review noted no change in the status of MG during pregnancy in 31.5% of cases, exacerbations in 41%, and remissions in 29%.

Several pregnancy-related factors may influence the management or expression of MG. Nausea, vomiting, altered gastrointestinal absorption, expanded plasma volume, and increased renal clearance may affect medications. Increased metabolic demand and exertion required by pregnancy (especially in labour) may worsen symptoms, requiring alterations in medication dosages.

The influence of MG on pregnancy

The available data suggest that MG may adversely affect pregnancy outcome. In a summary of cases and small series by Plauche, the incidence of pre-term delivery was 41% (Plauche, 1983). The reason for this apparently high rate of pre-term birth is unknown. Ten to 20% of infants born to women with MG developed neonatal myasthenia gravis (NMG), a transient condition due to the transplacental passage of anti-AChR antibodies (Morel et al, 1988; Tzartos et al, 1990). NMG is characterized by flat facies, difficulty in feeding and crying, and respiratory distress (Namba et al, 1970; Fenichel, 1978; Morel et al, 1988). Symptoms commonly begin 12–48 hours after birth, usually last 3 weeks (range 5–60 days), and respond well to anticholinesterase therapy (Fenichel, 1978). Rarely, the symptoms of MG appear in utero. These may include hydramnios, decreased movement, and contractures (Shepard, 1971; Holmes et al, 1980; Morel et al, 1988). The delayed onset of NMG and the rarity of in utero MG has been ascribed to the inhibitory effect of α-fetoprotein on the binding of AChR antibodies (Abramsky et al, 1979; Brenner et al, 1980) and differences between fetal and adult AChR (Mishina et al, 1986). Unfortunately, neither the clinical nor antibody status in the mother can predict the occurrence of NMG.

Since uterine smooth muscle contraction is not affected by MG, the course of the first stage of labour is normal. On the other hand, the voluntary muscles involved in expulsion may be weakened.

Management of MG in pregnancy

Anticholinesterase drugs, the mainstay of treatment for MG in non-pregnant patients, are also used in pregnancy (Fennel and Ringel, 1987). Most patients are treated with pyridostigmine (Mestinon), 240–1500 mg per day in divided doses given every 3–8 hours. If the patient requires more medication, as is often the case in advancing pregnancy, it is best to decrease the medication interval prior to increasing the dosage. The most common side-effects of the anticholinesterase drugs are nausea, vomiting, diarrhoea, and increased oral and bronchial secretions. Overdose can result in paradoxical weakness and respiratory failure (cholinergic crisis).

Corticosteroids are also beneficial to most patients with MG (Johns, 1987) and should be maintained in pregnancy if they are already being used. Thymectomy has also been used as a treatment for MG, and one centre reported fewer complications in pregnant women with MG who were thymectomized (Eden and Gall, 1983). However, the period from thymectomy to improvement is highly variable and the surgery is not without risk (Plauche, 1983). It is not recommended during pregnancy (Plauche, 1983). Plasmapheresis is effective in the acute management of life-threatening MG (Levine and Keesey, 1986) and may be used in pregnancy in such cases. The management of labour in patients with MG does not require significant modification. Undue stress and extreme exhaustion should be avoided. Outlet forceps may be useful in the second stage to limit the fatigue caused by expulsive efforts. Caesarean birth should be reserved for obstetric indications. During labour, anticholinesterase drugs should be administered by parenteral route to avoid erratic absorption. Regional anaesthesia is a safe option if preanaesthetic evaluation with an experienced anaesthesiologist is available (Rolbin et al, 1978).

Certain medications should be avoided in patients with MG. These are summarized in Table 7 and include aminoglycosides, lithium salts,

Table 7. Medications that may exacerbate or cause muscle weakness in patients with MG.

Penicillamine	Cholistin
Lithium salts	Polymixin B
β-Adrenergic drugs	Tetracycline
Procainamide	Lincomycin
Quinine	Propranolol
Neomycin	Ether
Streptomycin	Halothane
Kanamycin	Trichloroethylene
Gentamicin	Barbiturates
Magnesium salts	

β-mimetics, penicillamine, and several other antibiotics that may exacerbate MG. In particular, magnesium sulphate should be avoided as it may precipitate myasthenic crisis (Cohen et al, 1976). In patients with pre-eclampsia, seizure prophylaxis and treatment can be accomplished with phenytoin (Ryan et al, 1988).

Breast-feeding should be avoided as these antibodies are present in breast milk (Varner, 1991).

AUTOIMMUNE THYROID DISEASE

Graves' disease and chronic autoimmune thyroiditis (Hashimoto's thyroiditis) are the two main forms of autoimmune thyroid disease. They represent a spectrum of disorders that includes hyperthyroid, euthyroid, and hypothyroid states. Each is mediated by autoimmune processes that alter thyroid function (Utiger, 1991a). The terminology of the involved autoantibodies has been confusing due to inconsistencies in laboratory assays. Currently, Graves' disease is felt to be mediated by thyroid stimulating immuno-globulins (TSI). These antibodies bind to thyroid stimulating hormone (TSH) receptors and either stimulate or inhibit thyroid function (Utiger, 1991a). Those antibodies which stimulate the thyroid, function like TSH and have been termed thyroid stimulating antibodies (TSAb) while those that suppress thyroid activity are referred to as thyrotropin inhibitor immuno-globulins (TBII) (Mariotti et al, 1989). Patients with Hashimoto's disease have antithyroglobulin and antimicrosomal (antithyroid peroxidase) auto-antibodies (Utiger, 1991a; Mariotti et al, 1989). Some patients with auto-immune thyroid disease have both TSI (TSAb, TBII) and antimicrosomal and antithyroglobulin antibodies—the final expression of their thyroid disease depends upon the interplay of the various autoimmune influences.

A complete review of thyroid physiology in normal pregnancy is beyond the scope of this text. Briefly, serum thyroxine (T_4) and tri-iodothyronine (T_3) concentrations rise during normal pregnancy (Burrow, 1988). This is due to an elevation of thyroid binding globulin (TBG), the main thyroid hormone carrier protein. Although total T_4 and T_3 levels are elevated, free hormone levels are unchanged in pregnancy. As only the small percentage of hormone that is unbound (free) is metabolically active, normal pregnancy is a euthyroid state. Due to the increase in TBG, T_3 resin uptake (RT_3U) is decreased in normal pregnancy while the free thyroxine index (FTI) is unchanged. TSH is also unaffected by pregnancy (Table 8). Recent studies utilizing cordocentesis have revealed a progressive increase in fetal thyroid function from the end of the first trimester through 36 weeks' gestation (Thorpe-Beeston et al, 1991). Compared with adults, the term fetus has higher TSH concentrations, lower total and free T_3 levels, and similar TBG, total T_4, and free T_4 levels (Lowe and Cunningham, 1991; Thorpe-Beeston et al, 1991). Iodine is actively concentrated on the fetal side of the placenta and is avidly taken up by the fetal thyroid in the last two trimesters (Lowe and Cunningham, 1991). TSH and T_3 are not thought to cross the placenta

Table 8. Thyroid function tests in pregnancy.[a]

Test	Normal non-pregnant	Normal pregnant[b]	Hyperthyroid pregnant	Hypothyroid pregnant
Total serum T_4 (mg/dl)	5–12	6–15	↑ ↑	NL ↓
Total serum T_3 (ng/dl)	75–200	90–250	↑	NL (↓)[c]
RT_3U (%)	25–37	20–25	NL or ↑	↓ ↓
FTI[d]	—	NL	↑	↓
Serum TSH (mv/ml)	0.4–4.5	NL	NL	↑
Serum free T_4 (ng/dl)	0.8–2.0	NL	↑	↓
Serum free T_3 (pg/ml)	1.4–4.4	NL	↑	NL (↓)[c]

NL, normal.
[a] Normal values for these tests vary greatly between laboratories and may vary with age.
[b] Women ingesting oestrogens (i.e. oral contraceptives) may have thyroid function tests consistent with pregnancy.
[c] Decreased only in severe cases of hypothyroidism.
[d] This is a calculation that can be done for either T_4 or T_3. It is based on the product of the total T_4 or T_3 and the RT_3U.

(Lowe and Cunningham, 1991), but placental transfer of T_4 has recently been demonstrated by the presence of thyroxine in the cord blood of neonates with congenital inability to produce T_4 (Mariotti et al, 1989).

The influence of pregnancy on thyroid disease

Hyperthyroidism occurs in 0.05–0.2% of gestations (Burrow, 1988; Davis et al, 1989). Graves' disease is the most common recognized hyperthyroid disorder in pregnancy, followed by multinodular goitre, and thyroiditis (Amino et al, 1982b; Burrow, 1988). Common symptoms include palpitations, tremor, weight loss, heat intolerance, and diarrhoea. Care must be taken to distinguish symptoms normally seen in pregnancy from those of hyperthyroidism. Tachycardia (heart rate greater than 100 beats/min), widened pulse pressure, failure to gain weight in pregnancy, and the ocular findings of Graves' disease (exophthalmos, lid lag, and chemosis) are reliable signs of hyperthyroidism in pregnancy (Thomas and Reid, 1987). Laboratory diagnosis usually reveals an elevation in free and total T_4, normal to elevated RT_3U (versus the normal decrease seen in pregnancy), and an elevated FTI.

Graves' disease has been thought to be more easily controlled during pregnancy, suggesting that pregnancy may favourably influence the disease (Burrow, 1988). However, recent clinical studies do not support this (Amino et al, 1982b; Davis et al, 1989). For example, in one series of 41 pregnancies in 35 women with Graves' disease in remission and receiving no therapy, 18 of 41 (44%) cases showed transient increases in FT_4I and FT_3I between 10 and 15 weeks' gestation. All of these patients had normal thyroid function in the second and third trimesters, but 32 of 41 (78%) developed postpartum thyrotoxicosis (Amino et al, 1982b). The postpartum period has been noted by others to be a common time for relapse (Amino et al, 1977).

Severe complications of hyperthyroidism include congestive heart failure (CHF) and thyroid storm. CHF occurred in 7 of 60 (12%) pregnant women with thyrotoxicosis in one series (Davis et al, 1989). The hyperthyroidism was untreated or undiagnosed in 6 of the 7 patients. CHF may be caused by cardiac hypertrophy from long-term sympathomimetic effects of T_4 (Davis et al, 1989). Thyroid storm is rare; manifestations include fever, central nervous system effects, dehydration, and hyperdynamic cardiac failure.

The most common causes of hypothyroidism in women of reproductive age are iatrogenic (surgery and irradiation) followed by Hashimoto's thyroiditis (Burrow, 1988; Davis et al, 1988). Severe cases are rarely seen in pregnancy (Davis et al, 1988). The reasons for this are uncertain, but it is widely believed that hypothyroidism results in anovulation and infertility (Lowe and Cunningham, 1991). This may be due to an elevation in TSH causing hyperprolactinaemia (Kinch et al, 1969). Symptoms of hypothyroidism include constipation, cold intolerance, coarse hair, and lethargy. As with hyperthyroidism, many of these symptoms are difficult to distinguish from symptoms in normal pregnancy. Severe cases result in myxoedema characterized by periorbital oedema, hypothermia, a large tongue, and delayed deep tendon reflexes. Although myxoedema is quite rare in pregnancy, cases have been reported (Lachelin, 1970). Pregnancy does not appear to influence the course of hypothyroidism.

The most reliable laboratory measurement of hypothyroidism in pregnancy is an elevated TSH. T_4 is also low but to a lesser degree than would be expected due to the elevation of TBG in pregnancy. Subclinical hypothyroidism (an elevation of TSH with normal T_4 and T_3 levels in asymptomatic patients) is probably underdiagnosed in pregnancy (Lowe and Cunningham, 1991).

The influence of thyroid disease on pregnancy

Fetal outcome in hyperthyroidism appears to be predominantly dependent upon metabolic control in the mother (Davis et al, 1989). Pre-term delivery, small-for-gestation fetuses, and perinatal mortality are all increased in women with inadequately treated or untreated thyrotoxicosis (Burrow, 1988; Davis et al, 1989). Even if the mother is euthyroid, the fetus is at risk for either hyper- or hypothyroidism. Neonatal thyrotoxicosis occurs in 1% of women with a history of Graves' disease (Munro, 1978). The fetus is at risk even when the mother is euthyroid because neonatal disease is thought to be mediated by the transplacental passage of TSAbs (Matsuura et al, 1988). In utero manifestations can include tachycardia, impaired growth, goitre, hydramnios, hydrops, hyperkinesis, and craniosynostosis (Belfar et al, 1991; Utiger, 1991b). Increased perinatal mortality has been noted (Belfar et al, 1991; Utiger, 1991b). Postnatal development may be impaired as well (Man et al, 1971; Hollingsworth, 1983). Serial cordocentesis illustrated the resolution of fetal hyperthyroidism in a case treated with maternal propylthiouracil (PTU) (Porreco and Bloch, 1990).

The effect of hypothyroidism on fetal outcome is less clear. Older studies reported an increase in spontaneous abortions, stillbirth, pre-term delivery, malformations, and perinatal mortality in infants born to women with hypothyroidism (Greenman et al, 1962; Man et al, 1971; Thomas and Reid, 1987). Later reports have been more favourable, suggesting that hypothyroidism has little, if any, effect on pregnancy outcome (Montoro et al, 1981; Pekonen et al, 1984). However, in one recent series of 16 pregnancies in 14 overtly hypothyroid women, complications included anaemia (31%), abruptio (19%), pre-eclampsia (44%), and postpartum haemorrhage (14%) (Davis et al, 1988). Perinatal morbidity was attributed to pre-eclampsia and abruptio and included small-for-gestational-age fetuses (31%) and stillbirths (12%). Additionally, two women suffered from cardiac dysfunction. It must be emphasized that these cases were overtly hypothyroid. Complications were less impressive in women with subclinical hypothyroidism (Davis et al, 1988). Further prospective trials will help to clarify the extent of perinatal risk in women with hypothyroidism.

Hypothyroidism can also occur in utero, most frequently due to transplacental passage of PTU. This is characterized by goitre and hydramnios (Belfar et al, 1991; Davidson et al, 1991). Hypothyroidism in utero is worrisome since fetal nervous system development may be dependent upon normal concentrations of thyroxine (Rovet et al, 1987; Calvo et al, 1990;

Lowe and Cunningham, 1991). Cordocentesis may be useful to ascertain fetal thyroid status in unclear cases (Perelman et al, 1990; Porreco and Bloch, 1990; Wenstrom et al, 1990; Davidson et al, 1991). An attempt has been made to use amniotic fluid thyroid indices for this purpose, but they do not reliably predict fetal thyroid status (Hollingsworth and Alexander, 1983). Successful in utero therapy with intra-amniotic thyroxine injections to treat fetal hypothyroidism has been reported (Davidson et al, 1991). At the time of delivery, and again at 7–10 days of life, all infants born to mothers with thyroid autoimmune antibodies should undergo thyroid testing. Neonatal hyperthyroidism has occurred 7–10 days after delivery due to the initial protective effects of PTU against TSAb. When the PTU is metabolized, the TSAbs may then cause thyrotoxicosis for up to 3 months (Thomas and Reid, 1987). Many advocate universal screening of all newborns for hypothyroidism. Clinical diagnosis is difficult, most likely due to the initially protective effect of maternal thyroxine (Vulsma et al, 1989). Early treatment with thyroxine is crucial to prevent intellectual impairment (Lowe and Cunningham, 1991).

Management of thyroid disease in pregnancy

Thioamides, which inhibit thyroid hormone synthesis, are the primary medical therapy for Graves' disease in pregnancy. Propylthiouracil (PTU) and methimazole are both effective choices. Each drug crosses the placenta and may suppress fetal thyroid function. Some physicians prefer to use PTU rather than methimazole during pregnancy because it crosses the placenta less readily (Marchant et al, 1977), blocks the peripheral conversion of T_4 to T_3, and methimazole has been associated with aplasia cutis in the fetus (Stephan et al, 1982). In mild-to-moderate Graves' disease, PTU is started at 300–450 mg per day given in divided doses every 8 hours. In more severe cases, initial doses of up to 600 mg per day may be required. Once the symptoms have improved and the total T_4 or free T_4 has started to fall (usually within 2–4 weeks of starting therapy), the dose of PTU is reduced. As a rule of thumb, the dose can be halved. Follow-up thyroid studies are then done 2–4 weeks later to guide any further changes in the dose of PTU. Because PTU may suppress fetal thyroid function, the minimum effective dose should be utilized. Thus, the aim of therapy is the lowest dose of PTU required to maintain the FTI or free T_4 at the upper limits of normal.

Thioamides require several weeks to exert their maximum effect. In the meantime, patients with prominent adrenergic symptoms of thyrotoxicosis can be treated with β-blockers. Propranolol, 20–80 mg daily, can be adjusted to keep the maternal heart rate at or slightly below 100 beats/min.

Thyroid storm demands aggressive therapy with treatment that includes: (1) intravenous hydration (Mariotti et al, 1989), control of fever (Burrow, 1988), PTU 1000–1200 mg daily in divided doses (Thorpe-Beeston et al, 1991), propranolol, 1–2 mg i.v. up to three doses, to control the heart rate (Lowe and Cunningham, 1991), sodium iodide, 1 g in 500 ml of i.v. fluid administered over 2–4 hours, and dexamethasone, 1 mg i.m. every 6 hours (Vulsma et al, 1989). The patient should be managed in an intensive care unit, and invasive cardiac monitoring may be required. Precipitating causes such as infection, pre-eclampsia, and anaemia should be aggressively treated.

Thyroxine replacement is standard therapy for most pregnant patients with hypothyroidism regardless of aetiology. A reasonable initial dosage is 0.1–0.15 mg of thyroxine daily for a 3-week period. The dose is then adjusted until the serum TSH is normal and the patient is asymptomatic. Dosage can be increased by 0.05 mg increments as needed. Serial thyroid function tests should be performed during the course of pregnancy in women requiring replacement therapy. Two recent prospective studies have shown a need for an increase in thyroxine dosage in women during the course of pregnancy (Pekonen et al, 1984; Davidson et al, 1991).

Postpartum thyroid dysfunction

Postpartum thyroid dysfunction is an increasingly recognized problem which is now noted to occur in 5–10% of women (Amino et al, 1982a; Jansson et al, 1984; Fung et al, 1988; Hayslip et al, 1988). This disorder has been underdiagnosed in the past, possibly due to the presence of vague symptoms often attributed to the emotional and physical demands of the postpartum period. However, postpartum hypothyroidism results in carelessness, depression, impaired concentration, and an increase in total complaints compared with normal controls (Hayslip et al, 1988).

The clinical course is variable, and these women may be either hyperthyroid alone, become hyperthyroid and then hypothyroid, or be hypothyroid alone. The symptoms of hyperthyroidism usually begin between 1 and 4 months postpartum. Since the disorder is caused by the release of preformed thyroid hormone secondary to glandular disruption rather than stimulation of excessive hormone production, treatment with thioamides is not helpful (Tamaki et al, 1987). The disorder is usually self-limited (Amino et al, 1982a), but β-blockade with propranolol (20–80 mg per day) may be needed temporarily for severe symptoms. Symptoms of hypothyroidism typically develop between 3 and 8 months postpartum, and resolve by 6–9 months after delivery. However, one study of women followed for at least 5 years noted persistent hypothyroidism in 10 of 59 cases (Tachi et al, 1988b). Severe cases can be treated with thyroid replacement using thyroxine.

Postpartum thyroid dysfunction is an immune disorder. Lymphocytic thyroiditis was found in each of nine women who underwent fine needle biopsy due to postpartum hypothyroidism (Jansson et al, 1984). Furthermore, several investigators have noted an association with antimicrosomal antibodies and postpartum thyroid dysfunction (Amino, 1982a; Jansson, 1984; Vargas, 1988) and an association between antimicrosomal antibodies and lymphocytic infiltration (Yoshida et al, 1978). Amino noted antimicrosomal antibodies in 12.2% of postpartum patients versus 7.8% in non-pregnant controls (Amino et al, 1982a) which he proposes as the reason for the high prevalence of postpartum thyroid dysfunction (Amino et al, 1982a).

Because most women who develop postpartum thyroid dysfunction have antimicrosomal antibodies, testing for their presence may be useful in screening for the development of postpartum thyroid disease. Hayslip et al (1988) screened 1034 women for antimicrosomal antibodies on the second postpartum day. Of 51 women with antimicrosomal antibodies followed for at least 6 months, 34 (67%) developed biochemical thyroid dysfunction. Twenty (44%) required thyroxine therapy for hypothyroidism. Elevations in anti-DNA antibody titres and certain HLA types may be associated with postpartum thyroid disease, but data are preliminary (Yoshida et al, 1978; Tachi et al, 1988a,b; Vargas et al, 1988).

The obstetrician should be alert for symptoms of postpartum thyroid dysfunction, including depression, memory loss, and malaise, as well as traditional symptoms of hyper- and hypothyroidism. Thyroid function tests and antimicrosomal antibodies should be obtained to confirm the diagnosis in suspected cases. Symptomatic patients may benefit from treatment as outlined above.

RHEUMATOID ARTHRITIS

Rheumatoid arthritis (RA) is a systemic disorder characterized by inflammation of the synovial joints. The adult form of the disease affects three times as many women as men and RA is estimated to occur in 0.1–0.05% of all pregnancies (Varner, 1991). Typically, disease onset is gradual with involvement of the diarthrodial (synovial) joints including the metacarpophalangeal (MCP) joints, the proximal interphalyngeal (PIP) joints, the wrists, and the shoulders. Fibrous joints are rarely affected. A cycle of damage leading to joint instability leading to further damage often ensues, resulting in a slowly progressive course. This may eventually lead to joint deformities especially in the MCP and PIP joints. Systemic manifestations may include subcutaneous nodules (rheumatoid nodules), fatigue, pulmonary granulomas, vasculitis, pleurisy, and pericarditis. Juvenile rheumatoid arthritis (JRA) is a related disorder that begins in individuals under 16 years of age. The clinical course of JRA is usually more benign than adult RA and is self-limited in 75% of patients.

RA is thought to be an autoimmune disorder. Evidence of an immunological origin for the disease includes the presence of a characteristic IgM and IgG autoantibody which reacts with antigens on the Fc portion of immunoglobulins. This antibody can be measured in the serum and is termed rheumatoid factor (RF). The synovial fluids of patients with RF contain immune complexes with immunoglobulin as well as decreased complement levels. Furthermore, the synovium in affected joints is infiltrated with lymphocytes and monocytes. RA is more prevalent in women with HLA-D4 (Stobo, 1982).

The influence of pregnancy on RA

RA has consistently been reported to improve during pregnancy in approximately 75% of women (Oka, 1958a; Flebo and Snorrason, 1961; Kaplan and Diamond, 1965; Oka and Vainio, 1966; Persillin, 1977; Ostensen and

Husby, 1983) (Table 9). Most remissions begin in the first trimester (Ostensen and Husby, 1983) with a peak improvement in symptoms towards the end of gestation. In addition to improvement of arthritic symptoms, rheumatoid nodules may disappear during pregnancy (Ostensen and Husby, 1984). Unfortunately, over 90% of patients with gestational remissions suffer exacerbations within the first 6 months postpartum (Persillin, 1977).

Table 9. The effect of pregnancy on RA.

Authors	Patients	Pregnancies	Pregnancies with improvement in RA
Hench, 1938	22	37	33 (89%)
Oka, 1958a	93	114	88 (77%)
Smith and West, 1960	12	12	9 (75%)
Betson and Dorn, 1964	21	21	13 (62%)
Ostensen et al, 1983	31	49	37 (76%)
Ostensen and Husby, 1983*	10	10	9 (90%)

* Prospective study. All others were retrospective.

There are no laboratory tests or clinical features that predict the course of RA in pregnancy, and pregnancy does not appear to alter the long-term course for women with RA. In a study of 100 consecutive patients with RA during pregnancy, there was no evidence of worse disease when compared with matched controls (Oka and Vainio, 1966).

The reasons for the ameliorating effect of pregnancy on RA are unclear. Initially, hormonal changes associated with pregnancy were thought perhaps to affect the disease. However, cortisol elevations have not been found to correlate with symptoms (Oka, 1958b; Smith and West, 1960). Nor do oestrogens affect the disease in non-pregnant patients (Gilbert et al, 1964; Bijlsma et al, 1987). More compelling data implicate pregnancy specific serum proteins in the amelioration of RA. Transfusion of non-pregnant RA patients with serum obtained from pregnant women has improved RA symptoms (Josephs, 1964). Specifically, pregnancy α-glycoprotein (PAG) has been shown to improve arthritis in experimental models (Kasukawa et al, 1979). Others suggest that the placenta may be involved with the improvement of RA by the removal of immune complexes (Klippel and Cerere, 1989).

The influence of RA on pregnancy

RA does not appear to have a significant adverse effect on pregnancy. Reports suggest a rate of spontaneous abortion of 15–25% in women with RA (Kaplan and Diamond, 1965; Ostensen and Husby, 1983; Siamopoulou-Mavridou et al, 1988), which is similar to the rate in the general population. The two studies with controls found contrary results. One noted a slight increase in spontaneous abortions in women with RA (Kaplan, 1986), but the other did not (Silman et al, 1988). One case of fetal growth retardation presumed due to vasculitis has been reported in a woman with RA (Duhring, 1970), but this case represents an isolated report. Increased risks of dystocia, pre-eclampsia, and preterm birth have not been noted (Morris, 1969).

Management of RA in pregnancy

Patients should be seen more frequently in cases of active disease. Rest should be advised and physical therapy may be of benefit in difficult cases. Simple analgesia is best accomplished with paracetamol (acetaminophen *USP*) or low doses of narcotics. Salicylates and NSAIDs should be avoided if at all possible (see discussion above under SLE). Glucocorticoids, such as prednisone, are usually effective and are relatively safe in pregnancy (see discussion above under SLE). Data are less clear on other medications used to treat RA. Gold salts may be safe (Cohen et al, 1981), but they cross the placenta and theoretically could cause fetal immunosuppression. Antimalarials, D-penicillamine, and cytotoxic agents should be avoided. In the absence of gross contractures potentially interfering with the mechanics of vaginal birth, no special intrapartum care is required. Patients with gross hip contractures are rare, and management of these cases must be individualized.

REFERENCES

Abramowsky CR, Vegas ME, Swinehart G & Gyves MT (1980) Decidual vasculopathy of the placenta in lupus erythematosus. *New England Journal of Medicine* **303(12):** 668–672.

Abramsky O, Lisak RP, Brenner T, Zeidman A & Beyth Y (1979) Preliminary communications: significance in neonatal myasthenia gravis of inhibitory effect of amniotic fluid on binding of antibodies to acetylcholine receptor. *Lancet* **ii:** 1333–1335.

Amino N, Miyai K, Yamamoto T et al (1977) Transient recurrence of hyperthyroidism after delivery in Graves' disease. *Journal of Clinical Endocrinology and Metabolism* **44:** 130.

Amino N, Mori H & Iwatani Y (1982a) High prevalence of transient post-partum thyrotoxicosis and hypothyroidism. *New England Journal of Medicine* **306(14):** 849–852.

Amino N, Tanizawa O, Mori H et al (1982b) Aggravation of thyrotoxicosis in early pregnancy and after delivery in Graves' disease. *Journal of Clinical Endocrinology and Metabolism* **55:** 108–112.

Ariga H, Edwards J & Sullivan DA (1989) Androgen control of autoimmune expression in lacrimal glands of MRL/Mp-*lpr/pr* mice. *Clinical Immunology and Immunopathology* **53:** 499–508.

Aster RH (1990) 'Gestational' thrombocytopenia: a plea for conservative management. *New England Journal of Medicine* **323(4):** 264–266.

Ayromlooi J (1978) A new approach to the management of immunologic thrombocytopenic purpura in pregnancy. *American Journal of Obstetrics and Gynecology* **130:** 235.

Ballageer V, Spitz B, Kieckens L, Moreau H, Van Assche A & Collen D (1989) Predictive value of increased plasma levels of fibronectin in gestational hypertension. *American Journal of Obstetrics and Gynecology* **161(2):** 432–436.

Bear RA (1976) Pregnancy in patients with renal disease. *Obstetrics and Gynecology* **48(1):** 13–18.

Belfar HL, Foley TP, Hill LM & Kislak S (1991) Sonographic findings in maternal hyperthyroidism; fetal hyperthyroidism/fetal goiter. *Journal of Ultrasound Medicine* **10:** 281–284.

Besinger RE, Niebyl JR, Keyes WG & Johnson TRB (1991) Randomized comparative trial of indomethacin and ritodrine for the long-term treatment of preterm labor. *American Journal of Obstetrics and Gynecology* **164:** 981–988.

Betson JR & Dorn RV (1964) Forty cases of arthritis and pregnancy. *Journal of the International College of Surgeons* **42:** 521.

Bierman FZ, Baxi L, Jaffe I & Driscoll J (1988) Fetal hydrops and congenital complete heart block: response to maternal steroid therapy. *Journal of Pediatrics* **112:** 646–648.

Bijlsma WJ, Huger-Bruning O & Thijssen JHH (1987) Effect of estrogen treatment on clinical and laboratory manifestations of rheumatoid arthritis. *Annals of the Rheumatic Diseases* **46**: 777.

Billingham RE & Beer AE (1984) Reproductive immunology: past, present, and future. *Perspectives in Biology and Medicine* **27**: 259–275.

Blanford AT & Murphy BEP (1977) In vitro metabolism of prednisolone, dexamethasone, betamethasone, and cortisol by the human placenta. *American Journal of Obstetrics and Gynecology* **127**: 264–267.

Bobrie G, Liote F, Houillier P, Grunfeld JP & Jungers P (1987) Pregnancy in lupus nephritis and related disorders. *American Journal of Kidney Diseases* **9**: 339–343.

Branch DW & Scott JR (1991) Clinical implications of antiphospholipid antibodies: the Utah experience. In Harris EN, Exner T, Hughes GRV & Asherson RA (eds) *Phospholipid-binding Antibodies*, pp 335–346. Boca Raton, FL: CRC Press.

Branch DW, Scott JR, Kochenour NK & Hershgold E (1985) Obstetric complications associated with the lupus anticoagulant. *New England Journal of Medicine* **313**: 1322–1326.

Brenner T, Beyth Y & Abramsky O (1980) Inhibitory effect of α-fetoprotein on the binding of myasthenia gravis antibody to acetylcholine receptor. *Proceedings of the National Academy of Sciences (USA)* **77**: 3635–3639.

Bresnihan B, Oliver M, Grigor RR, Leukonia RM & Hughes GRV (1977) Immunological mechanism for spontaneous abortion in systemic lupus erythematosus. *Lancet* **ii**: 1205–1207.

Burkett G (1985) Lupus nephropathy and pregnancy. *Clinical Obstetrics and Gynecology* **28(2)**: 310–323.

Burrow GN (1988) Thyroid diseases. In Burrow GN & Ferris TF (eds) *Medical Complications during Pregnancy*, 3rd edn, pp 224–253. Philadelphia: W. B. Saunders.

Burrows RF & Kelton JG (1990a) Low fetal risks in pregnancies associated with idiopathic thrombocytopenic purpura. *American Journal of Obstetrics and Gynecology* **163**: 1147–1150.

Burrows RF & Kelton JG (1990b) Thrombocytopenia at delivery: a prospective survey of 6715 deliveries. *American Journal of Obstetrics and Gynecology* **162**: 731–734.

Buyon JP, Cronstein BN, Morris M, Tanner M & Weissman G (1986) Serum complement values (C3 and C4) to differentiate between systemic lupus activity and pre-eclampsia. *American Journal of Medicine* **81**: 194–200.

Buyon JP, Swersky SH, Fox HE, Bierman FZ & Winchester RJ (1987) Intrauterine therapy for presumptive fetal myocarditis with acquired heart block due to systemic lupus erythematosus. *Arthritis and Rheumatism* **30(1)**: 44–49.

Calvo R, Obregon MJ, de Ona CR, del Rey E & de Escobar GM (1990) Congenital hypothyroidism, as studied in rats. *Journal of Clinical Investigation* **86**: 889–899.

Carr RE, Henkin DP, Rothfield N et al (1968) Ocular toxicity of antimalarial drugs: long term follow-up. *American Journal of Ophthalmology* **66**: 738–742.

Chambers DC, Hall JE & Boyce J (1967) Views and reviews: myasthenia gravis and pregnancy. *Obstetrics and Gynecology* **29(4)**: 597–603.

Chameides L, Truex RC, Vetter V, Rashking WJ, Galioto FM & Noonan JA (1977) Association of maternal systemic lupus erythematosus with congenital complete heart block. *New England Journal of Medicine* **297**: 1204–1207.

Christiaens GCML & Helmerhorst FM (1987) Validity of intrapartum diagnosis of fetal thrombocytopenia. *American Journal of Obstetrics and Gynecology* **157**: 864–865.

Cohen BA, London RS & Goldstein PJ (1976) Myasthenia gravis and preeclampsia. *Obstetrics and Gynecology* **43(supplement 1)**: 355.

Cohen DL, Orzel J & Taylor A (1981) Infants of mothers receiving gold therapy. *Arthritis and Rheumatism* **24**: 104.

Cook RL, Miller RC, Katz VL & Cefalo RC (1991) Immune thrombocytopenic purpura in pregnancy: a reappraisal of management. *Obstetrics and Gynecology* **78(4)**: 578–583.

Cote CJ, Meuwissen HJ & Pickering RJ (1974) Effects on the neonate of prednisone and azathioprine administered to the mother during pregnancy. *Journal of Pediatrics* **85**: 324.

Cowchock FS, Reece EA, Balaban D, Branch DW & Plouffe L (1992) Repeated fetal losses associated with antiphospholipid antibodies: a collaborative randomized trial comparing prednisone to low dose heparin treatment. *American Journal of Obstetrics and Gynecology* in press.

Crowley P, Chalmers I & Kierse MJNC (1990) The effects of corticosteroid administration before preterm delivery: an overview of the evidence from controlled trials. *British Journal of Obstetrics and Gynaecology* **97**: 11–25.

Daffos F, Capella-Pavlovsky M & Forestier (1985) Fetal blood sampling during pregnancy with the use of a needle guided by ultrasound: a study of 606 cases. *American Journal of Obstetrics and Gynecology* **153(6)**: 655–660.

Daffos F, Forestier F, Kaplan C & Cox W (1988) Prenatal diagnosis and management of bleeding disorders with fetal blood sampling. *American Journal of Obstetrics and Gynecology* **158(4)**: 939–946.

Davidson KM, Richards DS, Schatz DA & Fisher DA (1991) Successful in utero treatment of fetal goiter and hypothyroidism. *New England Journal of Medicine* **324(8)**: 543–546.

Davis LE, Leveno KJ & Cunningham FG (1988) Hypothyroidism complicating pregnancy. *Obstetrics and Gynecology* **72**: 108–112.

Davis LE, Lucas MJ, Hankins GDV, Roark ML & Cunningham FG (1989) Thyrotoxicosis complicating pregnancy. *American Journal of Obstetrics and Gynecology* **160**: 63–70.

Deng JS, Bair LW, Shen-Schwarz S, Ramsey-Goldman R & Medsger T (1987) Localization of Ro (SS-A) antigen in the cardiac conduction system. *Arthritis and Rheumatism* **30(11)**: 1232–1238.

Derksen RHWM, Bouma BN & Kater L (1986) The striking association between the lupus anticoagulant and fetal loss in systemic lupus erythematosus. *Arthritis and Rheumatism* **29**: 695.

Derue GJ, Englert HG, Harris EN et al (1985) Fetal loss in systemic lupus; association with anticardiolipin antibodies. *Obstetrics and Gynecology* **5**: 207.

Devoe LD & Loy GL (1984) Serum complement levels and perinatal outcome in pregnancies complicated by systemic lupus erythematosus. *Obstetrics and Gynecology* **63**: 796–800.

Devoe LD & Taylor RL (1979) Systemic lupus erythematosus in pregnancy. *American Journal of Obstetrics and Gynecology* **135**: 473–479.

Druzin ML, Lockshin M, Edersheim TG, Hutson JM, Krauss AL & Kogut E (1987) Second-trimester fetal monitoring and preterm delivery in pregnancies with systemic lupus erythematosus and/or circulating anticoagulant. *American Journal of Obstetrics and Gynecology* **157**: 1503–1510.

Duhring JL (1970) Pregnancy, rheumatoid arthritis, and intrauterine growth retardation. *American Journal of Obstetrics and Gynecology* **108**: 325.

Eden RD & Gall SA (1983) Myasthenia gravis and pregnancy: a reappraisal of thymectomy. *Obstetrics and Gynecology* **62**: 328–333.

Engel AG, Sakakibara H, Sahashi K et al (1979) Passively transferred experimental auto-immune myasthenia gravis. *Neurology* **29**: 179–188.

Fenichel GM (1978) Clinical syndromes of myasthenia in infancy and childhood. *Archives of Neurology* **35**: 97–103.

Fennell DF & Ringel SP (1987) Myasthenia gravis and pregnancy. *Obstetrical and Gynecological Survey* **41(7)**: 414–421.

Fine LG, Barnett EV, Danovitch GM et al (1981) Systemic lupus erythematosus in pregnancy. *Annals of Internal Medicine* **94**: 667–677.

Flebo M & Snorrason E (1961) Pregnancy and the place of therapeutic abortion in rheumatoid arthritis. *Acta Obstetrica et Gynecologica Scandinavica* **40**: 116.

Fraga A, Mintz G, Orozco J & Orozco JH (1974) Sterility and fertility rates, fetal wastage and maternal morbidity in systemic lupus erythematosus. *Journal of Rheumatology* **1(3)**: 293–298.

Friedman EA & Rutherford JW (1956) Pregnancy in lupus erythematosus. *Obstetrics and Gynecology* **8(5)**: 601–610.

Fries JF & Holman MR (1975) Systemic lupus erythematosis: a clinical analysis. In Smith LM Jr (ed.) *Major Problems in Internal Medicine*, pp 127–129. Philadelphia: W. B. Saunders.

Fung HYM, Kologlu M, Collison K et al (1988) Postpartum thyroid dysfunction in Mid Glamorgan. *British Medical Journal* **296**: 241–244.

Garenstein M, Pollach VE & Kark RM (1962) Systemic lupus erythematosus and pregnancy. *New England Journal of Medicine* **267**: 165–169.

Gilbert M, Kotstein J & Cunningham C (1964) Norethynodrel with mestranol in the treatment of rheumatoid arthritis. *Journal of the American Medical Association* **190**: 235.

Gimovsky ML, Montoro M & Paul RH (1984) Pregnancy outcome in women with systemic lupus erythematosus. *Obstetrics and Gynecology* **63(5)**: 686–692.

Gounder MP, Baker D, Saletan S, Monheit AG, Hultin MB & Coller BS (1986) Intravenous gammaglobulin therapy in the management of a patient with idiopathic thrombocytopenic purpura and a warm autoimmune erythrocyte panagglutinin during pregnancy. *Obstetrics and Gynecology* **67(5):** 741–746.

Greenman GW, Gabrielson MO, Howard-Flanders J et al (1962) Thyroid dysfunction in pregnancy. *New England Journal of Medicine* **267:** 426.

Grennan DM, McCormick JN, Wojtacha D, Carty M & Behan W (1978) Immunological studies of the placenta in systemic lupus erythematosus. *Annals of the Rheumatic Diseases* **37:** 129–134.

Grouse LD & Young RK (1983) Myasthenia gravis: a clinical and basic science review. *Journal of the American Medical Association* **250(18):** 2516–2521.

Guzman L, Avalos E, Ortiz R, Gurrola R, Lopez E & Herrera R (1987) Placental abnormalities in systemic lupus erythematosus: *in situ* deposition of antinuclear antibodies *Journal of Rheumatology* **14(5):** 924–928.

Hanly JG, Gladman DD, Rose TH, Laskin CA & Urowitz MB (1988) Lupus pregnancy: a prospective study of placental changes. *Arthritis and Rheumatism* **31(3):** 358–366.

Hardin JA (1986) The lupus autoantigens and the pathogenesis of systemic lupus erythematosus. *Arthritis and Rheumatism* **29(4):** 457–460.

Harris EN (1990) A reassessment of antiphospholipid syndrome. *Journal of Rheumatology* **17(6):** 733–735.

Harris EN & Spinnato JA (1991) Should anticardiolipin tests be performed in otherwise healthy pregnant women? *American Journal of Obstetrics and Gynecology* **165:** 1272–1277.

Harris EN & the Kingston Anti-Phospholipid Groups (KAPS) The second anti-cardiolipin standardization workshop. *American Journal of Clinical Pathology* **94:** 476–484.

Hart C & Naughton RF (1964) The ototoxicity of chloroquine phosphate. *Archives of Otolaryngology* **80:** 407–412.

Hayslett JP & Lynn RI (1980) Effect of pregnancy in patients with lupus nephropathy. *Kidney International* **18:** 207–220.

Hayslip C, Fein HG, O-Donnell VM, Friedman DS, Klein TA & Smallridge RC (1988) The value of serum antimicrosomal antibody testing in screening for symptomatic postpartum thyroid dysfunction. *American Journal of Obstetrics and Gynecology* **159:** 203–209.

Hench PS (1938) The ameliorating effect of pregnancy on chronic atrophic (infectious) rheumatoid arthritis, fibrositis, and intermittent hydrarthritis. *Proceedings of the Staff Meetings of the Mayo Clinic* **13:** 161.

Hollingsworth DR (1983) Graves' disease. *Clinical Obstetrics and Gynecology* **26:** 615–634.

Hollingsworth DR & Alexander NM (1983) Amniotic fluid concentrations of iodothyronines and thyrotropin do not reliably predict fetal thyroid status in pregnancies complicated by maternal thyroid disorders or anencephaly. *Journal of Clinical Endocrinology and Metabolism* **57:** 349–355.

Holmes LB, Driscoll SG & Bradley WG (1980) Contractures in a newborn infant of a mother with myasthenia gravis. *Journal of Pediatrics* **96:** 1067.

Hou S (1985) Pregnancy in women with chronic renal disease. *New England Journal of Medicine* **312(13):** 836–839.

Houser MT, Fish AJ, Tagatz GE, Williams PP & Michael AF (1980) Pregnancy and systemic lupus erythematosus. *American Journal of Obstetrics and Gynecology* **138:** 409–413.

Imbasciati E, Surian M, Bottino W et al (1984) Lupus nephropathy and pregnancy. *Nephron* **36:** 46–51.

Imperiale TF & Petrulis AS (1991) A meta-analysis of low dose aspirin for the prevention of pregnancy induced hypertensive disease. *Journal of the American Medical Association* **266(2):** 260–264.

Infante-Rivard C, David M, Gauthier R & Rivard GE (1991) Lupus anticoagulants, anticardiolipin antibodies, and fetal loss. *New England Journal of Medicine* **325:** 1063–1066.

Jackson R & Gulliver M (1979) Neonatal lupus erythematosus progressing into systemic lupus erythematosus. *British Journal of Dermatology* **101:** 81–86.

Jansson R, Bernander S, Karlsson A, Levin K & Nilsson G (1984) Autoimmune thyroid dysfunction in the postpartum period. *Journal of Clinical Endocrinology and Metabolism* **58:** 681–687.

Johns TR (1987) Long-term corticosteroid treatment of myasthenia gravis. *Annals of the New York Academy of Sciences* **505:** 568–583.

Jones RW, Asher MI, Rutherford CJ & Munro HM (1977) Autoimmune (idiopathic) thrombocytopenic purpura in pregnancy and the newborn. *British Journal of Obstetrics and Gynaecology* **84:** 679–683.

Josephs C (1964) Observations on the treatment of rheumatoid arthritis by transfusions of blood from pregnant women. *British Medical Journal* **2:** 134.

Jungers P, Dougados M, Pellissier C et al (1982a) Influence of oral contraceptive therapy on the activity of systemic lupus erythematosus. *Arthritis and Rheumatism* **25(6):** 618–623.

Jungers P, Dougados M, Pelissier C et al (1982b) Lupus nephropathy and pregnancy. *Archives of Internal Medicine* **142:** 771–776.

Kaplan C, Daffos F, Forestier F et al (1990) Fetal platelet counts in thrombocytopenic pregnancy. *Lancet* **336:** 979–982.

Kaplan D (1986) Fetal wastage in patients with rheumatoid arthritis. *Journal of Rheumatology* **13:** 875.

Kaplan D & Diamond H (1965) Rheumatoid arthritis and pregnancy. *Clinical Obstetrics and Gynecology* **8:** 286.

Karpatkin M, Porges RF & Karpatkin S (1981) Platelet counts in infants of women with autoimmune thrombocytopenia. *New England Journal of Medicine* **305(16):** 936–939.

Karpatkin S (1980) Autoimmune thrombocytopenic purpura. *Journal of the American Society of Hematology* **56(3):** 329–343.

Kasukawa R, Ohara M, Yoshida H & Yoshida T (1979) Pregnancy-associated α_2-glycoprotein in rheumatoid arthritis. *International Archives of Allergy and Applied Immunology* **58:** 67.

Katz AI & Lindheimer MD (1985) Does pregnancy aggravate primary glomerular disease? *American Journal of Kidney Diseases* **VI(4):** 261–265.

Kinch RA, Plunkett ER & Devlin MC (1969) Postpartum amenorrhea galactorrhea of hypothyroidism. *American Journal of Obstetrics and Gynecology* **105:** 766.

Klippel GL & Cerere FA (1989) Rheumatoid arthritis and pregnancy. *Rheumatic Disease Clinics of North America* **15:** 213.

Lachelin GC (1970) Myxoedema and pregnancy; a case report. *Journal of Obstetrics and Gynaecology of the British Commonwealth* **77:** 77.

Lahita RG, Bradlow HL, Kunkel HG & Fishman J (1979) Alterations of estrogen metabolism in systemic lupus erythematosus. *Arthritis and Rheumatism* **22(11):** 1195–1198.

Lahita RG, Bradlow HL, Fishman J & Kunkel HG (1982) Abnormal estrogen and androgen metabolism in the human systemic erythematosus. *American Journal of Kidney Diseases* **1(4):** 206–210.

Lanham JG, Walport MJ & Hughes GRV (1983) Congenital heart block and familial connective tissue disease. *Journal of Rheumatology* **10:** 823–825.

Lee LA, Bias WB, Arnett FC et al (1983) Immunogenetics of the neonatal lupus syndrome. *Annals of Internal Medicine* **99:** 592–596.

Lee LA, Coulter S, Erner S & Chu H (1987) Cardiac immunoglobulin deposition in congenital heart block associated with maternal anti-Ro autoantibodies. *American Journal of Medicine* **83:** 793–796.

Levine SE & Keesey JC (1986) Successful plasmapheresis for fulminant myasthenia gravis during pregnancy. *Archives of Neurology* **43:** 197–198.

Lindstrom JM, Seybold ME, Lennon VA, Whittingham S & Duane DD (1976) Antibody to acetylcholine receptor in myasthenia gravis. *Neurology* **26:** 1054–1059.

Lockshin MD (1985) Lupus pregnancy. *Clinics in Rheumatic Diseases* **11(3):** 611–632.

Lockshin MD (1989) Pregnancy does not cause systemic lupus erythematosus to worsen. *Arthritis and Rheumatism* **32(6):** 665–670.

Lockshin MD (1990) Pregnancy associated with systemic lupus erythematosus. *Seminars in Perinatology* **14(2):** 130–138.

Lockshin MD, Reinits E, Druzin ML, Murrman M & Estes D (1984) Case-control prospective study demonstrating absence of lupus exacerbation during or after pregnancy. *American Journal of Medicine* **77:** 893–898.

Lockshin MC, Harpel PC, Druzin ML et al (1985) Lupus pregnancy II. Unusual pattern of hypocomplementemia and thrombocytopenia in the pregnant patient. *Arthritis and Rheumatism* **28(1):** 58–65.

Lockshin MD, Qamar T & Druzin ML (1987a) Hazards of lupus pregnancy. *Journal of Rheumatology* **14:** 214–217.

Lockshin MD, Qamar R, Druzin ML & Goei S (1987b) Antibody to cardiolipin, lupus anticoagulant, and fetal death. *Journal of Rheumatology* **14:** 259–262.

Lockshin MD, Bonfa E, Elkon D & Druzin ML (1988) Neonatal lupus risk to newborns of mothers with systemic lupus erythematosus. *Arthritis and Rheumatism* **31(6):** 697–701.

Lockshin MD, Druzin ML & Qamar R (1989) Prednisone does not prevent recurrent fetal death in women with antiphospholipid antibody. *American Journal of Obstetrics and Gynecology* **160:** 439–443.

Lockwood CJ & Peters JH (1990) Increased plasma levels of ED1+ cellular fibronectin precede the clinical signs of preeclampsia. *American Journal of Obstetrics and Gynecology* **162(2):** 358–362.

Lom-Orta H, Diaz-Jouanen E & Alarcon-Segovia D (1979) Lymphocytotoxic antibodies during pregnancy in systemic lupus erythematosus. *Lancet* **i:** 1034.

Lowe TW & Cunningham FG (1991) Thyroid disease in pregnancy. *Williams Obstetrics Supplement* **9:** 1–15.

Lubbe WF, Palmer SJ, Butler WS & Liggins GC (1983) Fetal survival after prednisone suppression of maternal lupus-anticoagulant. *Lancet* **i:** 1361–1363.

Luster MI, Hayes HT, Korach K et al (1984) Estrogen immunosuppression is regulated through estrogenic responses in the thymus. *Journal of Immunology* **133:** 110–116.

McCune AB, Weston WL & Lee LA (1987) Maternal and fetal outcome in neonatal lupus erythematosus. *Annals of Internal Medicine* **106:** 518–523.

McGee CD & Makowski EL (1970) Systemic lupus erythematosus in pregnancy. *American Journal of Obstetrics and Gynecology* **107(7):** 1008–1012.

Mackworth-Young CG, Parke AL, Morley KD, Fotherby K & Hughes GRV (1983) Sex hormones in male patients with systemic lupus erythematosus: a comparison with other disease groups. *European Journal of Rheumatism Inflammation* **6:** 228–232.

McMillan R (1981) Chronic idiopathic thrombocytopenic purpura. *New England Journal of Medicine* **304(19):** 1135–1147.

Man EB, Holden RH & Jones WS (1971) Thyroid function in human pregnancy, VII, development and retardation of 4-year old progeny of euthyroid and of hypothyroxinemic women. *American Journal of Obstetrics and Gynecology* **109:** 12.

Marchant B, Brownlie BEW, Hart DM et al (1977) The placental transfer of propylthiouracil, methimazole and carbamizole. *Journal of Clinical Endocrinology and Metabolism* **45:** 1187.

Mariotti S, Chiovato L, Vitti P et al (1989) Recent advances in the understanding of humoral and cellular mechanisms implicated in thyroid autoimmune disorders. *Clinical Immunology and Immunopathology* **50:** S73–S84.

Martin JN, Morrison JC & Files JC (1984) Autoimmune thrombocytopenic purpura: current concepts and recommended practices. *American Journal of Obstetrics and Gynecology* **150:** 86–96.

Matsuura N, Fujieda K, Iida Y et al (1988) TSH-receptor antibodies in mothers with Graves' disease and outcome in their offspring. *Lancet* **i:** 14–17.

Meehan RT & Dorsey JK (1987) Pregnancy among patients with systemic lupus erythematosus receiving immunosuppressive therapy. *Journal of Rheumatology* **14(2):** 252–258.

Metz KA, Boegel WA & Steinberg AD (1980) Therapeutic studies in New Zealand mice. *Arthritis and Rheumatism* **23:** 41–47.

Mintz R, Niz J, Gutierrez G, Garcia-Alonso A & Karchmer S (1986) Prospective study of pregnancy in systemic lupus erythematosus. Results of a multidisciplinary approach. *Journal of Rheumatology* **13(4):** 732–739.

Mishina M, Takai T, Imoto K, Noda M, Takahashi T & Numa S (1986) Molecular distinction between fetal and adult forms of muscle acetylcholine receptor. *Nature* **321:** 406–411.

Moise Jr KJ, Carpenter Jr RJ, Cotton DB, Wasserstrum N, Kitshon B & Cano L (1988a) Percutaneous umbilical cord blood sampling in the evaluation of fetal platelet counts in pregnant patients with autoimmune thrombocytopenic purpura. *Obstetrics and Gynecology* **72(3):** 346–350.

Moise KJ, Huhta JC, Sharif DF et al (1988b) Indomethacin in the treatment of premature labor: effects of the fetal ductus arteriosus. *New England Journal of Medicine* **319:** 327–331.

Montoro M, Collea JV, Frasier SD & Mestman JH (1981) Successful outcome of pregnancy in women with hypothyroidism. *Annals of Internal Medicine* **94(1):** 31–34.

Morel E, Eymard B, Garabedian BV, Pannier C, Culac O & Bach JF (1988) Neonatal myasthenia gravis: a new clinical and immunologic appraisal on 30 cases. *Neurology* **38:** 138–142.

Morris WIC (1969) Pregnancy in rheumatoid arthritis and systemic lupus erythematosus. *Australia and New Zealand Journal of Obstetrics and Gynaecology* **9:** 136.

Mund A, Simson J & Rothfield N (1963) Effect of pregnancy on course of systemic lupus erythematosus. *Journal of the American Medical Association* **183(11):** 917–920.

Munro DS, Dirmikis SM, Humphries H, Smith T & Broadhead GD (1978) The role of thyroid stimulating immunoglobulins of Graves' disease in neonatal thyrotoxicosis. *British Journal of Obstetrics and Gynaecology* **85:** 837.

Namba T, Brown SB & Grob D (1970) Neonatal myasthenia gravis: report of two cases and review of the literature. *Pediatrics* **45(3):** 488–504.

Nossent HC & Swaak TJG (1990) Systemic lupus erythematosus. VI. Analysis of the inter-relationship with pregnancy. *Journal of Rheumatology* **17(6):** 771–776.

Oka M (1958a) Effect of pregnancy on onset and course of rheumatoid arthritis. *Annals of the Rheumatic Diseases* **12:** 222.

Oka M (1958b) Activity of rheumatoid arthritis and plasma 17 hydroxycorticosteroids during pregnancy and following parturition. *Acta Rheumatologica Scandinavica* **4:** 243.

Oka M & Vainio V (1966) Effect of pregnancy on the prognosis and serology of rheumatoid arthritis. *Acta Rheumatologica Scandinavica* **12:** 47.

Olson NY & Lindsley CB (1987) Neonatal lupus syndrome. *American Journal of Diseases of Children* **141:** 908–910.

Ostensen M & Husby G (1983) A prospective clinical study of the effect of pregnancy on rheumatoid arthritis and ankylosing spondylitis. *Arthritis and Rheumatism* **26:** 1155.

Ostensen M & Husby G (1984) Pregnancy and rheumatic disease. A review of recent studies in rheumatoid arthritis and ankylosing spondylitis. *Klinische Wochenschrift* **62:** 891–895.

Ostensen M, Aune B & Husby G (1983) Effect of pregnancy and hormonal changes on the activity of rheumatoid arthritis. *Scandinavian Journal of Rheumatology* **12:** 69.

Parke A (1988) Antimalarial drugs and pregnancy. *American Journal of Medicine* **85:** 30–33.

Pearson HA & McIntosh S (1978) Neonatal thrombocytopenia. *Clinical Haematology* **7:** 111.

Pekonen F, Teramo K, Ikonen E, Osterlund K, Makinen T & Lamberg B-A (1984) Women on thyroid hormone therapy: pregnancy course, fetal outcome, and amniotic fluid thyroid hormone level. *Obstetrics and Gynecology* **63:** 635–638.

Perelman AH, Johnson RL, Clemons RD, Finberg HJ, Clewell WH & Trujillo L (1990) Intrauterine diagnosis and treatment of fetal goitrous hypothyroidism. *Journal of Clinical Endocrinology and Metabolism* **71:** 618–621.

Persillin RH (1977) The effect of pregnancy on rheumatoid arthritis. *Bulletin of the Rheumatic Diseases* **27:** 922.

Petri M, Howard D & Repke J (1991) Frequency of lupus flare in pregnancy; the Hopkins Lupus Pregnancy Center experience. *Arthritis and Rheumatism* **34(12):** 1538–1545.

Plauche WC (1983) Myasthenia gravis. *Clinical Obstetrics and Gynecology* **26(3):** 592–604.

Porreco RP & Bloch CA (1990) Fetal blood sampling in the management of intrauterine thyrotoxicosis. *Obstetrics and Gynaecology* **76(3):** 509–512.

Provost TT, Watson R, Gammon WR, Radowsky M, Harley JB & Reichlin M (1987) The neonatal lupus syndrome associated with U$_1$RNP (nRNP) antibodies. *Medical Intelligence* **316(18):** 1135–1138.

Purtilo DT & Sullivan SL (1979) Immunological bases for superior survival of females. *American Journal of Diseases of Children* **133:** 1251–1253.

Ramsey-Goldman R (1988) Pregnancy in systemic lupus erythematosus. *Rheumatic Disease Clinics of North America* **14(1):** 169–185.

Ramsey-Goldman R, Hom D, Deng JS et al (1986) Anti-SS-A antibodies and fetal outcome in maternal systemic lupus erythematosus. *Arthritis and Rheumatism* **29(10):** 1269–1273.

Rauch AE, Mycek JA, Mills CR et al (1990) Risk of thrombocytopenia in offspring of mothers with presumed immune thrombocytopenic purpura. *New England Journal of Medicine* **323(26):** 1841 (letter).

Reece EA, Romero R, Clyne LP et al (1984) Lupus like anticoagulant in pregnancy. *Lancet* i: 344.

Richards DS, Wagman AJ & Cabaniss ML (1990) Ascites not due to congestive heart failure in a fetus with lupus-induced heart block. *Obstetrics and Gynecology* **76:** 957–959.

598   R. M. SILVER AND D. WARE BRANCH

Rolbin SH, Levinson G, Shnider SM & Wright RG (1978) Anesthetic considerations for myasthenia gravis and pregnancy. *Anesthesia and Analgesia* **57**: 441.

Rosove MH, Tabsh K, Wassertrum N, Howard P, Hahn BH & Kalunian KC (1990) Heparin therapy for pregnant women with lupus anticoagulant or anticardiolipin antibodies. *Obstetrics and Gynecology* **75**: 630–634.

Roubinian JR, Talai N, Greenspan JS, Goodman JR & Siiteri PK (1978) Effect of castration and sex hormone treatment on survival, anti-nucleic acid antibodies, and glomerulonephritis in NZB/NZW F₁ mice. *Journal of Experimental Medicine* **147**: 1568–1582.

Rovet J, Ehrlich R & Sorbara D (1987) Intellectual outcome in children with fetal hypothyroidism. *Journal of Pediatrics* **110**: 700–704.

Ryan G, Lange IR & Naugler-Colville MA (1988) Phenytoin prophylaxis in severe pre-eclampsia and eclampsia. *Proceedings of the Fifth Congress of the International Society for the Study of Hypertension in Pregnancy*, Montreal.

Samuels P, Bussel JB, Braitman LE et al (1990) Estimation of the risk of thrombocytopenia in the offspring of pregnant women with presumed immune thrombocytopenia purpura. *New England Journal of Medicine* **323(4)**: 229–235.

Schur PH (1989) Clinical features of SLE. In Kelley WN, Harris ED, Ruddy S & Sledge CB (eds) *Textbook of Rheumatology*, p 1101. Philadelphia: W. B. Saunders.

Scioscia AL, Brannum PAT, Copel JA & Hobbins JC (1988) The use of percutaneous umbilical blood sampling in immune thrombocytopenic purpura. *American Journal of Obstetrics and Gynecology* **159**: 1066–1068.

Scopelitis E, Biundo JJ & Alspaugh MA (1980) Anti-SS-A antibody and other antinuclear antibodies in systemic lupus erythematosus. *Arthritis and Rheumatism* **23(3)**: 287–293.

Scott JR (1977) Fetal growth retardation associated with maternal administration of immuno-suppressive drugs. *American Journal of Obstetrics and Gynecology* **128**: 668.

Scott JR, Cruikshank DP, Kochenour NK, Pitkin RM & Warenski JC (1980) Fetal platelet counts in the obstetric management of immunologic thrombocytopenic purpura. *American Journal of Obstetrics and Gynecology* **136**: 495–499.

Scott JS, Maddison PJ, Taylor PV et al (1983) Connective-tissue disease, antibodies to ribonucleoprotein, and congenital heart block. *New England Journal of Medicine* **309**: 209–212.

Scott JR, Rote NS & Cruikshank DP (1983) Antiplatelet antibodies and platelet counts in pregnancies complicated by autoimmune thrombocytopenic purpura. *American Journal of Obstetrics and Gynecology* **145**: 932–939.

Shepard MK (1971) Arthrogryposis multiplex congenital in sibs. *Birth Defects* **7**: 127.

Siamopoulou-Mavridou A, Manoussakis MN, Mavridis AK & Moutsopoulos HM (1988) Outcome of pregnancy in patients with autoimmune rheumatic disease before the disease onset. *Annals of the Rheumatic Diseases* **47**: 982.

Silman AJ, Roman E, Beral V & Brown A (1988) Adverse reproductive outcomes in women who subsequently develop rheumatoid arthritis. *Annals of the Rheumatic Diseases* **47**: 979.

Smith WD & West HF (1960) Pregnancy in rheumatoid arthritis. *Acta Rheumatologica Scandinavica* **6**: 189.

Soliven BC, Lange DJ, Penn AS et al (1988) Seronegative myasthenia gravis. *Neurology* **38**: 514–517.

Steinberg AD, Melez KA, Raveche ES et al (1979) Approach to the study of the role of sex hormones in autoimmunity. *Arthritis and Rheumatism* **22**: 1170–1176.

Stephan MJ, Smith DW, Ponzi JW & Alden ER (1982) Origin of scalp vertex aplasia cutis. *Journal of Pediatrics* **101**: 850.

Stern R, Fishman J, Brusman H & Kunkel HG (1977) Systemic lupus erythematosus associated with Klinefelter's syndrome. *Arthritis and Rheumatism* **20(1)**: 18–22.

Stobo JD (1982) Rheumatoid arthritis—from Rubens to restriction maps. *Western Journal of Medicine* **137**: 109.

Stuart MJ, Gross SJ, Elrad H & Graeber JE (1982) Effects of acetylsalicylic acid injection on maternal and neonatal hemostasis. *New England Journal of Medicine* **307**: 909–912.

Tachi J, Amino N, Iwatani Y et al (1988a) Increase in antideoxyribonucleic acid antibody titer in postpartum aggravation of autoimmune thyroid disease. *Journal of Clinical Endocrinology and Metabolism* **67**: 1049–1053.

Tachi J, Amino M, Tamaki H, Aozasa M, Iwatani Y & Miyai K (1988b) Long term follow-up and HLA association in patients with postpartum hypothyroidism. *Journal of Clinical Endocrinology and Metabolism* **66:** 480–484.

Talal N (1989) Autoimmunity and sex revisited. *Clinical Immunology and Immunopathology* **53:** 355–357.

Tamaki H, Amino N, Aozasa M, Mori M, Tanizawa O & Miyai K (1987) Serial changes in thyroid stimulating antibody and thyrotropin binding inhibitor immunoglobulin at the time of postpartum occurrence of thyrotoxicosis in Graves' disease. *Journal of Clinical Endocrinology and Metabolism* **65:** 324–330.

Tan EM, Cohen AS, Fries JF et al (1982) The 1982 revised criteria for the classification of systemic lupus erythematosus. *Arthritis and Rheumatism* **25(11):** 1271–1277.

Taufield PA, Ales KL, Resnick LM et al (1987) Hypocalcuria in preeclampsia. *New England Journal of Medicine* **316(12):** 715–718.

Taylor PV, Scott JS, Gerlis LM, Path FRC, Esscher E & Scott O (1986) Maternal antibodies against fetal cardiac antigens in congenital complete heart block. *New England Journal of Medicine* **315:** 667–672.

Tervila L, Goecke C & Timonen S (1973) Estimation of gestosis of pregnancy (EPH-gestosis). *Acta Obstetrica et Gynecologica Scandinavica* **52:** 235.

Thomas R & Reid RL (1987) Thyroid disease and reproductive dysfunction: a review. *Obstetrics and Gynecology* **70:** 789–798.

Thorpe-Beeston JG, Nicolaides KH, Felton CV, Butler J & McGregor AM (1991) Maturation of the secretion of thyroid hormone and thyroid-stimulating hormone in the fetus. *New England Journal of Medicine* **324:** 532–536.

Tzartos SJ, Efthimiadis A, Morel E, Eymard B & Back JF (1990) Neonatal myasthenia gravis: antigenic specificities of antibodies in sera from mothers and their infants. *Clinical and Experimental Immunology* **80:** 376–380.

Utiger RD (1991a) The pathogenesis of autoimmune thyroid disease. *New England Journal of Medicine* **325(4):** 278–279.

Utiger RD (1991b) Recognition of thyroid disease in the fetus. *New England Journal of Medicine* **324:** 559–561.

Vanhaesebrouck P, Thiery M, Leroy JG et al (1988) Oligohydramnios, renal insufficiency, and ileal perforation in preterm infants after intrauterine exposure to indomethacin. *Journal of Pediatrics* **113:** 738–743.

Vargas MT, Briones-Urbina R, Gladman D, Papsin FR & Walfish PG (1988) Antithyroid microsomal autoantibodies and HLA-DR5 are associated with postpartum thyroid dysfunction; evidence supporting an autoimmune pathogenesis. *Journal of Clinical Endocrinology and Metabolism* **67:** 327.

Varner MW (1991) Autoimmune disorders and pregnancy. *Seminars in Perinatology* **15(3):** 238–250.

Varner MW, Meehan RT, Syrop CH, Strottman MP & Goplerud CP (1983) Pregnancy in patients with systemic lupus erythematosus. *American Journal of Obstetrics and Gynecology* **145(8):** 1025–1037.

Vulsma T, Gons MH & de Vijlder JJM (1989) Maternal–fetal transfer of thyroxine in congenital hypothyroidism due to a total organification defect or thyroid agenesis. *New England Journal of Medicine* **321:** 13–16.

Watson RM, Lane AT, Barnett NK et al (1984) Neonatal lupus erythematosus: a clinical, serological and immunogenetic study with review of the literature. *Medicine* **63(6):** 362–378.

Weiner CP, Kwaan HC, Xu C, Paul M, Burmeister L & Hauck W (1985) Antithrombin III activity in women with hypertension during pregnancy. *Obstetrics and Gynecology* **65(3):** 301–306.

Wenstrom KD, Weiner DP, Williamson RA & Grant SS (1990) Prenatal diagnosis of fetal hyperthyroidism using funipuncture. *Obstetrics and Gynecology* **76(3):** 513–517.

Wong KL, Chan FY & Lee CP (1991) Outcome of pregnancy in patients with systemic lupus erythematosus. *Archives of Internal Medicine* **151:** 269–273.

Yin CS & Scott JR (1985) Failure of maternal dexamethasone treatment to prevent immunological thrombocytopenia in the infant. *Obstetrics and Gynaecology* **152:** 316.

Yoshida H, Amino N, Yagawa K et al (1978) Association of serum antithyroid antibodies with lymphocytic infiltration of the thyroid gland: studies of seventy autopsied cases. *Journal of Clinical Endocrinology and Metabolism* **46:** 859–862.

Zulman JI, Talal N, Hoffman GS & Epstein WV (1979) Problems associated with the management of pregnancies in patients with systemic lupus erythematosus. *Journal of Rheumatology* **7(1):** 37–49.

Zurier RB, Argyros TG, Urman JD, Warren J & Rothfield NF (1978) Systemic lupus erythematosus. *Obstetrics and Gynecology* **51(2):** 178–180.

10

Immunological aspects of pre-eclampsia

C. W. G. REDMAN

Pre-eclampsia is primarily a placental disease, but its precise cause is unknown (Redman, 1991). It appears to develop in three stages: the first is deficient placentation (Brosens et al, 1972) which results in placental ischaemia. This ultimately leads to the maternal syndrome which is thought to be the result of a factor or factors released by the ischaemic placenta which cause generalized endothelial dysfunction (Roberts et al, 1989). Poor placentation affects the spiral arteries—the end arteries of the uteroplacental circulation—which fail to undergo the adaptive dilatation of pregnancy so that they retain the musculoelastic structure that is otherwise normally lost in the terminal segments. Subsequently the ability of these arteries to maintain an adequate uteroplacental blood flow is further compromised by an obstructive lesion called acute atherosis (Zeek and Assali, 1950), which comprises endothelial deposits of fibrin, aggregated platelets and fat-filled macrophages (foam cells).

Whereas poor placentation is a problem of the first half of pregnancy (6–18 weeks), the time course of the evolution of acute atherosis is not known. There is some evidence for its occurrence early in pregnancy (Lichtig et al, 1984) and it has been suggested that it might be a lesion with immune origins (Lichtig et al, 1985).

IMMUNE MECHANISMS AND THE PATHOGENESIS OF PRE-ECLAMPSIA

There is no unequivocal evidence that the cause of pre-eclampsia involves immune mechanisms. Pre-eclampsia is mainly a disorder of first pregnancy (MacGillivray, 1958); but not exclusively so, because a similar syndrome appears in multiparae, particularly those with a previous history of the condition (Campbell and MacGillivray, 1985). That the protective effect of parity might have an immunological basis has been considered for many years. However, it is not the only possible explanation. It could be that the connective tissue of the uterus and the structure of its arteries could be permanently altered by a pregnancy in a way that prevented poor placentation subsequently. However, a small number of studies have suggested that the protective effect of multiparity may be lost after a change of partner

(Feeney and Scott, 1980; Ikedife, 1980; Chng, 1982). If there is partner specificity then the only possible explanation would be immunological.

If the protective effect of parity has an immune basis, the implication is that pregnancy provokes a beneficial maternal immune response to the conceptus. This is the converse of Rhesus disease where the immune reaction is harmful, and the disease gets worse rather than better with succeeding pregnancies.

But what could be the nature of the acquired protection? The simplest hypothesis would be that a pre-eclamptic factor, presumably originating in the ischaemic placenta and directly 'toxic' to the mother, is neutralized by the formation of maternal antibodies. This would be plausible if the time course of pre-eclampsia were short and confined to the stage when overt signs are evident.

But pre-eclampsia is a disorder of placentation, and placentation involves a fetal–maternal interaction, occurring much earlier than the overt disease— at 6–18 weeks of gestation, immediately after implantation. This is an interesting time because if the fetus is an allograft this must be when it consolidates its position. It is therefore likely that immune mechanisms are involved in, if not control, placentation.

The essential feature of placentation is infiltration of a maternal tissue (the placental bed) by fetal cells (invasive trophoblast). This process that extends outwards from the basal plate into the decidua and myometrium alters the spiral arteries, turning them from thick-walled, small-bored vessels into thin-walled, widely dilated conduits.

If maternal immune responses controlled placentation, and at present there is no direct evidence that they do, then they would need to generate tolerance to prevent the otherwise inevitable immune rejection of the invasive fetal cells. Pre-eclampsia would arise because of a partial failure of this permissive response and hence of the adaptations that depend on adequate infiltration of the placental bed by trophoblast: although the pregnancy continued it would be compromised, particularly with respect to the ultimate provision of an adequate uteroplacental blood flow. There is an important corollary, namely, if maternal immune regulation were not merely partly deficient but failed completely there would be early fetal immune rejection and abortion; that is, the immune mechanisms for pre-eclampsia and recurrent spontaneous abortions could be the same.

Central to this hypothesis is the role of maternal–fetal incompatibility in determining whatever maternal immune responses might control the success or otherwise of placentation. This leads immediately to the related subject of preimmunization: can the adverse immune effects of maternal–fetal incompatibility be ameliorated by prior exposure to paternal antigens stimulating a protective immune response? Is this how a previous pregnancy protects women from pre-eclampsia? If so, are all pregnancies equally protective, regardless of gestational maturity, and are there other modes of preimmunization that are also protective? It should be noted parenthetically that preimmunization is the central (and contentious) issue concerning the prevention of recurrent spontaneous abortions by immunotherapy.

Previous exposure to paternal antigens in a pregnancy ending in induced abortion appears to confer some protection from pre-eclampsia (Strickland et al, 1986; Seidman et al, 1989) although not everyone can detect this effect (Campbell and MacGillivray, 1985). Prior exposure to paternal antigens on sperm seems to give similar protection (Klonoff-Cohen et al, 1989) as the incidence of pre-eclampsia is higher amongst women who use barrier methods of contraception. Conception by donor insemination creates a converse situation of little or no prior exposure where the incidence of pre-eclampsia might be predicted to be unduly high. Unfortunately there are no good controlled studies although the largest uncontrolled study showed an apparently high incidence of pre-eclampsia (Need et al, 1983). A previous blood transfusion has also been reported to be protective (Feeney et al, 1977).

If maternal–fetal immune incompatibility were important in the origins of pre-eclampsia then it would be expected to be a genetic condition, perhaps involving the HLA system which is the strongest known determinant of immune incompatibility between individuals.

GENETIC FACTORS AND MATERNAL–FETAL INCOMPATIBILITY

Pre-eclampsia is well known to be familial. There is an increased frequency of the disease in the mothers but not the mothers-in-law of pre-eclamptic women (Sutherland et al, 1981) and in the daughters of eclamptic women. In one study the daughters of pre-eclamptic women were affected particularly if they themselves were the offspring of the affected pregnancy (Cooper et al, 1988), in another this was irrelevant (Arngrimsson et al, 1990). The familial pattern can be explained by postulating a recessive maternal gene with an estimated population frequency of about 25% (Chesley and Cooper, 1986). The data from family studies are best explained if both the mother and the offspring share the recessive gene (Liston and Kilpatrick, 1991).

The exceptionally high incidence of pre-eclampsia and eclampsia in one inbred family (Brocklehurst and Ross, 1960) is consistent with the recessive gene hypothesis. On the other hand, less, not more, pre-eclampsia was observed in an inbred Turkish community (Stevenson et al, 1971), and more of the disease was reported with marriages involving racial mixes, that is, more outbred than usual (Alderman et al, 1986).

If the maternal genotype were the only factor then identical twin sisters would be expected always to have concordant pregnancy histories. A recent report of a well authenticated pair, with severely affected and normal first pregnancies respectively (Thornton and Sampson, 1990), underlines the point that this may not be a simple inherited condition. The analogy is with Rhesus disease: identical twin sisters, both Rh negative, could differ in their pregnancy histories depending on the rhesus types of their partners.

There are some hints that the fetal genotype may contribute. For example pre-eclampsia occurs more commonly with the fetal chromosomal abnormalities of triploidy (Toaff and Peyser, 1976) and trisomy 13 (Bower et al, 1987; Boyd et al, 1987). However, when immune mechanisms controlling placentation are under consideration then the role of the fetal genotype may be that it is a factor determining maternal–fetal incompatibility. Cases that have been described where a particular male partner seemed to confer the susceptibility to severe disease (Astin et al, 1981), lend support to this concept. The genetics of maternal–fetal incompatibility are complex (Penrose, 1947) and may simulate straightforward maternal inheritance, as is observed with pre-eclampsia.

There is evidence that male fetuses are more immunogenic than females: in one-way reactions, maternal lymphocytes respond more vigorously to a son's stimulating cells than to those of HLA-identical female siblings (Komlos et al, 1990). Some have reported a modest excess of male fetuses in pre-eclamptic pregnancies (Toivanen and Hirvonen, 1970), not confirmed by others (Juberg et al, 1976); but in a recent analysis of all the reports a significant association with male fetuses was found (James, 1987).

Pre-eclampsia is commoner with multiple pregnancies. A report of a higher incidence with the more incompatible dizygous twins (Stevenson et al, 1976) was refuted (McFarlane and Scott, 1976), to be later followed by a claim to the contrary—of more pre-eclampsia with the less incompatible monozygous twins (McMullan et al, 1984).

The most extreme incompatibility occurs with in vitro fertilization of a donated oocyte (Tait et al, 1984). There are no good data, but early reports comment on an apparently high incidence of pre-eclampsia (Serhal and Craft, 1987).

PRE-ECLAMPSIA AND THE HLA SYSTEM

If maternal–fetal incompatibility is important in determining an aberrant immune relationship leading to poor placentation and later pre-eclampsia, then it is most likely to involve the HLA system.

Excessive HLA compatibility between partners has been considered to underlie immunologically mediated recurrent abortions (Gill, 1983) although it is not consistently observed (see Redman, 1990a for a review). The same association has been claimed in pre-eclamptic couples (Jenkins et al, 1978; Bolis et al, 1987) although, once again, others cannot confirm the finding (Johnson et al, 1988). Recently pre-eclampsia has been associated with increased maternal–fetal sharing of HLA–DR4 (Kilpatrick et al, 1990), which has reactivated the concept.

An excess of HLA homozygosity, particularly at the B locus (Redman et al, 1978) was also not confirmed (Johnson et al, 1988) although a similar pattern was reported in women with recurrent spontaneous abortions (Johnson et al, 1984). If the association were real it would have the effect of reducing incompatibility between mother and fetus without increasing the degree of sharing.

The emphasis on HLA incompatibility as a possible determinant of success of the fetal allograft is historical rather than logical—arising from the belief that the fetal allograft should be like other allografts. In fact the engrafted tissue is trophoblast which does not express HLA-A, B, C or D, the polymorphic strong histocompatibility determinants. Instead, some forms of trophoblast, particularly those in direct contact with maternal tissues rather than blood, express a novel, non-polymorphic HLA antigen—HLA-G (Ellis, 1990). HLA-G has no known function, immune or otherwise, but, it must be supposed, is involved in some way in interactions with maternal cells in the decidua.

The unusual HLA expression by trophoblast precludes the possibility that maternal T cells, cytotoxic or helper, can respond directly to trophoblast—reviewed elsewhere (Redman, 1990b). This explains why maternal sensitization to fetal HLA is a sporadic event (Sargent et al, 1988), possibly the result of random breaks in the integrity of the syncytiotrophoblast either temporarily exposing underlying placental stromal cells, or permitting small fetomaternal bleeds, such as are known to provoke Rhesus sensitization. But the lack of classical HLA may increase the susceptibility of trophoblast to non-adaptive immunity, for example, mediated by natural killer cells (Ljunggren and Karre, 1990).

Thus it is likely that the immune interaction between mother and fetus is more analogous to that of a host–tumour than host–graft relationship.

An association with HLA may be unrelated to maternal–fetal immune incompatibility, but instead may reflect the importance of other, closely linked genes which predispose to, or cause, pre-eclampsia and account for its familial incidence. Although pre-eclampsia has been associated with HLA-DR4 (Simon et al, 1988; Kilpatrick et al, 1990) this has now been excluded by detailed genetic analysis of the restriction fragment length polymorphisms of HLA-DRB in informative pedigrees (Wilton et al, 1990) and the association probably indicates an underlying tendency to autoimmune disease with which HLA-DR4 is linked.

In summary, there is little consistent evidence that HLA genes are involved in pre-eclampsia although maternal–fetal incompatibility could still be relevant. HLA antigens are not the only determinants of immune reactivity so there is still the need to consider the more direct evidence of how the maternal immune system recognizes and responds to the fetus in pre-eclampsia.

Virtually all of the rest of our knowledge of immune disturbances in pre-eclampsia related to the end stages of the disease, in particular, to changes in maternal peripheral blood cells, immunoglobulins and the complement system. But before these are summarized, it is appropriate (in relation to a placental disease) to consider whether the histopathology of the placentas of pre-eclamptic women suggests immunological disturbances.

IMMUNE CAUSES FOR THE PLACENTAL PATHOLOGY

It is to be expected that at delivery the placentas of pre-eclamptic women would show features more of ischaemia than of immunologically mediated processes. This is, in general, the case although some reports seek to emphasize the possibility that immune damage is occurring in the placenta during the second stage of the illness.

Placentas of pre-eclamptic women contain more intense deposits of C1q, C3d and C9, distributed in the same way as in normal placentas: patchily in the larger fetal stem vessels (C1q and C9); or focally in the trophoblast basement membrane (C3d and C9). There are no differences in the amount or distribution of C4 and C6 (Sinha et al, 1984). A quantitative rather than qualitative difference in distribution was also seen using an antibody detecting C9 bound to the cytolytic terminal complement complex (Tedesco et al, 1990). These observations provide some evidence for an inflammatory process, but none that it is immunologically mediated. It could still be the result, for example, of ischaemic tissue damage.

There is more evidence of a possible immune process in the lesion of chronic villitis of unknown origin (Altshuler and Russell, 1975). The tertiary and terminal villi are infiltrated with a mixture predominantly of histiocytes and lymphocytes, amongst which there may also be fibroblasts, polymorphonuclear leukocytes, plasma cells and multinucleate giant cells. All of one villus, or a cluster of villi, are diffusely involved; there may be secondary obliterative vasculitis of the fetal vessels and perivillous deposition of fibrin occluding the intervillous space. In a proportion of cases, the intervillous space may also contain inflammatory cells and the decidua, focal lymphocytic infiltrates (Russell, 1980).

Although the problem is associated with pre-eclampsia (Labarrere and Althabe, 1986) it has been more closely linked to intrauterine growth retardation (Labarrere et al, 1982). Since both clinical syndromes may be separate consequences of the same primary placental disturbance, this need not be evidence that the villitis is merely an inconstantly associated feature. Nevertheless, it is questioned that the associations with pre-eclampsia or intrauterine growth retardation exist at all (Knox and Fox, 1984) and on the present evidence it is hard to conclude that this sort of lesion demonstrates that a disturbance of maternal immune tolerance of the placenta underlies pre-eclampsia.

Thus although the processes affecting the maternal spiral arteries may have immune origins, there is little convincing evidence of direct immune pathology in the placenta. Most of the changes in peripheral blood components in pre-eclampsia were sought in relation to the concept that the second stage of the illness is immunologically mediated. This does not fit the model being presented here. If the placental ischaemia theory is correct then any changes detected would be secondary, perhaps contributing to the total pathology but not essential for its initiation. However, the observations concerning peripheral blood leukocytes, immunoglobulins and complement components will be briefly examined.

PERIPHERAL BLOOD LEUKOCYTES

During normal pregnancy there is a significant leukocytosis, owing mainly to an increased number of neutrophils (Pitkin and Witte, 1979), but also of monocytes (Plum et al, 1978). The absolute numbers of lymphocytes, particularly T cells, are either unchanged (Cornfield et al, 1979) or reduced slightly (Moore et al, 1983a). Although some have suggested that normal pregnancy is associated with a relative reduction of CD4+ helper T cells (Sridama et al, 1982) this has not been confirmed (e.g. Moore et al, 1983a).

In pre-eclampsia the composition of peripheral blood leukocytes is largely unchanged. No consistent pattern emerges from various reports. There have been suggestions that the proportion of T cells is reduced (Sridama et al, 1983), and that of T helper cells is increased (Moore et al, 1983b), or, conversely, reduced (Bardeguez et al, 1991); the numbers of monocytes have been reported to be increased (Gusdon et al, 1984)—but not in all studies (Moore et al, 1983b).

MATERNAL CELL-MEDIATED IMMUNITY IN PRE-ECLAMPSIA

There is also no clear evidence that immune cell function is altered in peripheral blood. At first, evidence of maternal sensitization to paternal or fetal HLA was sought with the hypothesis that pre-eclampsia resulted from alloimmune rejection of the conceptus. In three studies abnormal sensitization was found using different assay systems and measuring maternal responses to placental antigens (Toder et al, 1979), paternal cells (Halbrecht and Komlos, 1974) or fetal cells (Gille et al, 1977). In contrast, depressed one-way MLR between maternal and paternal or fetal cells (Jenkins et al, 1978), or normal one- or two-way responses (Curzen et al, 1977; Sargent et al, 1982) were also reported. No evidence was found for paternal-specific cytotoxic cells in the immediate postpartum period (Redman et al, 1984).

There has been one report of significant increases in serum interleukin 2 concentrations in pre-eclampsia interpreted as evidence for maternal immune cell stimulation by fetal alloantigens (Sunder-Plassmann et al, 1989). Another, of increased but otherwise undefined mitogenic activity, measured with fibroblasts, has been presented as possible evidence for maternal endothelial cell damage, perhaps secondary to increased release of platelet derived growth factor, a product of endothelium as well as platelets (Musci et al, 1988).

Studies of peripheral blood natural killer (NK) cell activity have yielded conflicting results. Significantly increased (Toder et al, 1983), unchanged (Hill et al, 1986) or decreased (Alanen and Lassila, 1982) activity has been reported in pre-eclampsia.

POLYMORPHONUCLEAR CELL FUNCTION

Not only are the numbers of peripheral blood neutrophils increased during normal pregnancy but their functions are altered. Phagocytosis (Kvarstein and Gjonnaess, 1981) and spontaneous migration (Gleicher et al, 1980) are enhanced and there is metabolic activation (Mitchell et al, 1970).

There are no reports of altered granulocyte counts in pre-eclampsia but it has been proposed that the neutrophils are abnormally activated (Greer et al, 1989). This concept is based on the observation that, although neutrophil elastase immunoreactivity in peripheral blood plasma is increased in normal pregnancy, it is significantly higher in pre-eclampsia, but not in proportion to the clinical grading of the condition. The same authors suggest that neutrophil activation could lead to endothelial damage, the putative mechanism of end-stage pre-eclampsia suggested by Roberts et al (1989).

SERUM IMMUNOGLOBULINS

Normal pregnancy is associated with reduced serum concentrations of IgG and IgA but increases in IgD (Studd, 1971). Serum IgM concentrations have been reported to fall during the second trimester but return to normal levels towards term (Best et al, 1969) but others have not confirmed this pattern (Studd, 1971).

Maternal serum concentrations of IgG but not IgA are significantly reduced in pre-eclampsia (Benster and Wood, 1970; Studd, 1971). The pattern with respect to IgM is inconsistent, but its concentration is unaccountably increased in the cord sera of infants born to pre-eclamptic or eclamptic women (Yang et al, 1973). There are single reports of significantly reduced IgD (Studd, 1971) and increased IgE (Alanen, 1984) concentrations in pre-eclamptic sera. The fall in IgG has been ascribed to losses in urine associated with proteinuria but this cannot account for the different patterns of changes in serum IgA and IgE. A full explanation of the mechanisms and relevance of what is observed has yet to be given.

HLA ANTIBODIES

The hypothesis that lymphocytotoxic HLA antibodies might stimulate rejection of the fetal allograft is now known to be inappropriate. But the functions of maternal HLA antibodies as blocking antibodies have been emphasized, and an absolute or relative deficiency postulated when pregnancy fails such as with recurrent abortions or pre-eclampsia. Most investigators have examined the occurrence of lymphocytotoxic antibodies, rather than B cell antibodies or non-complement fixing antibodies. In pre-eclampsia, increased (Carretti et al, 1974), unchanged (Harris and Lordon, 1976) or reduced (Jenkins et al, 1977) concentrations have been reported. In only one study have HLA-DR antibodies been examined (Balasch et al, 1981), which showed no differences between pre-eclamptic and normal women.

It is most probable that HLA antibodies are formed sporadically, as a result of fetomaternal bleeding, usually at delivery, and have no significance. They do not affect the fetus for two reasons: because trophoblast does not express the relevant HLA antigens and because after they are transported across the trophoblast barrier, they are absorbed by the placental stroma (Doughty and Gelsthorpe, 1976).

OTHER ANTIBODIES

Since HLA antibodies are not involved, abnormal antibodies generated directly against trophoblast or other components of the placenta have been sought. If present, they could generate circulating immune complexes which might account for some of the features of pre-eclampsia, or render trophoblast cells susceptible to lysis by cytolytic cells. Such antibodies have been detected but none of the reports has been confirmed. For example, pre-eclampsia has been associated with maternal antibodies to placental polysaccharides (Kaku, 1953), to a placental microsomal fraction (Gaugas and Curzen, 1974), to trophoblast cells (Hulka and Brinton, 1963), to retroviral antigens contained within the placenta (Thiry et al, 1981) or to placental basement membrane (Bieglmayer et al, 1986).

An alternative approach is that at least some aspects of the pre-eclampsia syndrome may be caused by autoantibodies. It is well known, for example, that autoimmunity is a predisposing factor particularly when associated with systemic lupus erythematosus and either the lupus anticoagulant or anti-phospholipid antibodies (Branch et al, 1989) although such antibodies are not found in the majority of cases (Taylor et al, 1991). An increased prevalence of autoantibodies to endothelium (Rapaport et al, 1990), laminin (Foidart et al, 1986), smooth muscle (Alanen, 1984) or platelets (Samuels et al, 1987) in pre-eclamptic women has been reported.

IMMUNE COMPLEXES IN PRE-ECLAMPSIA

Circulating immune complexes may activate blocking or aggressive immune mechanisms and their possible presence in the blood of either normal or pre-eclamptic pregnant women is therefore of some interest. Unfortunately, there is no agreement between different investigators on this issue (summarized by Redman and Sargent, 1986). In pre-eclampsia deposits of immune complexes have been found in skin (Houwert-de Jong et al, 1982) and renal biopsies (Petrucco et al, 1974). But the renal histology is not consistent, nor comparable to that seen in unequivocal immune complex disease (Kincaid-Smith and Fairley, 1976). However, changes in the complement system include one feature that is typical of immune complex disorders.

THE COMPLEMENT SYSTEM

Changes in the serum concentrations of components of the complement system would be expected in an illness with highly disturbed coagulation function and diffuse endothelial dysfunction. Total haemolytic complement and C1q concentrations remain unchanged (Kitzmiller et al, 1973, for example). Plasma C3 concentrations are normal (Yang et al, 1973) or increased (Thomson et al, 1976) and there are increases in the products of its activity—C3a and C5a (Haeger et al, 1989). However, the changes do not precede the onset of the clinical syndrome (Haeger et al, 1991). Serum concentrations of C4 are reduced relative to normal (Houwert-de Jong et al, 1985; Hofmeyr et al, 1991) as they are in conditions such as active lupus erythematosus characterized by circulating immune complexes.

SUMMARY

The first pregnancy preponderance and apparent partner specificity of pre-eclampsia suggest that it might have an immune aetiology. The pathogenesis of pre-eclampsia is undefined although it is clear that it is a placental disorder. The maternal syndrome appears to be mediated by placental ischaemia secondary to spiral artery insufficiency. This leads to a hypothesis that pre-eclampsia is a two-stage disease. The first comprises processes that limit the size of the spiral arteries (poor placentation) or obstruct them (acute atherosis). Either or both may have immunological causes although there is no direct evidence. Factors limiting placentation could involve maternal immune intolerance of the fetal allograft, which in their most extreme expression could lead to immunologically mediated abortion. Thus pre-eclampsia may be part of a wider spectrum of pregnancy loss secondary to poor maternal immune accommodation of her genetically disparate fetus.

The second stage involves the consequences of the ensuing placental ischaemia. The syndrome is currently tentatively ascribed to diffuse maternal endothelial dysfunction. There is less reason to invoke immunological mechanisms in the second stage although neutrophil activation could explain generalized endothelial damage.

It should be clear that these conclusions are provisional and that the greatest need is for more investigation to eliminate the uncertainty which clouds our concepts.

REFERENCES

Alanen A (1984) Serum IgE and smooth muscle antibodies in preeclampsia. *Acta Obstetrica et Gynecologica Scandinavica* **63:** 581–582.
Alanen A & Lassila O (1982) Deficient natural killer cell function in pre-eclampsia. *Obstetrics and Gynecology* **60:** 631–634.
Alderman BW, Sperling RS & Daling JR (1986) An epidemiological study of the immunogenetic aetiology of pre-eclampsia. *British Medical Journal* **292:** 372–374.
Altshuler G & Russell P (1975) The human placental villitides: a review of chronic intrauterine infection. *Current Topics in Pathology* **60:** 63–112.
Arngrimsson R, Bjornsson S, Geirsson RT, Bjornsson H, Walker JT and Snaedal G (1990) Genetic and familial predisposition to eclampsia and pre-eclampsia in a defined population. *British Journal of Obstetrics and Gynaecology* **97:** 762–769.
Astin M, Scott JR & Worley RJ (1981) Pre-eclampsia/eclampsia: the fatal father factor. *Lancet* **ii:** 533.
Balasch J, Ercilla G, Vanrell JA, Vives J & Gonzalez-Merlo J (1981) Effects of HLA antibodies on pregnancy. *Obstetrics and Gynecology* **57:** 444–446.
Bardeguez AD, McNerney R, Frieri M, Verma UL & Tejani N (1991) Cellular immunity in preeclampsia: alterations in T-lymphocyte subpopulations during early pregnancy. *Obstetrics and Gynecology* **77:** 859–862.

Benster B & Wood EJ (1970) Immunoglobulin levels in normal pregnancy and pregnancy complicated by hypertension. *Journal of Obstetrics and Gynaecology of the British Commonwealth* **77:** 518–522.

Best JM, Bannatvala JE & Watson D (1969) Serum IgM and IgG responses in postnatally acquired rubella. *Lancet* **ii:** 65–68.

Bieglmayer C, Rudelstorfer R, Bartl W & Janisch H (1986) Detection of antibodies in pregnancy serum reacting with isolated placental basement membrane collagen. *British Journal of Obstetrics and Gynaecology* **93:** 815–822.

Bolis PF, Bianchi MM, La Fianza A, Franchi M & Belvedere MC (1987) Immunogenetic aspects of pre-eclampsia. *Biological Research in Pregnancy* **8:** 42–45.

Bower C, Stanley F & Walters BNJ (1987) Pre-eclampsia and trisomy 13. *Lancet* **ii:** 1032.

Boyd PA, Lindenbaum RH & Redman CWG (1987) Pre-eclampsia and trisomy 13: a possible association. *Lancet* **ii:** 425–427.

Branch DW, Andres R, Digre KB, Rote NS & Scott JR (1989) The association of antiphospholipid antibodies with severe preeclampsia. *Obstetrics and Gynecology* **73:** 541–545.

Brocklehurst JC & Ross R (1960) Familial eclampsia. *Journal of Obstetrics and Gynaecology of the British Commonwealth* **67:** 971–974.

Brosens IA, Robertson WB & Dixon HG (1972) The role of the spiral arteries in the pathogenesis of pre-eclampsia. In Wynn RM (ed.) *Obstetrics and Gynecology Annual*, pp 177–191. New York: Appleton Century-Crofts.

Campbell DM & MacGillivray I (1985) Pre-eclampsia in second pregnancy. *British Journal of Obstetrics and Gynaecology* **82:** 131–140.

Carretti N, Chiaramonte P, Pasini C, Zanetti M & Fagiolo U (1974) Association of anti-HLA antibodies with toxemia in pregnancy. In Centaro A, Carretti N & Addison GM (eds) *Immunology in Obstetrics and Gynecology*, pp 221–225. Amsterdam: Excerpta Medica.

Chesley LC & Cooper DW (1986) Genetics of hypertension in pregnancy: possible single gene control of preeclampsia and eclampsia in the descendants of eclamptic women. *British Journal of Obstetrics and Gynaecology* **93:** 898–908.

Chng PK (1982) Occurrence of pre-eclampsia in pregnancies to three husbands. Case report. *British Journal of Obstetrics and Gynaecology* **89:** 862–863.

Cooper DW, Hill JA, Chesley LC & Bryans CI (1988) Genetic control of susceptibility to eclampsia and miscarriage. *British Journal of Obstetrics and Gynaecology* **95:** 644–653.

Cornfield DB, Jemcks J, Binder RA & Rath CE (1979) T and B lymphocytes in pregnant women. *Obstetrics and Gynecology* **53:** 203–206.

Curzen P, Jones E & Gaugas JM (1977) Maternal–fetal mixed lymphocyte reactivity in pre-eclampsia. *British Journal of Experimental Pathology* **58:** 500–503.

Doughty RW & Gelsthorpe K (1976) Some parameters of lymphocyte antibody activity through pregnancy and further eluates of placental material. *Tissue Antigens* **8:** 43–48.

Ellis S (1990) HLA G: at the interface. *American Journal of Reproductive Immunology* **23:** 84–86.

Feeney JG & Scott JS (1980) Pre-eclampsia and changed paternity. *European Journal of Obstetrics, Gynecology and Reproductive Biology* **11:** 35–38.

Feeney JG, Tovey LAD & Scott JS (1977) Influence of previous blood transfusions on incidence of pre-eclampsia. *Lancet* **i:** 874–877.

Foidart JM, Hunt J, Lapiere C-M et al (1986) Antibodies to laminin in preeclampsia. *Kidney International* **29:** 1050–1057.

Gaugas JM & Curzen P (1974) Complement fixing antibody against solubilized placental microsomal fraction in pre-eclampsia sera. *British Journal of Pathology* **55:** 570–573.

Gill TJ (1983) Immunogenetics of spontaneous abortion in humans. *Transplantation* **35:** 1–6.

Gille J, Williams JH & Hoffman CP (1977) The feto-maternal lymphocyte interaction in pre-eclampsia and in uncomplicated pregnancy. *European Journal of Obstetrics, Gynecology and Reproductive Biology* **7:** 227–238.

Gleicher N, Beers P, Kerenyi TD, Cohen CJ & Gusberg SB (1980) Leukocyte migration enhancement as an indicator of immunologic enhancement. I. Pregnancy. *American Journal of Obstetrics and Gynecology* **136:** 1–4.

Greer IA, Haddad NG, Dawes J, Johnstone FD & Calder AA (1989) Neutrophil activation in pregnancy-induced hypertension. *British Journal of Obstetrics and Gynaecology* **96:** 978–982.

Gusdon JP, Heise ER, Quinn KJ & Matthews LC (1984) Lymphocyte subpopulations in normal and preeclampsia pregnancies. *American Journal of Reproductive Immunology* **5:** 28–31.

Haeger M, Bengstson A, Karlsson K & Heideman M (1989) Complement activation and anaphylatoxin (C3a and C5a) formation in preeclampsia and by amniotic fluid. *Obstetrics and Gynecology* **73:** 551–556.

Haeger M, Unander M & Bengtsson A (1991) Complement activation in relation to development of preeclampsia. *Obstetrics and Gynecology* **78:** 46–49.

Halbrecht IG & Komlos L (1974) Mixed wife–husband leukocyte cultures in disturbed and pathological pregnancies. *Israel Journal of Medical Science* **10:** 1100–1105.

Harris RE & Lordon RE (1976) The association of maternal lymphocytotoxic antibodies with obstetric complications. *Obstetrics and Gynecology* **48:** 302–304.

Hill JA, Hsia S, Doran DM & Bryans CI (1986) Natural killer cell activity and antibody dependent cell-mediated cytotoxicity in preeclampsia. *Journal of Reproductive Immunology* **9:** 205–212.

Hofmeyr GJ, Wilkins T & Redman CWG (1991) C4 and plasma protein in hypertension during pregnancy with and without proteinuria. *British Medical Journal* **302:** 218.

Houwert-de Jong MH, Te Velde ER, Nefkens MJJ & Schuurman HJ (1982) Immune complexes in skin of patient with pre-eclamptic toxaemia. *Lancet* **ii:** 387.

Houwert-de Jong MH, Claas FHJ, Gmelig-Meyling FHJ et al (1985) Humoral immunity in normal and complicated pregnancy. *Journal of Reproductive Immunology* **19:** 205–214.

Hulka JF & Brinton V (1963) Antibody to trophoblast during early postpartum period in toxemic pregnancy. *American Journal of Obstetrics and Gynecology* **86:** 130–134.

Ikedife D (1980) Eclampsia in multiparae. *British Medical Journal* **280:** 985–986.

James WH (1987) The human sex ratio. Part 1: a review of the literature. *Human Biology* **59:** 721–752.

Jenkins DM, Need JA & Rajah SM (1977) Deficiency of specific HLA antibodies in severe pregnancy pre-eclampsia/eclampsia. *Clinical and Experimental Immunology* **27:** 485–486.

Jenkins DM, Need JA, Scott JS, Morris H & Pepper M (1978) Human leukocyte antigens and mixed lymphocyte reaction in severe preeclampsia. *British Medical Journal* **1:** 542–544.

Johnson N, Moodley J & Hammond MG (1988) Human leucocyte antigen status in African women with eclampsia. *British Journal of Obstetrics and Gynaecology* **95:** 877–879.

Johnson PM, Barnes RM, Hart CA & Francis WJA (1984) Determinants of immunological responsiveness in recurrent spontaneous abortion. *Transplantation* **38:** 280–284.

Juberg RC, Gaar DG, Humphries JR, Cenac PL & Zambie MF (1976) Sex ratio in the progeny of mothers with toxemia of pregnancy. *Journal of Reproductive Medicine* **16:** 299–302.

Kaku M (1953) Placental polysaccharide and the aetiology of the toxaemia of pregnancy. *Journal of Obstetrics and Gynaecology of the British Empire* **60:** 148–156.

Kilpatrick DC, Liston WA, Jazwinska EC & Smart GE (1990) Histocompatibility studies in pre-eclampsia. *Tissue Antigens* **29:** 232–236.

Kincaid-Smith P & Fairley KC (1976) The differential diagnosis between pre-eclamptic toxemia and glomerulo-nephritis in patients with proteinuria during pregnancy. In Lindheimer MD, Katz AI & Zuspan FP (eds) *Hypertension in Pregnancy* pp 157–168. Chichester: John Wiley.

Kitzmiller JL, Stoneburner L, Yelenosky PF & Lucas WE (1973) Serum complement in normal pregnancy and pre-eclampsia. *American Journal of Obstetrics and Gynecology* **117:** 312–315.

Klonoff-Cohen HS, Savitz DA, Cefalo RC & McCann MF (1989) An epidemiologic study of contraception and preeclampsia. *Journal of the American Medical Association* **262:** 3143–3147.

Knox WF & Fox H (1984) Villitis of unknown aetiology: its incidence and significance in placentae from a British population. *Placenta* **5:** 393–402.

Komlos L, Vardimon D, Notmann J et al (1990) Role of children's sex in mixed lymphocyte culture reactivity. *American Journal of Reproductive Immunology* **22:** 4–8.

Kvarstein B & Gjonnaess H (1981) The influence of pregnancy and contraceptive pills upon oxygen consumption during phagocytosis by human leukocytes. *Acta Obstetrica et Gynaecologica Scandinavica* **60:** 505–506.

Labarrere C & Althabe O (1986) Chronic villitis of unknown aetiology and decidual maternal vasculopathies in sustained chronic hypertension. *European Journal of Obstetrics, Gynecology and Reproductive Biology* **21:** 27–32.

Labarrere C, Althabe O & Telenta M (1982) Chronic villitis of unknown aetiology in placentae of idiopathic small for gestational age infants. *Placenta* **3:** 309–317.

Lichtig C, Deutsch M & Brandes J (1984) Vascular changes of endometrium in early pregnancy. *American Journal of Clinical Pathology* **81:** 702–707.

Lichtig C, Deutsch M & Brandes J (1985) Immunofluorescent studies of the endometrial arteries in the first trimester of pregnancy. *American Journal of Clinical Pathology* **83:** 633–636.

Liston WA & Kilpatrick DC (1991) Is genetic susceptibility to pre-eclampsia conferred by homozygosity for the same single recessive gene in mother and fetus? *British Journal of Obstetrics and Gynaecology* **98:** 1079–1086.

Ljunggren H-G & Karre K (1990) In search of 'missing self': MHC molecules and NK cell recognition. *Immunology Today* **11:** 237–244.

McFarlane A & Scott JS (1975) Pre-eclampsia/eclampsia in twin pregnancies. *Journal of Medical Genetics* **13:** 208–211.

MacGillivray I (1958) Some observations on the incidence on pre-eclampsia. *Journal of Obstetrics and Gynaecology of the British Commonwealth* **65:** 536–539.

McMullan PF, Norman RJ & Marivate M (1984) Pregnancy-induced hypertension in twin pregnancy. *British Journal of Obstetrics and Gynaecology* **91:** 240–243.

Mitchell GW, Jacobs AA, Haddad V, Paul BB, Strauss RR & Sbarra AJ (1970) The role of phagocyte in host–parasite interactions. XXV. Metabolic and bactericidal activities of leukocytes from pregnant women. *American Journal of Obstetrics and Gynecology* **108:** 805–813.

Moore MP, Carter NP & Redman CWG (1983a) Lymphocyte subsets defined by monoclonal antibodies in human pregnancy. *American Journal of Reproductive Immunology* **3:** 161–164.

Moore MP, Carter NP & Redman CWG (1983b) Lymphocyte subsets in normal and pre-eclamptic pregnancies. *British Journal of Obstetrics and Gynaecology* **90:** 326–331.

Musci TJ, Roberts JM, Rodgers GM & Taylor RN (1988) Mitogenic activity is increased in the sera of preeclamptic women before delivery. *American Journal of Obstetrics and Gynecology* **159:** 1446–1451.

Need JA, Bell B, Meffin E & Jones WR (1983) Pre-eclampsia in pregnancies from donor inseminations. *Journal of Reproductive Immunology* **5:** 329–338.

Penrose LS (1947) On the familial appearances of maternal and foetal incompatibility. *Annals of Eugenics* **13:** 141–145.

Petrucco OM, Thomson NM, Lawrence JR & Weldon MW (1974) Immunofluorescent studies in renal biopsies in pre-eclampsia. *British Medical Journal* **1:** 473–476.

Pitkin RM & Witte DL (1979) Platelet and leukocyte counts in pregnancy. *Journal of the American Medical Association* **242:** 2696–2698.

Plum J, Thiery M & Sabre L (1978) Distribution of mononuclear cells during pregnancy. *Clinical and Experimental Immunology* **31:** 45–49.

Rapaport VJ, Hirata G, Yap HK & Jordan SC (1990) Anti-vascular endothelial cell antibodies in severe preeclampsia. *American Journal of Obstetrics and Gynecology* **162:** 138–146.

Redman CWG (1990a) Does immune abortion exist? Are there immunologically mediated mechanisms? If so, which mechanisms? *Research in Immunology* **141:** 169–175.

Redman CWG (1990b) The fetal allograft. *Fetal Medicine Review* **2:** 21–43.

Redman CWG (1991) Pre-eclampsia and the placenta. *Placenta* **12:** 301–308.

Redman CWG & Sargent IL (1986) Immunological disorders of human pregnancy. *Oxford Reviews of Reproductive Biology* **8:** 223–265.

Redman CWG, Bodmer JG, Bodmer WF, Beilin LJ & Bonnar J (1978) HLA antigens in severe pre-eclampsia. *Lancet* **ii:** 397–399.

Redman CWG, Sargent IL & Sutton L (1984) Immunological aspects of human pregnancy and its disorders. In Crighton DB (ed.) *Immunological Aspects of Reproduction in Mammals*, pp 219–250. London: Butterworth Scientific Ltd.

Roberts JM, Taylor RN, Musci TJ, Rodgers DM, Hubel CA & McLaughlin MK (1989) Preeclampsia: an endothelial cell disorder. *American Journal of Obstetrics and Gynecology* **161:** 1200–1204.

Russell P (1980) Inflammatory lesions of the human placenta. III. The histopathology of villitis of unknown aetiology. *Placenta* **1:** 227–244.

Samuels P, Main EK, Tomaski A, Mennuti MT, Gabbe SG & Cines DB (1987) Abnormalities in platelet antiglobulin tests in preeclamptic mothers and their neonates. *American Journal of Obstetrics and Gynecology* **157:** 109–113.

Sargent IL, Redman CWG & Stirrat GM (1982) Maternal cell-mediated immunity in normal and pre-eclamptic pregnancy. *Clinical and Experimental Immunology* **50:** 601–609.

Sargent IL, Wilkins T & Redman CWG (1988) Maternal immune responses to the fetus in early pregnancy and recurrent miscarriage. *Lancet* **ii:** 1099–1104.

Seidman DS, Ever-Hadani P, Stevenson DK & Gale R (1989) The effect of abortion on the incidence of pre-eclampsia. *European Journal of Obstetrics, Gynecology and Reproductive Biology* **33:** 109–114.

Serhal PF & Craft I (1987) Immune basis for preeclampsia: evidence from oocyte recipients. *Lancet* **ii:** 744.

Simon P, Fauchet R, Pilorge M et al (1988) Association of HLA-DR4 with the risk of recurrence of pregnancy hypertension. *Kidney International* **34(supplement):** S125–S128.

Sinha D, Wells M & Faulk WP (1984) Immunological studies in human placentae: complement components in pre-eclamptic chorionic villi. *Clinical and Experimental Immunology* **56:** 175–184.

Sridama V, Pacini F, Yang S-L, Moawad A, Reilly M & DeGroot LJ (1982) Decreased levels of helper T cells. A possible cause of immunodeficiency in pregnancy. *New England Journal of Medicine* **307:** 352–356.

Sridama V, Yang S-L, Moawad A & DeGroot LJ (1983) T-cell subsets in patients with preeclampsia. *American Journal of Obstetrics and Gynecology* **147:** 566–569.

Stevenson AC, Davison BCC, Say B, Ustuoplus LD, Einen MA & Toppozada HK (1971) Contribution of fetal/maternal incompatibility to aetiology of pre-eclamptic toxaemia. *Lancet* **ii:** 1286–1289.

Stevenson AC, Say B, Ustaoglu S & Durmus Z (1976) Aspects of pre-eclamptic toxaemia of pregnancy, consanguinity and twinning in Ankara. *Journal of Medical Genetics* **13:** 1–8.

Strickland DM, Guzick DS, Cox K, Gant NF & Rosenfeld CR (1986) The relationship between abortion in the first pregnancy and development of pregnancy-induced hypertension in the subsequent pregnancy. *American Journal of Obstetrics and Gynecology* **154:** 146–148.

Studd JWW (1971) Immunoglobulins in normal pregnancy, pre-eclampsia and pregnancy complicated by nephrotic syndrome. *Journal of Obstetrics and Gynaecology of the British Commonwealth* **78:** 786–790.

Sunder-Plassmann G, Derfler K, Wagner L et al (1989) Increased serum activity of interleukin-2 in patients with pre-eclampsia. *Journal of Autoimmunity* **2:** 203–205.

Sutherland A, Cooper DW, Howie PW, Liston WA & MacGillivray I (1981) The incidence of severe pre-eclampsia amongst mothers and mothers-in-law of pre-eclamptics and controls. *British Journal of Obstetrics and Gynaecology* **88:** 785–791.

Tait BD, Mraz G, Lutjen P & Leeton J (1984) HLA typing to establish maternity. *Lancet* **i:** 732–733.

Taylor PV, Skerrow S & Redman CWG (1991) Pre-eclampsia and antiphospholipid antibody. *British Journal of Obstetrics and Gynaecology* **98:** 604–606.

Tedesco F, Radillo O, Candussi G, Nazzaro A, Mollnes TE & Pecorari D (1990) Immunohisto-chemical detection of terminal complement complex and S protein in normal and pre-eclamptic placentae. *Clinical and Experimental Immunology* **80:** 236–240.

Thiry L, Yane F, Sprecher-Goldberger S, Cappel R, Bossens M & Neuray F (1981) Expression of retrovirus related antigen in pregnancy. II. Cytotoxic and blocking specificities in immunoglobulins eluted from the placenta. *Journal of Reproductive Immunology* **2:** 323–330.

Thomson NC, Stevenson RD, Behan W, Sloar D & Horne C (1976) Immunological studies in pre-eclamptic toxaemia. *British Medical Journal* **1:** 1307–1309.

Thornton JG & Sampson J (1990) Genetics of pre-eclampsia. *Lancet* **336:** 1319–1320.

Toaff R & Peyser MR (1976) Midtrimester preeclamptic toxemia in triploid pregnancies. *Israel Journal of Medical Science* **12:** 234–239.

Toder V, Eichenbrenner I, Amit S, Serr D & Nebel L (1979) Cellular hyperreactivity to placenta in toxemia of pregnancy. *European Journal of Obstetrics, Gynecology and Reproductive Biology* **9:** 379–384.

Toder V, Blank M, Gleicher N, Voljovich I, Mashiah S & Nebel L (1983) Activity of natural killer cells in normal pregnancy and edema-proteinuria hypertension gestosis. *American Journal of Obstetrics and Gynecology* **145:** 7–10.

Toivanen P & Hirvonen T (1970) Sex ratio of newborns: preponderance of males in toxemia of pregnancy. *Science* **170:** 186–187.

Wilton AN, Cooper DW, Brennecke SP, Bishop SM & Marshall P (1990) Absence of close linkage between maternal genes for susceptibility to pre-eclampsia/eclampsia and HLA DR beta. *Lancet* **336:** 653–657.

Yang S-L, Kleinman AM & Wei P-Y (1973) Immunologic aspects of term pregnancy toxemia. A study of immunoglobulins and complement. *American Journal of Obstetrics and Gynecology* **122:** 727–731.

Zeek PM & Assali NS (1950) Vascular changes in the decidua associated with eclamptogenic toxemia of pregnancy. *American Journal of Clinical Pathology* **20:** 1099–1109.

11

HIV infection in women

LOUISE PRIOLO
HOWARD L. MINKOFF

INTRODUCTION

As the percentage of women of reproductive age who are infected with HIV has increased, counselling about HIV testing has become a part of standard prenatal care. Obstetricians must be prepared therefore, to deal with the legal, ethical, clinical and infection control issues that revolve around the care of pregnant women infected with HIV.

Additionally obstetrician/gynaecologists are the primary care providers dealing with sexual risks. Since the heterosexual spread of HIV is an increasingly important vector of disease transmission obstetrician/gynaecologists will be called upon to develop and institute programmes to counsel all their sexually active patients about the risks of unsafe sex and techniques to minimize them.

All of these tasks require an understanding of the basic immunology, pathophysiology and epidemiology of HIV. Additionally a knowledge of the unique clinical consequences of this infection on women, both pregnant and non-pregnant, is required. This chapter will attempt to be a clinician's primer on these issues.

IMMUNOLOGY

Individuals infected with HIV develop symptoms as a result of a progressive disruption of cell-mediated immune responses. Numerous laboratory findings are associated with the progression of HIV disease and the development of AIDS. These markers can be divided into four categories: (1) measures of viral production; (2) the specific immune response to HIV; (3) non-specific immune system activation; and (4) measurements of immune system damage (Sheppard et al, 1991).

A variable degree of viraemia is seen in most individuals and can be measured directly or indirectly as infectious virus in the circulation or as the level of circulating antigens or immune complexes. HIV specific immunity is reflected in the levels of neutralizing antibody and antibody to various HIV components and in markers of cell-mediated immunity such as cellular or antibody-dependent cellular cytotoxicity. Non-specific activity of the immune system is reflected in elevation of β_2-microglobulin, neopterin, IL-2 receptor, immunoglobulins (Igs), serum IgA, immune complexes, immune mediators such as interleukin 1 (IL-1), interleukin 6 (IL-6) and tumour necrosis factor (TNF), and lymphocytes with cell surface markers associated with activation. In addition to some of the clinical features of HIV disease, such as weight loss, persistent fevers and diarrhoea, which are probably due to elevated lymphokine levels, direct measures of immune system damage include the loss of circulating CD4 cells, abnormalities in other lymphocyte subsets, functional anergy, and the patient's susceptibility to opportunistic infections (Sheppard et al, 1991).

Sheppard et al (1991) demonstrated a relationship between one laboratory marker for specific immunity (antibody to the p24 core protein), one marker for non-specific activation (serum neopterin) and the subsequent development of AIDS. The study concluded that the risk for the development of AIDS was greatest in subjects with both elevated neopterin levels and low p24 antibody titres (60% incidence of AIDS during follow-up). Patients with only one risk factor had intermediate outcomes. The groups with normal levels of neopterin and high p24 antibody had the best prognosis with a 9.6% incidence of AIDS. The low risk group continued to have CD4 levels above $700\,mm^3$ and remained asymptomatic throughout the follow-up period. The study demonstrated that p24 antibody titre and serum neopterin concentration, determined prospectively before the development of AIDS, were independent predictors of subsequent clinical outcome.

Individual variation in the levels of p24 antibody seen shortly after seroconversion have been reported and probably reflect variability in the HIV specific immune response capacity, influenced by classic immune response genes. Lymphokines produced in response to concomitant infections contribute to HIV disease by inducing viral replication and accelerated CD4 depletion, as well as cell death mediated by direct killing. It is also proposed that non-specific immune stimulation is caused by an interaction between the virus envelope glycoprotein (gp120) and the CD4 molecules on the surface of antigen activated helper T cells. The non-specific amplification of the immune response leads to the clinical manifestations of HIV disease (Sheppard et al, 1991). Thus, the three cardinal features of HIV disease, functional anergy, T cell loss, and clinical manifestations of chronic immune activation, are all produced by the same mechanism.

The highest incidence of AIDS occurs in patients with a weak HIV specific immune response and strong non-specific immune activation. Understanding the interaction between these two processes may improve the application of laboratory markers to the clinical management of HIV infected individuals and may suggest different approaches to chemotherapy and immune therapy. It is important to assess immune response capacity in advance of vaccine or immune therapy trials because high responders might have a better prognosis independent of the effects of immunization. Cytotoxic chemotherapeutic agents, including zidovidine (ZDV), might effect disease progression through non-specific suppression of immune activation rather than antiviral activities. Such an effect has been shown recently in the treatment of murine AIDS with cyclophosphamide (Sheppard et al, 1991).

For all adults with HIV infection routine immunization against influenza, *Pneumococcus*, *Haemophilus* influenza B, hepatitis B, tetanus and diphtheria is indicated and advised. The question of whether to immunize with live viral vaccines is more controversial. This is not as much an issue in adults with HIV infection, as it is in HIV infected children. The benefits of immunizing asymptomatic children against such common and potentially serious pathogens as measles, mumps, and rubella outweigh concerns about adverse effects from vaccination. Inactivated polio vaccine is advisable and preferable to live oral polio vaccine in these patients (Stiehm, 1990; Rhoads et al, 1991; Ruderman et al, 1991).

There is currently no clear evidence to support the concept that vaccination may accelerate HIV progression. Nor is there evidence that HIV infected patients developed chronic vaccine viral syndromes or persistent shedding of vaccine virus. The potential benefit of providing protection against current and future pathogens appears to outweigh the theoretical concern that vaccination may accelerate HIV disease.

PERINATAL HIV INFECTIONS

With an increasing shift in the epidemiology of HIV infection toward populations in which heterosexual activity and intravenous (i.v.) drug use predominate as modes of transmission, prevention of HIV transmission to women and of vertical transmission from mother to child have become urgent public health priorities.

As of July 1991, 18 648 cumulative cases of AIDS in women had been reported to the Centers for Disease Control (CDC). In 51% of women i.v. drug use was reported as the route of HIV exposure, and in an additional 33% heterosexual contact was reported as the route of HIV exposure (Centers for Disease Control, 1990a). The majority of these women are of childbearing age. National heel-stick surveys indicate that close to 6000 HIV-infected women give birth annually (Centers for Disease Control, 1990b). Assuming a 30% rate of HIV transmission from mother to child, this translates into 1800 infants born infected with HIV annually.

HIV infection numbers among the ten leading causes of death of children in the United States. The prevalence of HIV infection in children in the US can only be crudely estimated. Children currently account for 2% of the total number of individuals with AIDS reported to the CDC. As of 1990, estimates of the number of children with HIV infection in the US ranged between 5000 and 10 000 (Gwinn et al, 1991). Cumulatively, 3199 cases of paediatric AIDS have been reported. World wide the World Health Organisation (WHO) estimates that during the first decade of the AIDS pandemic approximately 500 000 AIDS cases occurred among women and children with an additional three million deaths in women and children anticipated during the 1990s (Chin, 1990). The WHO further estimates a 30% excess infant and child mortality in major American, western European, and sub-Saharan African cities where AIDS has become the leading cause of death for women aged 20–40, and expects not only hundreds of thousands of paediatric AIDS cases during the 1990s but also more than a million uninfected children orphaned because HIV infected mothers and fathers will die from AIDS.

The scope of the paediatric HIV epidemic is clearly linked to the prevalence of HIV infection in women of reproductive age. In the United States perinatal transmission (antepartum, intrapartum or postpartum, see below) accounts for over 80% of all reported cases of paediatric AIDS. Intrauterine HIV infection has been demonstrated by serological analysis and viral culture of the neonate's blood, cord blood and placental and fetal tissue samples. Intrapartum HIV infection, during passage through the birth canal, is suggested by the seroconversion of newborns in the neonatal period (Landesman et al, 1991) as well as the reportedly greater likelihood that the presenting twin, as opposed to its non-presenting sibling, will become infected (Goeddert et al, 1991). Postpartum HIV infection has been demonstated to occur through exposure to infected breast milk (Van de Perne et al, 1991).

Reported estimates of vertical transmission from mother to child range from 15–40% with the more recent studies (Newell et al, 1990; European Collaborative Study, 1991) noting transmission rates at the lower end of the range. Theoretically it is possible, however, that some apparently uninfected infants will harbour the virus in undetectable sites and may not be diagnosed as infected until many years after birth.

Short-term pregnancy outcomes do not appear to be markedly affected by HIV infections. After controlling for associated risk factors such as drug addiction, it has not been found, for example, that birth weights, or gestational ages are significantly influenced by maternal serostatus (Minkoff et al, 1990). Neither does the course of HIV disease appear to be markedly influenced by pregnancy. Several controlled studies have found that infected women who were pregnant had, at most, a very slight increase in the rate of depletion of CD4 cell counts and no influence on the rate of development of clinical illness was detected. Ryder, however, found that women with more advanced HIV disease or with lower CD4 counts were the patients most prone to the development of opportunistic infections during pregnancy (Crowe et al, 1991).

MANAGEMENT OF PREGNANT WOMEN WITH HIV INFECTION

Identification is the first step in management of the pregnant patient with HIV infection. Since 1985 the CDC has recommended HIV testing and counselling of pregnant patients who fall into high-risk groups for acquiring HIV infection, i.e. i.v. drugs users, patients who received blood transfusions between 1979 and 1985, and sexual partners of men who are HIV positive, i.v. drug users, bisexual, or haemophiliac (Centers for Disease Control, 1985). Also included in the CDC defined risk groups are men and women who emigrated from areas where HIV is widespread in the general population, such as Haiti and Central Africa. More recently recommendations for screening have reflected an understanding of both the increasing prevalence of HIV in women and the failure of programmes dependent on patient acknowledged risks. It is currently suggested that all women of reproductive age be offered HIV testing and that those who reside in high prevalence communities should have that testing recommended.

Heterosexual transmission is probably a significant source of infection in women who test positive without known specific risk factors. In some areas with a significant prevalence of HIV infection there is a trend in obstetric practice toward incorporation of HIV screening into the routine of first prenatal visit laboratory work (with informed consent). Patients who are in high risk groups but who test HIV negative, should be retested at 36 weeks' gestation. In all circumstances patients should be informed that they are being tested for HIV and they should be given the opportunity to decline such testing if they wish.

Patients who are identified as HIV positive on repeated ELISA testing with confirmation by Western blot, should be counselled appropriately and with extreme sensitivity about their status and its potential impact on their fetus. Patients should be strongly encouraged to refer their sexual partners for counselling, and to use condoms to avoid transmitting the HIV virus to sexual partners who are not already infected. Those patients who are drug users should be advised to enter drug treatment programmes and to avoid sharing needles and syringes. In addition to referring patients for psychiatric counselling if required, other consultations may be indicated for patients with clinical and laboratory abnormalities.

Management of pregnant patients with HIV infection must include careful and repeated testing for other sexually transmitted diseases (STDs) (Minkoff, 1987). As is recommended for all prenatal patients, these women should be tested for gonorrhoea, syphilis and hepatitis B at their first prenatal visit. The clinical manifestations of all STDs may be more severe and infections may recur more often. In addition to routine prenatal screening, patients should be assessed for *Chlamydia* infection and *Mycobacterium tuberculosis*. Since cytomegalovirus (CMV) and toxoplasmosis frequently occur in HIV-infected individuals, base-line antibody titres against these organisms should be obtained.

Many of the early symptoms that may indicate progression from asymptomatic HIV infection to AIDS, such as fatigue, shortness of breath, and anaemia, are non-specific and common in pregnancy. Obstetricians must be alert to these subtle symptoms as well as anorexia and weight loss, and begin treatment or seek consultation at the earliest opportunity. The patient's immune status should be monitored at regular intervals. It should be recognized that pregnancy itself produces significant changes in cell-mediated immunity. These changes are characterized by an apparent depression of CD4 cells whereas CD8 cell numbers are unchanged, producing an alteration in CD4/CD8 ratio. Biggar has demonstrated that CD4 cell levels fall to a nadir at approximately 7 months' gestation, and then rise by term to prepregnancy levels, independent of HIV antibody status (Biggar et al,

1989). At 7 months' gestation, however, the CD4 levels are 10–20% lower in HIV-seropositive women and start to decline again in these women immediately after delivery. Poor nutrition and abuse of drugs and alcohol are also known to affect T lymphocyte function.

Measurement of CD4 levels are helpful in determining an individual's risk for opportunistic infections and in choosing appropriate candidates for *Pneumocystis carinii* pneumonia (PCP) prophylaxis regimens and should be obtained each trimester. If a pregnant patient develops opportunistic infections during pregnancy, management should be co-ordinated with an infectious disease specialist and should reflect the optimal therapy for the entity under consideration independent of the patient's pregnancy status unless there is convincing evidence that standard therapy could compromise fetal well-being (see below). Under those circumstances the mother should be engaged in discussions regarding the risks and benefits of the therapeutic alternatives. There are few circumstances under which standard therapy needs to be modified because of pregnancy.

The intrapartum management of HIV-infected women is not substantially altered because of their serostatus. The mode of delivery is still based upon obstetrical indications. Although recent evidence suggests that intrapartum events may relate to vertical transmission, there are no empirical data that caesarean section can reduce viral transmission. There are, however, no appropriately designed studies on that subject. Since vaginal secretions can be HIV infected, and since intact skin is a potential barrier to infection, it is recommended that routine use of scalp electrodes be avoided in the setting of HIV infection. Again, no studies have actually demonstrated risk related to these devices. Finally the intrapartum period has been associated with the transmission of nosocomial infections to and from health care workers. The assiduous use of universal precautions is recommended. These precautions include the use of wall suction in place of mouth suction to clear the neonate's airway. Suction should be maintained below 140 mmHg.

Perhaps the most important task for the obstetricians in the postpartum period is to establish the optimal linkage between the patient and providers with expertise in HIV for both the mother and the child. New therapeutic and prophylactic regimens are being introduced on a regular basis for adults and children and all patients should have access to them. Beyond that, patients should be advised to avoid breast-feeding since infection clearly can occur through that mechanism and since safe alternatives to breast milk are readily available in the developed world. Universal precautions should be extended to the child at birth but bonding should be encouraged.

TREATMENT OF INFECTIONS DURING PREGNANCY

The most common opportunistic infection is *Pneumocystis carinii* pneumonia (PCP). The usual treatment for PCP, trimethoprim/sulphamethoxazole, has theoretical teratogenic risks, because trimethoprim is a folic acid inhibitor and sulpha derivatives may elevate unconjugated bilirubin levels in the blood of newborns. It is felt, however, that the benefits of these drugs during pregnancy outweigh the risks and kernicterus has never been documented in newborns who did not receive sulpha derivatives in the neonatal period (Baskin et al, 1980). Pentamidine may be used as a second line of therapy. It is also recommended that prophylaxis with pyrimethamine and sulphadiazine be used following the first episode of PCP even if CD4 levels are not below 200 mm^3.

Patients with AIDS who develop focal neurological findings, changes in sensorium, and fever must be suspected of having toxoplasmosis which is a common cause of CNS symptoms among these patients. Serological tests are of limited value in the diagnosis of acute toxoplasmosis in patients with AIDS, unless base-line titres were previously obtained.

Antibody to *Toxoplasma* is prevalent in the general population and therefore has a low predictive value for active infection. Serological testing of CSF is often negative in proven cases, but the demonstration of intrathecal production of antibody to *Toxoplasma* may be helpful.

The most useful diagnostic test has been the CT scan (Glatt et al, 1988). Lesions are often multiple, ring-enhancing with contrast, associated with oedema, and located in the cortical and subcortial regions of the brain, such as the basal ganglia. CT scans can produce false negative results. In pregnancy the diagnosis can sometimes be made without contrast media. Lumbar puncture procedures have not been proven to be of benefit. The clinical and radiological picture of toxoplasmosis of the CNS can be mimicked by several other conditions, including lymphoma, fungal infections, progressive multifocal leukoencephalopathy, tuberculosis, CMV, Kaposi's sarcoma and haemorrhage. Definitive diagnosis requires biopsy of the brain either by open biopsy or by stereotactically guided needle. The demonstration of tachyzoites (i.e. the invasive form of the protozoon) is necessary to establish the diagnosis.

Because of potential morbidity resulting from brain biopsy and the possibility of false negative results, some centres favour empirical therapy in patients with positive serological findings and a clinical picture compatible with toxoplasmosis. Improvement is usually seen clinically and on CT scan in 1–2 weeks.

Transmission of *Toxoplasma gondii* across the placenta can occur, and if it occurs early in fetal life, results in stillbirth, fetal damage, or delivery of a child with congenital toxoplasmosis (Remington and Desmonts, 1983). Transmission rates of 14%, 29% and 59% have been seen in the first, second and third trimester, respectively. These rates may be higher in the immunocompromised patient; the patient with very high titres and seroconverting patients are at particular risks. If seroconversion is noted, counselling about fetal risks should be given. If termination of pregnancy is not desired, treatment with sulphadiazine (6–8 g/day) and pyrimethamine (25–50 mg daily) should be administered; folic acid supplementation should be given to these patients.

Although percutaneous umbilical blood sampling (PUBS) has been helpful in fetal diagnosis, a theoretic risk of inoculating the fetus with maternal blood and enhancing the risk of congenital infection with HIV exists. Recurrence of toxoplasmosis in the HIV infected patient is common when treatment is discontinued. Therefore 6–8 weeks of suppressive therapy is recommended.This therapy then is followed with maintenance therapy for the life of the patient. Preventive measures also play a role. Patients should be educated to avoid contact with cats and soil, to wash hands well, and to cook all meat thoroughly.

Oropharyngeal candidiasis is the most common fungal infection seen in patients with AIDS and is predictive of progressive immunosuppression. Pregnant women, however, will more frequently have vaginal candidiasis. Recurrent maternal symptomatology may necessitate prophylactic courses of a topical antifungal, or in extreme circumstances a therapeutic course of oral ketoconazole 400 mg p.o. daily for 14 days followed by 5 days per month for 6 months of 400 mg of ketoconazole (Rawlinson et al, 1984). Though topical application of antifungal agents are effective, most patients develop recurrent infection when therapy is discontinued.

Mycobacterium tuberculosis occurs in up to 10% of AIDS patients, principally Haitians and i.v. drug users. Treatment is recommended for HIV-seropositive patients when there is a positive tuberculin skin test or radiological evidence of old tuberculosis. Preventive therapy with isoniazid for at least 12 months is recommended regardless of age. Biopsy may be required for diagnosis. For symptomatic patients therapy with standard antitubercular agents is usually effective.

Neurological complications of syphilis seem to occur more often in patients with HIV infection (Tramont. 1987). HIV-infected patients with syphilis should receive a regimen of antibiotics appropriate for neurosyphilis.

In addition to the treatment of specific infections, the medical management of HIV-infected individuals includes the use of antiretroviral agents for individuals whose CD4 count has declined to 500/mm^3. The first line drug is zidovidine (ZDV). Currently, there are no specific recommendations for the use of ZDV in pregnancy. Most clinicians would recommend the use of this agent, beyond the first trimester, for women with extreme immune compromise (CD4 less than 200/mm^3) and discuss its appropriateness with women whose counts are in a borderline range (between 200 and 500/mm^3).

PREVENTING VERTICAL TRANSMISSION OF HIV

A large number of research efforts are being undertaken in an effort to interrupt the vertical transmission of HIV. The first large-scale trial to go into the field involved the use of ZDV. Theoretically, ZDV given to the mother during pregnancy and to the infant immediately after birth could decrease vertical transmission by lowering the maternal viral load, preventing viral replication in placental cells and/or preventing viral replication in newly infected fetal cells.

Other trials that are just beginning or are being contemplated include the use of false receptors for the virus (soluble CD4 linked to IgG), monoclonal antibody to various portions of the viral envelope, HIVIg and vaccine trials. It is hoped that one or a combination of the above will be able to reduce perinatal transmission rates.

The care of patients who are both pregnant and have HIV disease brings together some of the most difficult ethical issues confronting clinicians. These issues include appropriateness of counselling, balancing confidentiality with the duty to warn and the obligation to provide care within the physician's realm of expertise. Physicians should consult freely with hospital counsel or ethics committees when trying to translate ethical constructs into clinical realities.

GYNECOLOGICAL CARE OF HIV-INFECTED WOMEN

Even when not pregnant, women are confronted by unique clinical dilemmas when HIV infected. These problems include cervical disease, genital infections and contraception concerns.

The findings that some members of the group of human papillomavirus (HPV) can transform cells in vitro and the detection of HPV DNA in cells from cervical cancer, suggest that HPV may be aetiologically involved in the development of cervical dysplasia and cancer (Reeves et al, 1989). A high prevalence of cervical dysplasia among women with HIV infection has been observed and linked to the frequent occurrence of HPV infection in HIV-infected women. The previously reported occurrence of cervical cancer and cervical intraepithelial neoplasia (CIN) in immunocompromised women points to a role for immune depletion in the development of cancer. An investigation of T lymphocyte subsets in women who manifest genital HPV infection showed a lower percentage of CD4 cells and a higher percentage of CD8 cells compared with women with normal cervical cytological evaluations. A decrease in natural killer cell activity could also be demonstrated in patients with condyloma acuminata.

During the course of HIV infection, peripheral T lymphocyte cells and cell-mediated immune responses are progressively diminished. HIV-induced immunodeficiency has been shown to increase not only the risk for opportunistic infections but also the risk for the development of various neoplasia including squamous, rectal and oral carcinoma. A study performed by Sehafer demonstrated that HIV-infected women had a tenfold higher prevalence of dysplasia. In addition to co-factors such as sexual activity, frequent genital infections and smoking, HIV-induced immunosuppression is now considered another important risk factor for the development of dysplasia (Sehafer et al, 1991).

Several studies have now shown that the impairment of lymphocyte function significantly correlates with an increasing risk for cervical dysplasia. It is now speculated that the HIV-induced immunodeficiency may lead to an active chronic HPV infection and thereby to persistence or progression of dysplasia (Byrne et al, 1989). As a consequence, clinical surveillance of HIV-infected women should include cytological investigation of the uterine cervix at regular intervals; the frequency should depend on the stage of HIV disease with biannual smears having been recommended as the routine (Minkoff and DeHovitz, 1991). The high proportion of suspicious colposcopic findings and the observed severity of CIN in HIV-infected women suggest that liberal use of colposcopic examinations should be utilized and immediate directed biopsies be performed for all suspicious lesions (Maiman et al, 1991).

Several gynaecological infections have been reported to have their natural history modified by HIV infection. Pelvic inflammatory disease (PID), for example, has been reported to manifest differently in the setting of HIV infection. In one study, women who had PID and who were HIV infected were significantly less likely to manifest a leukocytosis and showed a trend toward more abscesses and more surgical intervention (Hoegsberg et al, 1990). It has been suggested that immunocompromise *per se* is sufficient justification for the in-patient management of PID (Peterson et al, 1990). Since the causative organisms have not been shown to vary with serostatus, however, there is currently no basis to suggest treatment regimens other than those recommended by the CDC for all women with PID.

The association of HIV infection with vaginal candidiasis was discussed under the heading of infections in pregnancy.

HIV-infected individuals may have unique manifestations of genital ulcer disease. Women with genital ulcers ascribed to HIV infection have been reported (Covino and McCormack, 1990). More frequent shedding of herpes simplex virus might also be anticipated. Finally, in regard to ulcerative diseases, it has been reported that chancroid may be more refractory to single dose therapy in HIV-infected individuals. If single dose therapy with a quinoline or trimethoprim–sulphamethazole fails, a 3-day regimen of fluorquinolone (such as ciprofloxacin) should be considered (MacDonald et al, 1989).

Since fertility rates are not linked to serostatus, contraceptive considerations are important components of the care of HIV-infected women. Clearly all discussions must reflect an understanding that HIV can be transmitted sexually so that if the woman's sexual partner is not known to be HIV seropositive then a primary focus must be on the prevention of viral transmission. If contraception is the primary concern it must be recognized that barrier techniques have a higher failure rate than hormonal contraception. Empirical data about the possible interaction of HIV disease and oral contraception have been limited to reports from endemic areas suggesting enhanced HIV acquisition by prostitutes who used oral contraceptives (Plummer et al, 1991). Those data do not address issues of relevance to prevalent seropositive women. A reported 'sexual dimorphism' in immune response leaves open the possibility of an altered natural history among women using oral contraceptives, though the direction of that effect is uncertain (Grossman, 1984). Current information does not seem sufficient to contraindicate the use of oral contraceptives in the setting of HIV disease so long as issues of disease transmission are separately addressed.

CONCLUSION

Women comprise an increasing percentage of individuals with HIV infection and will continue to do so if epidemiological trends persist. The responsibilities of individuals concerned with the health of women will be to develop and implement strategies both to reduce risks for the uninfected and to diagnose and appropriately manage the infected. It is clear therefore that obstetrician/gynaecologists, if they are successfully to accomplish both of these goals, need to be not only informed, compassionate clinicians but advocates as well. They must assist their patients in confronting the barriers to care that currently exist for women. In meeting these multiple responsibilities, physicians will help to continue a trend towards an improved duration and quality of life for HIV-infected individuals.

REFERENCES

Baskin CG, Law S & Wenger NK (1980) Sulfadiazine rheumatic fever prophylaxis during pregnancy: does it increase the risk of kernicterus in the newborn? *Cardiology* **65:** 222–225.

Biggar RJ, Pahava S, Minkoff HL et al (1989) Immunosuppression in pregnant women infected with human immunodeficiency virus. *American Journal of Obstetrics and Gynecology* **161:** 1239–1244.

Byrne MA, Taylor-Robinson D, Munday PE & Harris JRW (1989) The common occurrence of human papillomavirus infection and intraepithelial neoplasia in women infected by HIV. *AIDS* **3:** 379–389.

Centers for Disease Control (1985) Recommendations for assisting in the prevention of perinatal transmission of human T lymphotrophic virus type II/lymphadenopathy associated virus and acquired immunodeficiency syndrome. *Morbidity and Mortality Weekly Report* **34:** 721–731.

Centers for Disease Control (1990a) AIDS in women—U.S. *Morbidity and Mortality Weekly Report* **39:** 850–853.

Centers for Disease Control (1990b) HIV prevalence estimates and AIDS case projection for the United States, report based upon a workshop. *Morbidity and Mortality Weekly Report* **39(RR-16):** 1–31.

Chin J (1990) Current and future dimension of the HIV-AIDS pandemic in women and children. *Lancet* **336:** 221–224.

Covino JP & McCormack W (1990) Vulvar ulcer of unknown etiology in human immunodeficiency virus infected women: response to treatment with zidovidine. *American Journal of Obstetrics and Gynecology* **163:** 116–118.

Crowe S, Carlin J, Stewart K, Lucas R & Hoy J (1991) Predictive value of CD4 lymphocyte numbers for the development of opportunistic infections and malignancies in HIV infected persons. *Journal of Acquired Immune Deficiency Syndrome* **4:** 770–775.

European Collaborative Study (1991) Children born to women with HIV-1 infection: natural history and risk of transmission. *Lancet* **337:** 253–260.

Glatt AE, Chirgwin K & Landesman SH (1988) Treatment of infections associated with human immunodeficiency virus. *New England Journal of Medicine* **318:** 1439–1448.

Goeddert JJ, Duliege AM, Amos CI, Felton S & Biggar RJ (1991) High risk of HIV-1 infection for first-born twins. *Lancet* **338:** 1471–1475.

Grossman C (1984) Possible underlying mechanisms of sexual dimorphism in the immune response: fact and hypothesis. *Journal of Steroid Biochemistry* **34:** 241–251.

Gwinn M, Pappaioanov M, George JR et al (1991) Prevalence of HIV infection in child bearing women in the United States. *Journal of the American Medical Association* **265:** 1704–1708.

Hoegsberg B, Abulafia O, Sedlis A et al (1990) Sexually transmitted diseases and human immunodeficiency virus infection among women with pelvis inflammatory diseases. *American Journal of Obstetrics and Gynecology* **163:** 1135–1139.

Landesman S, Weiblem B, Mendez H et al (1991) Clinical utility of HIV-1gA immunoblot assay in the early diagnosis of perinatal HIV infection. *Journal of the American Medical Association* **266:** 3443–3446.

MacDonald KS, Cameron DW, D'Costa L, Mdinya-Achola JO, Plummer FA & Ronald AR (1989) Evaluation of fleroxacine (R023–6240) as single oral dose therapy of culture proven chancroid in Nairobi, Keyna. *Antimicrobial Agents and Chemotherapy* **33:** 612–614.

Maiman M, Tarriare N, Vierra J, Svarez J, Serur E & Boyce JG (1991) Colposcopic evaluation of human immunodeficiency virus in seropositive women. *Obstetrics and Gynecology* **78:** 84–88.

Minkoff HL (1987) Care of pregnant women infected with human immunodeficiency virus. *Journal of the American Medical Association* **258:** 2714–2717.

Minkoff HL & DeHovitz JA (1991) The care of HIV infected women. *Journal of the American Medical Association* **266:** 2253–2258.

Minkoff HL, Henderson C, Mendez H et al (1990) Pregnancy outcomes among women infected with HIV and matched controls. *American Journal of Obstetrics and Gynecology* **163:** 1598–1603.

Newell ML, Pedcham CS & Lepaje P (1990) HIV infection in pregnancy: implications for women and children. *AIDS* **4(1):** S111–S117.

Peterson HB, Cealand E & Zenilman J (1990) Pelvic inflammatory disease: review of treatment options. *Review of Infectious Diseases* **12:** 656–664.

Plummer FA, Simonon JH, Cameron DW et al (1991) Co-factors in male–female sexual transmission of human immunodeficiency virus type 1. *Journal of Infectious Diseases* **163:** 233–239.

Rawlinson K, Subrow A, Harris M et al (1984) Disseminated Kaposi's sarcoma in pregnancy: a manifestation of acquired immune deficiency syndrome. *Obstetrics and Gynecology* **63:** 25.

Reeves WC, Rawis WE & Brinton LA (1989) Epidemiology of genital papillomavirus and cervical cancer. *Review of Infectious Diseases* **11:** 436–439.

Remington JS & Desmonts G (1983) Toxoplasmosis. In Remington JS & Klein JO (eds) *Infectious Diseases of the Fetus and Newborn Infant*, pp 143–263. Philadelphia: WB Saunders.

Rhoads J, Birx D & Wright C (1991) Safety and immunogencity of multiple conventional immunizations administered during early HIV infection. *Journal of Acquired Immune Deficiency Syndrome* **4:** 724–730.

Ruderman JW, Barka N, Peter JB et al (1991) Antibody response to MMR vaccination in children who received IVIG as neonates. *American Journal of Diseases of Children* **145:** 425–426.

Sehafer A, Friedman W, Mielke M, Schwaitlander B & Koch MA (1991) The increased frequency of cervical dysplasia neoplasia in women infected with the human immunodeficiency virus is related to the degree of immunosuppression. *American Journal of Obstetrics and Gynecology* **164:** 593–599.

Sheppard HW, Aschar MS, McRae B, Anderson RE, Long W & Jean-Pierre A (1991) The initial immune response to HIV and immune system activation determine the outcome of HIV disease. *Journal of Acquired Immune Deficiency Syndrome* **4:** 704–711.

Stiehm ER (1990) Role of immunoglobulin therapy in neonatal infections: where we stand today. *Review of Infectious Diseases* **12(4):** 439–442.

Tramont FC (1987) Syphilis in the AIDS era. *New England Journal of Medicine* **316:** 1600–1601.

Van de Perne P, Simonon A, Msellati P et al (1991) Postnatal transmission of human immunodeficiency virus type 1 from mother to infant. *New England Journal of Medicine* **325:** 593–598.

12

Contraception

WARREN R. JONES

INTRODUCTION

The principle of vaccination for contraceptive purposes is physiologically and clincally attractive and has major implications for fertility regulation in both developing and Western societies. Immunological influences on fertility may feasibly be deployed in the human reproductive process at stages leading up to and including implantation. This process has components that are both antigenically unique and immunogenic, and therefore potentially amenable to a precise immunological attack. This, therefore, is the basis of contraceptive vaccine development involving immunization against specific reproductive tract antigens (Jones, 1982; Ada and Griffin, 1991a). This chapter examines the current status of and realistic future possibilities for the use and deployment of contraceptive vaccines.

IMMUNOLOGICAL BASIS

The basis and rationale of fertility regulating vaccines has been underpinned historically by an extensive body of research involving the induction of infertility in immunized experimental animals and by the recognition of the role of immunological factors in a proportion of infertile men and women.

Advantages of immunological contraception

Immunological contraception has several well defined potential advantages:

1. The use of a non-pharmacologically active agent.
2. Ease and convenience of administration, making it suitable for distribution, if necessary, by paramedical personnel.
3. Long lasting (up to 12 months or more) but potentially reversible antifertility activity.
4. Acceptability of the 'vaccine' principle; of particular importance in developing countries where the method can be incorporated into primary health care programmes.
5. Reduced patient failure.
6. Large scale production at relatively low cost.

Baillière's Clinical Obstetrics and Gynaecology—
Vol. 6, No. 3, September 1992
ISBN 0–7020–1634–9

Selection of antigen(s)

A target antigen in a contraceptive vaccine should be specific to the reproductive process. In order to avoid cross-reactive autoimmunity, the antigen selected should not be present in other tissues in the vaccine recipient, and, preferably, should be present only transiently during the reproductive process (e.g. embryonic antigens, phase-specific antigens, antigens of the male gamete in the female genital tract). Based on these criteria, antigens (hormonal or otherwise) of the trophoblast and of the sperm are attractive targets for an immune attack in the female. On the other hand, ovarian oocytes in the female and sperm in the male are less attractive possibilities.

A vaccine antigen should have no physiological role outside the reproductive process. It should be amenable to chemical and structural characterization and should be potentially available in pure form from natural sources, or be capable of large-scale production by conventional synthesis or genetic engineering techniques. Immunization against the antigen should prevent or disrupt fertilization or implantation without undesirable side-effects. The antifertility effect of a contraceptive vaccine should preferably, but not necessarily, be potentially reversible.

Vaccine development

The strategic approach to the development of a contraceptive vaccine may involve the following:

1. The identification, isolation, characterization and production of reproductive tract antigens either by classical methods of analysis and synthesis or by recombinant DNA technology.
2. The possible modification of native target antigens to enhance immunogenicity.
3. The identification and use, where appropriate, of naturally occurring antibodies associated with reproductive failure, in the selection and, possibly, the preparation of target antigens.
4. The generation of monoclonal, and then polyclonal, antibodies to relevant antigens, and their use in identification, genetic characterization and preparative enrichment of antigen fractions.
5. The identification or development of acceptable carriers, adjuvants and/or delivery systems in the preparation of a vaccine for human use.
6. The establishment of appropriate experimental animal models, which often may need to involve infrahuman primates, for preclinical efficacy and safety studies.
7. Clinical trials of safety, immunogenicity, efficacy and reversibility.

The various components of this strategy have assumed differing degrees of importance and relevance depending on the antigen(s) selected and have been influenced by the dramatic advancs in vaccine technology and molecular genetics. Thus, for example, the identification of naturally occurring antibodies proved important in the early stages of research into sperm vaccine development, but more recently, hybridoma technology, DNA expression library probing and recombinant DNA techniques have played a central role. On the other hand, the extensive research underpinning the advanced strategy for a vaccine directed against human chorionic gonadotrophin (hCG) has required detailed attention to the development of peptide-carrier conjugation methods, the assessment of adjuvants and delivery systems suitable for use in man, and the selection of appropriate infrahuman primate models for efficacy and safety studies.

APPROACHES TO IMMUNOLOGICAL CONTRACEPTION

The immunological abrogation of fertility might, theoretically, involve a number of different stages or processes in the human reproductive system. However, in practice, logistic and safety considerations impose certain limits (Ada and Griffin, 1991b). At present these limits encompass potentially feasible approaches to immunological contraception involving target antigens in the gametes, the zygote and the placenta. Other approaches, though theoretically attractive, have serious practical disadvantages. Immunization against the pituitary gonadotrophins, gonadotrophin releasing hormone (GnRH), sex steroids and other physiological molecules in the hypothalamic–pituitary–gonadal axis may inhibit fertility. However, a contraceptive vaccine acting against these hormone targets would raise two potential serious risks:

1. The continuous physiological production of such hormones in the face of an immune response would lead to persistent immune complex formation with possible tissue damage.
2. Steroid hormones are necessary for the upkeep of their target reproductive organs and they also act on a variety of other target tissues. Depriving the body of the functions of these hormones would lead to menopause-like side-effects.

Some of the more feasible approaches to immunological fertility regulation will now be considered briefly. The most encouraging and advanced method, a vaccine directed against hCG, will be considered in more detail.

Spermatozoal antigens

There has been intense interest, over several decades, in the possibility of inducing infertility in females and, to a lesser extent, in males, by immunization against sperm. Unfortunately, until relatively recently, progress in antisperm vaccine development has been slow. This, at least in part, has been due to the fact that the antigens defined in experimental animals have sometimes been irrelevant outside a particular species, or that their human counterparts have proved difficult to identify/isolate and characterize. Despite this, the principle of inducing immunity to sperm for contraceptive purposes remains attractive, and more rapid advances in the field have accompanied the advent of new technologies in molecular biology, monoclonal antibody generation and immunochemistry. The historical background to sperm vaccine development has been a vast literature on experimental immunization against sperm in laboratory animals extending back for almost a century (Jones, 1982). Superficial clinical encouragement also arose from the somewhat curious reports in the 1920s and 1930s of the induction of infertility in women immunized with crude sperm extracts. Further support has derived from the demonstration of antisperm antibodies in the serum and reproductive tract of some infertile men and women. By and large these individuals are healthy, apart from their infertile state, and it seems reasonable to conclude from these experiments of nature, that safe and effective anti-sperm vaccination is a feasible proposition (Jones, 1974).

At least in theory, an antisperm vaccine might be designed to operate in several ways. In our current state of knowledge, the most feasible action is likely to be directed against the transport, viability or fertilizing capacity of the sperm or against its progenitor cells in the testis. It is also possible, but more difficult, to envisage the immunological manipulation of physiological events such as sperm maturation in the epididymis, decapacitation, capacitation and of the immunosuppressive mechanisms which modulate the exposure to, and recognition of, the immune response to sperm in the female.

This review will confine itself to the realistic prospects of achieving effective contraception by active immunization against sperm in both the female and the male. It must be stated, however, that the principle of vaccination against sperm would seem to be inordinately more difficult to apply to the male than to the female. In the female, immunity to sperm would be expected to operate against 'foreign' antigen(s) (i.e. sperm) when they are introduced at coitus. On the other hand, in the male, the contraceptive requirement of this approach involves an autoimmune reaction against antigens continuously present in the body. This inherently raises the spectre of possible untoward and permanent tissue damage, or disruption of hormonal function.

Notwithstanding this important and primary immunological consideration, it is still possible that a practical and safe sperm vaccine could be developed for use in the male. Such a vaccine would need to be directed against secluded, and presumably, phase-specific antigens on the cells involved in spermatogenesis, or would need to react selectively with post-testicular sperm during their sojourn in the male tract or in the ejaculate. It is known that circulating antisperm antibodies can enter the male genital tract via the rete testis and prostate, so that the use of specific and well defined sperm antigens (possible sperm-coating) may lead to the development of a vaccine which may 'inactivate' sperm in the absence of testicular damage.

Potential target antigens on sperm

Evidence from experimental immunization in laboratory animals, and studies of the biological significance of sperm antibodies in infertile individuals, indicates that the basic requirement of a target sperm antigen is that is should be accessible on the cell surface to an immune attack mediated within the female (and possibly the male) genital tract (Jones, 1974). In other words, it should be a cell membrane component, an intrinsic (internal) component expressed on the sperm surface, or a seminal plasma component bound to the sperm. When considering an antisperm vaccine for use in the female two potential problems become apparent. One is the extent of the antigen (sperm) load introduced at coitus and the second is the necessity for presence of an adequate level of antibody (either by transudation or local secretion) in the upper regions of the female genital tract. Immune cells may also need to be recruited to ensure an effective response.

A variety of sperm antigens of potential utility have now been identified and their antifertility effects described in laboratory animals (see Naz and Menge, 1990 and relevant chapter in Alexander et al, 1990). Most are species specific but others are not, or at least have primate homology. Progress in sperm vaccine research has been desultory; much has been promised over many decades but little has yet been delivered. One of the more hopeful of recently described sperm antigens is the differentiation antigen SP-10, (Herr et al, 1990), an intra-acrosomal protein which arises during spermatogenesis but is exposed during the acrosome reaction. It is highly conserved in humans and infrahuman primates, has a molecular weight of 28 kDa, has been cloned and sequenced, and provokes antibodies which appear to inhibit sperm–ovum fusion. Efficacy studies in baboons using the whole molecule or selected peptides should indicate whether or not this antigen has a future role in immunocontraception.

Antigens of the oocyte

The most extensively studied potential target component of the oocyte is the zona pellucida (ZP) (Jones, 1982; Henderson et al, 1988; Dean and Millar, 1990). The ZP is an acellular mucopolysaccharide layer which first appears in the pre-antral secondary follicle and encases the mature oocyte and zygote. It has a physiological role in sperm binding in the early stages of fertilization and it also blocks polyspermy and mechanically protects the developing zygote until just prior to implantation. Usually only one oocyte is produced in each cycle in the human, and therefore the ZP presents a theoretically attractive target for immunological contraception. This has provoked considerable and ongoing interest in the antigenicity of the ZP and its susceptibility to immunological attack (Shivers et al, 1972; Sacco, 1987; Dunbar, 1989).

The ZP is highly immunogenic and contains antigens that appear to be tissue-specific. Active or passive immunization of rodents against ZP antigens reduces fertility. Antisera to ZP block sperm penetration and can be demonstrated by phase contrast or immunofluorescence microscopy to coat the zona surface. There is also some evidence that egg 'hatching' can be inhibited. In addition, sera from infertile women with anti-ZP antibodies block in vitro fertilization involving human gametes, and ova from women exhibiting these antibodies are incapable of in vitro fertilization.

Antibodies to human ZP cross-react with pig ZP so that in early studies there has been an animal source of antigen for extensive analysis and possible vaccine development. Generally, however, antibodies (both mono-clonal and polyclonal) raised against ZP recognize antigens that are species-specific. However, ZP genes seem to be conserved across mammalian species so that results of experimental studies in homologous animal models, where the ZP genes have been isolated, can be extrapolated to higher animals.

Despite these encouraging considerations, there are some doubts as to whether ZP antigens will ultimately prove to be suitable targets for a contraceptive vaccine. Although immunization regimens involving reason-ably well characterized ZP antigens can be shown to inhibit fertility effectively in several species including infrahuman primates, these effects are invariably accompanied by altered ovarian function and/or autoimmune pathology in the ovary (Henderson et al, 1988). These findings are not unduly surprising since the target antigens involved are present on ovarian oocytes as well as mature ova. The data also suggest that the genesis of the ovarian immunopathology cannot adequately be explained by the relative impurity of the antigenic preparations, but that it is related to intrinsic properties of ZP proteins that provoke a cytotoxic response in ovarian tissue.

In view of the adverse effects provoked by immunization with purified ZP proteins containing both T and B cell epitopes, a desirable ZP immunogen should contain only B cell epitopes in order to elicit a selective antibody response and to avoid tissue pathology and irreversibility (Dean and Millar, 1990). These, of course, are general requirements of a contraceptive vac-cine, but they have become more visibly important in the experimental studies of ZP immunization. This approach has been adopted by Dean and colleagues (Millar et al, 1989; Dean and Millar, 1990) who have demon-strated relatively long-term, but reversible, antifertility effects in female mice, in the absence of immunopathology, following immunization with a B epitope containing synthetic peptide (ZP-3 peptide) coupled to a T epitope carrier molecule to stimulate helper T cell function. Another approach to safe immunization against the oocyte might involve the identification of phase-specific antigen(s) on the surface of the ovulated ovum. Such antigens would ideally be present, or at least expressed, during a brief period span-ning the events involved in sperm–ovum contact and sperm penetration.

Embryonic and placental antigens

The major interest in this group of antigens lies with hCG which will be considered below. Many other glycoproteins of trophoblast origin have now been described and proposed as target antigens for contraceptive vacci-nation.

Antigens that are intrinsic to, or present on the surface of trophoblast cells, have the advantage of being expressed at only one anatomical site following fertilization and they are in intimate contact with maternal blood. Much progress has been made in this area and both monoclonal antibodies and newer techniques in molecular genetics have been recruited to identify and isolate putatively specific antigens of the trophoblast surface (Mueller et al, 1986; Anderson et al, 1987). This approach should gain momentum over the next few years and should ultimately assume a place in the development of contraceptive vaccines despite the relative disadvantage of its mode of action which involves the interception of pregnancy at a peri-implantation stage.

HUMAN CHORIONIC GONADOTROPHIN

The antifertility vaccine that will most likely be applied first to family planning programmes is one directed against the pregnancy hormone hCG. This hormone is produced by the trophoblast cells of the conceptus and can be found on the trophectoderm as early as the blastocyst stage prior to implantation. It provides a signal of conception, at least in part, by its luteotrophic effect on the corpus luteum whereby it stimulates maternal ovarian secretion of progesterone which is necessary to establish and maintain a pregnancy in its earliest stages. A vaccine directed against hCG might therefore be expected to interrupt pregnancy at a very early (peri-implantation) stage by either neutralizing the physiological luteotrophic action of hCG or by immunologically destroying the trophoblast cells of the pre- or post-implantation blastocyst (Figure 1).

Immunization against the whole hCG molecule will provoke antibodies which cross-react strongly with human luteinizing hormone (hLH), from the anterior pituitary gland, since hCG and hLH have α-chains in common. For

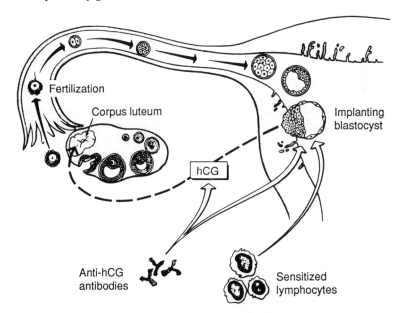

Figure 1. Possible modes of action of an anti-hCG vaccine. Antibodies capable of neutralizing hCG may inhibit its luteotrophic action on the corpus luteum. Cytotoxic anti-hCG antibodies or sensitized lymphocytes may disrupt the peri-implantation blastocyst.

practical purposes, therefore, efforts to develop an anti-hCG vaccine have been confined to the use of the β-chain and its natural or synthetic component peptides.

Whatever the mode of action, data in actively immunized marmosets (Hearn, 1976) and baboons (Stevens, 1976), indicate that an hCG vaccine is capable of blocking fertility at an early stage of pregnancy, with no discernible alterations in the menstrual cycle. These early data provided encouragement for the feasibility and acceptability of a contraceptive vaccine based on hCG.

Potential hCG antigens

hCG is a glycoprotein with a molecular weight of approximately 38 kDa and a carbohydrate content of 30%. The hCG molecule consists of two dissimilar covalently linked subunits designated α and β. These subunits have been dissociated and purified and their primary structures established. The α-subunit of hCG is similar in structure to its counterpart in hLH and other pituitary glycoprotein hormones except for its content of β-galactose and sialic acid. There are, however, chemical differences between the β-subunit of hCG (β-hCG) and those of the pituitary hormones. Notwithstanding this, β-hCG and the β-chain of hLH (β-hLH) have 94 (85%) of their first 110 amino acids in common. However, β-hLH has only 110 residues, whereas β-hCG has 145. Except for two positions, the 35 amino acid sequence of the carboxy-terminal (CT) end of β-hCG is not represented in β-hLH. These extra residues confer potentially unique antigenic properties on hCG and provide the basis of an immunogen capable of provoking antibodies with specificity for hCG.

Vaccine development

Intact hCG is unacceptable as a vaccine immunogen due to the potential hazards of immunity to the human α-subunit which is common to other hormones. However, vaccines have been formulated using the whole β-hCG subunit and have proved to be immunogenic and potentially efficacious in early human trials (Talwar et al, 1976, 1990; Nash et al, 1980). Although, contaminating immunity to hLH remains a theoretical concern in any vaccine approach using the β-hCG subunit, the available data fail to demonstrate any clinical evidence of overt immunological or endocrinological hazards.

A vaccine formulation has been prepared using the unique CT peptide portion of β-hCG as antigen (Lee et al, 1980; Stevens et al, 1981a). This approach was adopted by the World Health Organisation Task Force on Fertility Regulating Vaccines in order to achieve specificity and to avoid cross-reactive autoimmunity involving β-hLH. The antigen, a synthetic oligopeptide corresponding to the amino acid sequence 109–145 in β-hCG, was conjugated to diphtheria toxoid to enhance its immunogenicity. The remaining components of the vaccine were a water-soluble synthetic muramyl dipeptide (MDP) analogue as adjuvant and a saline–oil emulsion vehicle with an oil phase consisting of 4 parts squalene to 1 part mannide mono-oleate (Arlacel-A) as an emulsifying agent. The aim of this vaccine was to produce reversible immunity, and therefore contraception, for around 12 months, following which a booster injection would be required to maintain protection.

The prototype vaccine proved efficacious in baboons (Stevens et al, 1981b) and was subjected to detailed toxicological and immunological safety testing (Stevens and Jones, 1983). Preclinical assessment involved acute toxicology in the mouse and rat, subacute toxicology in the rat, and muscle irritancy studies in the rabbit. Immunosafety studies were conducted in baboons who received three intramuscular injections of 0.5 ml vaccine volume at 28-day intervals. Clinical, haematological, biochemical and urinary parameters were assessed together with in vivo testing for hypersensitivity, tissue autoantibodies, immune complexes, and hormone antibody cross-reactivity. Histopathology was assessed extensively following sacrifice 90 days after the last injection. Additional studies involved a separate group of baboons hyperimmunized with the vaccine or its individual components by six injections at fortnightly intervals.

A phase I clinical trial of the safety and immunogenicity of this vaccine was approved by the US Food and Drug Administration in 1984 and subsequently by the Australian Department of Health in 1985. The trial was conducted during 1986 and 1987, and details of its design and results were published subsequently (Jones et al, 1988). In brief, 30 premenopausal female subjects who had been surgically sterilized previously were assigned to five dosage groups of six subjects each and received the vaccine by intramuscular injection on two occasions 6 weeks apart. In each group four subjects received the full vaccine and two received the adjuvant and vehicle alone in a similar injection volume. The highest vaccine dose comprised 1.0 mg peptide–carrier conjugate in 0.5 ml vehicle. Immunogenicity and safety parameters were intensively monitored over a 6-month follow-up period, with further follow-up assessment as indicated.

The results of this trial confirmed the immunogenicity and potential safety of a vaccine based on the CT peptide of β-hCG. The vaccine was well tolerated and produced no unacceptable side-effects on clinical or laboratory assessment. Extensive longitudinal serological studies were performed on all subjects to assess the possibility of cross-reactive autoimmunity. The findings showed:

1. an increase in the level of pre-existing antibodies of mixed specificity resulting from the generalized stimulation of the immune system by the vaccine;
2. antibodies reacting with other tissues possibly as a result of molecular mimicry between the hCG peptide and diphtheria toxoid components of the vaccine.

None of the tissue cross-reactions observed was considered significant nor indicative of future immunopathology associated with the use of this particular hCG vaccine. However, these experiments did highlight the need to include such tests as an integral part of ongoing hCG vaccine development programmes and in the future clinical evaluations of these vaccines.

It has been estimated that approximately 0.26 nmol/l of hCG binding capacity will be needed to neutralize the level of hCG (135 mIU/ml) present in the maternal circulation at the time of implantation. However, preliminary data from the phase I trial indicate that the biological neutralizing capacity of the hCG antisera is approximately 50% of its in vitro binding capacity for the hormone, suggesting that an antibody titre of at least 0.52 nmol/l will be needed to achieve an antifertility effect if the vaccine works solely by neutralizing the biological action of the hormone. This threshold of antibody production was exceeded in all five subject groups, with the antibody titres in the higher dose groups reaching 5–7 times the level estimated to confer antifertility efficacy. In the majority of subjects in all dose groups, the hCG antibodies remained above the efficacy threshold for approximately 6 months and, in the case of the highest dose group, for more than 10 months.

FUTURE STUDIES

The prototype hCG peptide vaccine developed by the World Health Organisation is a complex formulation which requires careful but vigorous mixing immediately prior to injection. Although suitable for phase I and preliminary phase II clinical trials in a small number of volunteers, it is unsuitable, in its present form, for manufacture and clinical use on a large scale.

Ongoing studies are therefore aimed at the development of a second generation of the hCG vaccine which will consist of simpler components and formulations. These studies involve comparative evaluations of new hCG peptides, alternative carriers, adjuvants and vehicles in which the vaccine can be administered. Of particular interest in this regard is the development of biodegradable and biocompatible delivery systems that permit long-lasting antifertility immunity to be generated following a single injection of vaccine. The successful development of safe, effective and acceptable vaccines of this type will be particularly beneficial to both the users and providers of family planning methods in those countries where the storage and distribution of drugs and devices is difficult and access to health services is limited. Other approaches to contraceptive vaccine development will undoubtedly involve the use of expression vectors for antigen presentation by either parenteral or oral routes. The need to optimize the required immune response without undesirable effects of hypersensitivity reactions, hapten (antigen) suppression or T cell memory will require careful consideration for any new method of vaccine presentation.

There has been much interest, but little progress, in the selective establishment of local immunity in the genital tract as a desirable feature of antifertility vaccines, particularly, for example, one directed against sperm. A method which avoided or at least minimized systemic immunity would greatly reduce the likelihood of vaccine side-effects.

No doubt, new target antigens will be identified and polyvalent vaccines may be devised which inhibit fertility at more than one step in the reproductive process. Another feature of antifertility vaccines is the possibility of combining them with therapy for endemic infection so that co-immunization is achieved against disease and fertility.

The availability of antifertility vaccines will not eliminate the need for existing methods of birth control. The family planning requirements of a particular individual or population vary widely and no single method will be adequate for all. Contraceptive vaccines will be particularly attractive to persons where medical care is not easily accessible, where education and motivation to use a method frequently or precisely does not exist, where experience has shown unacceptable side-effects of other methods or where the cost of other methods greatly exceeds that of vaccine use on an annual basis.

SUMMARY

The principle of vaccination for the purposes of fertility regulation is scientifically elegant and socially compelling. Factors such as economic production, convenience of use, relatively long-lasting but reversible protection, low failure rate and the avoidance of mechanical devices or exogenous hormones make this approach a potentially attractive option for family planning programmes in both developing and developed countries.

The major efforts in research and development have involved the prospect of active immunization against specific antigens of sperm, oocyte, zygote and early embryo, and the pregnancy hormone human chorionic gonadotrophin (hCG). Several anti-hCG vaccines have entered clinical trials. They operate by preventing or interrupting pregnancy at the peri-implantation stage probably by neutralizing the luteotrophic effect of hCG. The most refined vaccine is one directed against the unique C-terminal peptide on the β-subunit of hCG. This vaccine provokes antibodies that are specific for hCG and do not cross-react with human luteinizing hormone (hLH). Preclinical studies in baboons and data from a phase I human trial indicate that this method is free of side-effects and provides the promise of a duration of effectiveness of up to 12 months.

Future research will optimize the anti-hCG approach, utilize new vaccine delivery systems and broaden the spectrum of target antigens of potential utility for contraceptive vaccines.

REFERENCES

Ada GL & Griffin PD (1991a) The process of reproduction in humans: antigens for vaccine development. In Ada GL & Griffin PD (eds) *Vaccines for Fertility Regulation: The Assessment of their Safety and Efficacy*, pp 13–26. Cambridge: Cambridge University Press.

Ada GL & Griffin PD (1991b) *Vaccines for Fertility Regulation: The Assessment of their Safety and Efficacy*. Cambridge: Cambridge University Press.

Alexander NJ, Griffin D, Spieler JM & Waites GMH (eds) (1990) *Gamete Interaction: Prospects for Immunocontraception*. New York: Wiley-Liss.

Anderson DJ, Johnson PM, Alexander NC et al (1987) Report of WHO-sponsored workshop on monoclonal antibodies to human sperm and trophoblast antigens. *Journal of Reproductive Immunology* **10**: 231–257.

Dean J & Millar SE (1990) Zona pellucida: target for a contraceptive vaccine. In Alexander NJ, Griffin D, Spieler JM & Waites GMH (eds) *Gamete Interaction: Prospects for Immunocontraception*, pp 313–326. New York: Wiley-Liss.

Dunbar BS (1989) Ovarian antigens and infertility. *American Journal of Reproductive Immunology* **21**: 28.

Hearn JB (1976) Immunisation against pregnancy. *Proceedings of the Royal Society for Medicine* **195**: 149–160.

Henderson CJ, Hulme MJ & Aitken RJ (1988) Contraceptive potential of antibodies to the zona pellucida. *Journal of Reproduction and Fertility* **83**: 325–343.

Herr JC, Wright RM, John E et al (1990) Monoclonal antibody MHS-10 and its cognate intra-acrosomal antigen SP-10. In Alexander NJ, Griffin D, Spieler JM & Waites GMH (eds) *Gamete Interaction: Prospects for Immunocontraception*, pp 13–36. New York: Wiley-Liss.

Jones WR (1974) The use of antibodies developed by infertile women to identify relevant antigens. In Diczfalusy E (ed.) *Immunological Approaches to Fertility Control*, p 376. Stockholm: Karolinska Institutet.

Jones WR (1982) *Immunological Fertility Regulation*. Melbourne: Blackwell Scientific.

Jones WR (1988) Immunology and infertility. In Behrman SJ, Kistner RW & Patton GW (eds) *Progress in Infertility* (3rd edn), p 751. Boston: Little, Brown & Co.

Jones WR, Bradley J, Judd SJ et al (1988) Phase I clinical trial of a World Health Organisation birth control vaccine. *Lancet* **i**: 1295–1298.

Lee AC, Powell JE, Tregear GW et al (1980) A method for preparing β-hCG COOH peptide-carrier conjugates of predictable composition. *Molecular Immunology* **17**: 749–756.

Millar SE, Chamow SM, Baur AW et al (1989) Vaccination with synthetic zona pellucida peptide produces long-term contraception in female mice. *Science* **246**: 935–938.

Mueller UW, Hawes CS & Jones WR (1986) Cell surface antigens of human trophoblast: definition of an apparently unique system with a monoclonal antibody. *Immunology* **59**: 135–138.

Nash H, Talwar GP, Segal SJ et al (1980) Observations on the antigenicity and clinical effects of a candidate anti-pregnancy vaccine. *Fertility and Sterility* **34**: 328–335.

Naz R & Menge A (1990) Development of antisperm contraceptive vaccine for humans: why and how? *Human Reproduction* **5**: 511–518.

Sacco AG (1987) The zona pellucida: current status as a candidate antigen for contraceptive vaccine development. *American Journal of Reproductive Immunology and Microbiology* **15**: 122–130.

Shivers CA, Dudkiewicz AB, Franklin LE & Fussell EN (1972) Inhibition of sperm–egg interaction by specific antibody. *Science* **178**: 1211–1213.

Stevens VC (1976) Perspective of development of a fertility control vaccine from hormonal antigens of trophoblast. In *Development of Vaccines for Fertility Regulation*, pp 93–110. Copenhagen: Scriptor.

Stevens VC & Jones WR (1983) Pre-clinical safety studies on an hCG vaccine. In Isojima S & Billington WD (eds) *Reproductive Immunology 1983*, pp 233–237. Amsterdam: Elsevier.

Stevens VC, Cinader B, Powell JE, Lee AC & Koh SW (1981a) Preparation and formulation of a human chorionic gonadotrophin antifertility vaccine: selection of adjuvant and vehicle. *American Journal of Reproductive Immunology* **1**: 315–321.

Stevens VC, Powell JE, Lee AC & Griffin PD (1981b) Anti-fertility effects from immunization of female baboons with C-terminal peptides of hCG beta subunit. *Fertility and Sterility* **36**: 98–105.

Talwar GP, Sharma NC, Dubey SK et al (1976) Isoimmunization against human chorionic gonadotrophin with conjugates of processed β-subunit of the hormone and tetanus toxoid. *Proceedings of the National Academy of Sciences (USA)* **73**: 218–222.

Talwar GP, Singh O, Pal R & Arunan K (1990) Experiences of the anti-hCG vaccine of relevance to development of other birth control vaccines. In Alexander NJ, Griffin D, Spieler JM & Waites GMH (eds) *Gamete Interaction: Prospects for Immunocontraception*, pp 579–593. New York: Wiley-Liss.

13

The immune system and gynaecological cancer

S. T. A. MALIK
A. A. EPENETOS

INTRODUCTION

The relationship of the immune system and cancer has traditionally been considered in terms of immune surveillance in the control of cancer and the potential for immunotherapy in cancer. There is little evidence to suggest that the frequency of gynaecological neoplasms is increased in immunosuppressed patients or in immunodeficient animals, with the possible exception of human papilloma virus (HPV) associated cervical cancer.

However, the prospects for effective immunotherapy of cancer have been considerably enhanced by the availability of biological molecules such as monoclonal antibodies and recombinant cytokines. Monoclonal antibodies that recognize putative tumour associated antigens have already had an impact on the immunodiagnosis of cancer and the development of assays for tumour markers and their clinical use as antitumour agents have been addressed (Hird et al, 1990). This review discusses the use of active immunotherapy and cytokine therapy in the treatment of gynaecological cancer and breast cancer.

ACTIVE IMMUNOTHERAPY IN GYNAECOLOGICAL CANCER

Non-specific active immunotherapy

The earliest recorded trials of non-specific immunostimulants in patients with advanced malignancies were reported by a New York surgeon, William Coley, at the turn of the century (Coley, 1896). Coley had observed objective tumour regression in cancer patients who had intercurrent infections, particularly erysipelas. On the basis of these observations patients with advanced cancer, including gynaecological cancers, were treated with preparations of erysipelas-inducing streptococci and *Serratia marcescens* with remarkable results (Nauts, 1987). However, therapy with 'Coley's toxins' was largely abandoned with the advent of radiotherapy and chemotherapy, and due to the problems associated with obtaining preparations of standardized activity.

Non-specific immunoadjuvants such as BCG and *Corynebacterium*

Baillière's Clinical Obstetrics and Gynaecology—
Vol. 6, No. 3, September 1992
ISBN 0–7020–1634–9

parvum were shown to have antitumour activity in animal tumour models, and have been investigated in patients with ovarian cancer. The most notable results of BCG therapy in gynaecological cancer were reported by Alberts et al (1979) in a randomized study of 121 patients treated with chemotherapy alone (cyclophosphamide and adriamycin), or chemotherapy combined with BCG given by scarification. There was a significantly higher response rate in the BCG group (18%) compared with the control group (3%), and this was reflected in the median survival of the two groups of 22.3 months and 13.7 months respectively. However, two subsequent studies from the same group of investigators failed to confirm any additional benefit of BCG in combination with cisplatin containing regimens (Alberts et al, 1989a,b). There are two reported randomized trials of intravenous *C. parvum* in combination with standardized chemotherapy in ovarian cancer. Wanebo et al (1979) noted no additional benefit, but a significantly higher response rate and progression free interval was noted in the immunotherapy group in the trial reported by Gall et al (1980). However, the design of the latter study has been criticized because all of the immunotherapy patients in this multicentre study were treated at a single institution. Therapy with multiple courses of intraperitoneal *C. parvum* alone led to two complete and three partial responses in a group of 11 patients with ovarian cancer (Bast et al, 1983).

Other immunoadjuvants such as levamisole and the heat and penicillin-treated preparation of the low virulence strain of *Streptococcus pyogenes* (OK-432) have been given to patients with ovarian cancer, but the value of these agents remains to be assessed in randomized clinical trials. Two randomized studies of adjuvant immunotherapy with OK-432 and the immunostimulant sizofuran have been reported (Okamura et al, 1989) in patients with cervical cancer. There was a statistically significant 3-year recurrence-free rate in the 221 patients in the OK-432 group (72%), compared with the 161 patients in the control group (58.6%). Sizofuran also led to a significantly greater 5-year survival rate in patients with stage II–III cancer, compared with the control group.

A series of studies of BCG immunotherapy in conjunction with cytotoxic chemotherapy were reported in patients with stage II breast cancer (Buzdar et al, 1979). The promising results were not substantiated in randomized controlled trials (Hubay et al, 1985). There are no convincing data that the use of levamisole, or other immunoadjuvants has any therapeutic benefit in patients with breast cancer. Intralesional BCG and purified protein derivative (PPD) have both been used to treat local chest wall recurrences of breast cancer with some success (Klein et al, 1976; Pardridge et al, 1979). For example, repeated injections of BCG led to tumour regressions in 8 of 11 patients. Five of these patients had complete tumour regressions that lasted from 12 to 33 months (Pardridge et al, 1979).

Specific active immunotherapy

Specific active immunotherapy entails the injection of tumour antigens in order to generate an antitumour immune response. There is increasing evidence that some human cancers express potentially highly immunogenic epitopes such as the polymorphic epithelial mucin (PEM). Ovarian cancer patients have been shown to mount an immune response to ovarian tumour cells (Levin et al, 1975). Graham and Graham (1962) reported that the injection of whole tumour homogenates, saline extracts, or unirradiated tumour cell suspensions given in conjunction with chemotherapy and radiotherapy, led to a higher survival rate. The significance of these results is dubious because the chemotherapy was not standardized and a small number of patients was studied.

A novel approach has been to inject viral oncolysates from ovarian cancer cell lines infected with the influenza virus. The infected cell lines express both ovarian cancer-associated and viral antigens. Viral oncolysates were administered intraperitoneally to 31 patients with ascites. Ascites disappeared in seven patients and was accompanied by a reduction of tumour mass in three of the patients (Freedman et al, 1988). In two out of five patients with solid intraperitoneal tumours only, objective tumour regression was noted. In most patients injected with viral oncolysates, antibodies and T cell responses to tumour cell surface antigens and viral antigens were detected (Freedman et al, 1990). Further studies of this approach are awaited.

CYTOKINE THERAPY

Many of the antitumour effects of non-specific immunostimulants are due to the release of cytokines. For example, the antitumour effect of endotoxin was shown to be mediated by a serum factor now known to be tumour necrosis factor (TNF) (Carswell et al, 1975). Lymphotoxin (LT or TNF-β) was identified as a soluble lymphocyte-derived mediator with antitumour effects in vitro, released in the course of delayed hypersensitivity reactions (Granger and Williams, 1968). Cytokines are peptide cell regulators, most of which were originally characterized as products of the immune system and termed lymphokines or monokines. However, it is now evident that many cytokines are produced by other cell populations and have roles that extend beyond their immunomodulatory effects. Table 1 lists some of the major cytokines that have been identified.

Several cytokines are thought to have in vitro and in vivo antitumour actions (Balkwill, 1989). The direct effects of cytokines on tumour growth may be cytotoxic or cytostatic and are occasionally related to the induction of cellular differentiation (Kelly et al, 1990). The antitumour actions of cytokines may also be mediated indirectly by activation of host antitumour responses and disruption of the host–tumour relationship, e.g. by toxic effects on tumour vasculature.

In addition to their use as antitumour agents, cytokines are likely to be used increasingly as adjuncts to existing standard therapies. The colony stimulating factors are already in clinical use as agents to alleviate the myelosuppressive effects of chemotherapy and bone marrow transplantation, and their use may allow further dose escalation of existing chemotherapy regimens (Peters, 1991). Experimental data suggest other potential

Table 1. List of major cytokines.

	Molecular weight (kDa)	Normal sources
Interferons		
Interferon-α	17–23	Leukocytes
Interferon-β	20	Fibroblasts
Interferon-γ	20	T, NK cells
Tumour necrosis factors		
TNF-α	17–26	Many cells
TNF-β	20–25	T and B cells
Colony stimulating factors		
G-CSF	19	Many cells
GM-CSF	45	Many cells
M-CSF	22	Many cells
Multi-CSF (IL-3)	25	Many cells
Interleukins		
IL-1	17.5	Many cells
IL-2	17.2	T cells
IL-4	20	Many cells
IL-5	18	T cells
IL-6	26	Many cells
IL-7	26	T cells
IL-8	8	Many cells
IL-9	8	Many cells
IL-10	8	T cells
IL-11	16	T cells
Transforming growth factors		
TGF-α	15	Many cells
TGF-β	25	Many cells

uses for cytokines in cancer therapy, e.g. modulation of oncogene expression (Marth et al, 1990), modulation of oestrogen and progesterone receptor expression (DeCicco et al, 1988), and enhancement of antibody localization (Smyth et al, 1988). The following section will review the status of cytokine therapy of gynaecological cancers with cytokines that have undergone clinical trials as antitumour agents, i.e. the interferons (IFNs), tumour necrosis factor, and interleukin 2 (IL-2).

Interferons

The three major classes of IFNs (α, β, and γ) have antiproliferative effects on tumour cells in vitro and in vivo (Balkwill, 1989). There is experimental evidence to suggest that their antitumour activity can be due to a direct effect on tumour cells, mediated by activation of effector cells such as natural killer cells and macrophages, or caused by alterations of the host–tumour relationship. Data from human ovarian cancer xenograft models indicate that a direct, dose-dependent cytostatic effect is their major mode of action (Balkwill et al, 1989; Malik et al, 1992). In general, IFN-α was noted to be more effective in the therapy of human cancer xenografts (Balkwill et al,

1989), but the precise mechanism of its antitumour effect remains to be elucidated. Recent data suggest that some of the antitumour activity of IFN-γ may be mediated by modulation of tryptophan metabolism (Malik et al, 1992) and by inhibition of c-*erb*-β$_2$ proto-oncogene expression in ovarian cancer cells (Marth et al, 1990). Since IFNs were originally described as virally induced proteins that inhibited the replication of viruses (Isaacs and Lindemann, 1957), their use in HPV-associated anogenital neoplasms is of potential therapeutic value.

Several trials of IFN-α in patients with ovarian cancer have been reported (reviewed in Bookman and Bast, 1991). Systemic administration of IFN-α, either intramuscularly or subcutaneously, has shown minimal activity in most studies (Einhorn et al, 1982, 1988; Freedman et al, 1983; Niloff et al, 1985). Following intraperitoneal instillation of IFN-α, 30–1000-fold higher levels of IFN-α were noted in the peritoneal fluid compared with serum. Berek et al (1985) reported complete and partial remissions in five of 11 patients treated with intraperitoneal IFN-α. An escalating dose regimen was used, starting at 5×10^6 to 50×10^6 units given weekly over a period of 16 weeks. Response was related to the residual amount of tumour prior to commencement of therapy, and none of the patients with a residual tumour mass of greater than 5 mm achieved a response. Five out of the seven patients (71%) with residual tumour less than 5 mm had surgically documented responses. The major side-effects were fever, vomiting and occasionally abdominal pain. Willemse et al (1990) treated 20 evaluable patients with minimal residual disease at second look laparotomy with IFN-α2b, administered at a dose of 50×10^6 units weekly for 8 weeks. Of the 17 patients re-evaluated at third look laparotomy, five were in complete remission, four had partial remissions, six had stabilization of disease, and in two patients there was progression of disease. Their findings confirmed those of Berek et al (1985) in that all responses were confined to patients with residual tumour less than 5 mm. The feasibility of combination therapy with IFN-α and chemotherapy has been demonstrated in patients with ovarian cancer (Nardi et al, 1990) but randomized trials are required to assess the contribution of IFN to IFN–cytotoxic drug combination regimens. Although IFN-β interacts with the same receptor as IFN-α, there are no studies assessing the relative antitumour effects of these cytokines in patients with solid tumours. There has been one study reporting the use of intraperitoneal IFN-β in patients with advanced bulky ovarian cancer. No objective responses were noted, although the reaccumulation of ascites was prevented in some patients (Rambaldi et al, 1985).

Several recent clinical trials of IFN-γ in the treatment of ovarian cancer have been reported. IFN-γ has a broader range of immunomodulatory actions compared with IFN-α and IFN-β, such as the induction of MHC class II antigens on tumour cells and the activation of antitumour macrophages. Allevana et al (1990) administered recombinant IFN-γ (rIFN-γ) to seven patients and noted the enhancement of MHC class II expression on tumour cells, and an increase in the cytotoxicity of tumour associated macrophages and lymphocytes. D'Aquisto et al (1988) conducted a phase I trial of intraperitoneal rIFN-γ in 27 patients with refractory ovarian cancer and noted minimal toxicity up to doses of 8×10^6 units. No responses were noted; however, most of the patients had advanced disease and only four patients were studied at each dose level. Pujade-Lauraine et al (1991) have reported the preliminary findings of a trial of intraperitoneal rIFN-γ in patients with ovarian cancer. Fifteen complete and two partial surgically documented responses were seen in 58 patients treated with intraperitoneal rIFN-γ at a dose of 20×10^6 units, twice weekly for 2–4 months. Most responses were seen in patients with small volume disease (<2 cm). Welander et al (1988), however, noted objective tumour regressions in 4 of 14 patients with relapsed ovarian carcinoma following intravenous administration of IFN-γ. This study needs to be confirmed because of the apparent efficacy of systemic IFN-γ in some patients with bulky chemotherapy-resistant disease.

The potential role of HPV in anogenital neoplasms, particularly cervical carcinoma, and the antiviral effect of IFNs suggest a possible therapeutic role for these cytokines. For example, selective suppression of HPV type 18 mRNA levels in HeLa cervical carcinoma cells was noted in vitro (Nawa et al, 1990). Significant antitumour effects of IFNs in advanced cervical carcinoma have, however, not been reported, and the data from clinical trials in early stage tumours are conflicting. Durham et al (1990) noted improvement in both the histology and HPV expression in six out of seven patients with cervical intraepithelial neoplasia (CIN) whilst no effect was noted in a double-blind study reported by Frost et al (1990). Both studies were conducted with intralesional injections of IFN-α2b. Other reports suggest the effect of IFNs may not be related solely to HPV infection. Yliskoski et al (1990) reported a placebo-controlled trial to assess the effect of leukocyte IFN cream on patients with HPV-associated CIN or vaginal intraepithelial neoplasia. Clinical evaluation showed that four out of nine patients treated with topical IFN over a period of 12 months showed clinical remissions (assessed by colposcopy and histological examination, and remained HPV negative. In the placebo group, seven of ten patients showed clinical improvement, but four of these patients also remained HPV positive. Whilst this study suggested that IFN was more effective at eliminating HPV infection than reversing malignant change, other studies suggest that IFN may eliminate dysplastic cells more effectively than virally infected cells (Davidovich et al, 1989). There is one study of the use of IFN-γ in the therapy of HPV-associated neoplasms (Kirby et al, 1988). A total of 28 patients with refractory genital warts were treated with intramuscular IFN-γ. A 53% response rate was noted and minimal side-effects were seen.

The use of interferons in the therapy of gynaecological cancers needs further investigation, particularly in the treatment of small volume residual ovarian cancer. Their efficacy needs to be assessed in randomized controlled studies either as single agents or in combination with chemotherapeutic agents. Experimental data suggest that additive antitumour effects with normal therapy may be seen, e.g. IFN-α has been shown to upregulate progesterone receptor expression in endometrial cancers in patients (Scambia et al, 1991), but there are no reported clinical trials of this combined approach to date. IFNs have shown some activity in experimental models of human breast cancer (Balkwill et al, 1989), but this has not been confirmed in clinical trials.

Tumour necrosis factor

Tumour necrosis factor was identified as the major cytokine that mediated the antitumour effects of endotoxin and other agents known to cause reticuloendothelial hyperplasia in experimental animal models (Carswell et al, 1975). However, subsequent studies have shown that TNF is a cytokine with multiple effects on a variety of cell populations, and that its antitumour activity in experimental models has to be interpreted with caution (Malik and Balkwill, 1992). Numerous clinical trials of recombinant TNF have been reported with uniformly disappointing results (Jones and Selby, 1989) in spite of extensive experimental evidence suggesting that it would be effective against human tumours in vivo (Malik and Balkwill, 1992). Some success has been noted with intratumoral injection of TNF but this is of limited clinical value (Diehl et al, 1987). Trials of intratumoral injection of crude lymphotoxin have shown objective tumour regressions of short duration in breast cancer patients with skin metastases (Papermaster et al, 1976; Pulley et al, 1986). Rath et al (1991) treated patients with malignant ascites, including ovarian cancer patients, and noted that intraperitoneal rTNF prevented the reaccumulation of ascites. The mechanism of this effect is unknown, but has been noted in experimental models of human ovarian cancer (Malik et al, 1989; Manetta et al, 1989). As discussed in the next section, Malik et al (1989) noted a paradoxical effect of TNF in three human ovarian cancer xenograft models, i.e. although TNF was effective in eradicating ascitic tumour, it also promoted the implantation of tumour cells in the abdominal cavity. It seems unlikely that TNF as a single agent will have significant antitumour effects in gynaecological malignancies, particularly as ovarian cancers have been shown to produce TNF (Naylor et al, 1990). However, the use of intraperitoneal TNF in combination with other cytokines, particularly IFN-γ, remains an attractive therapeutic option in view of their synergistic effects in experimental models (Balkwill et al, 1986).

Interleukin 2

The description of the lymphokine-activated killer (LAK) cell phenomenon has been a major stimulus to the development of adoptive specific immunotherapy, i.e. injection of immune cells activated in vitro to an antitumour state (Grimm et al, 1982). Autologous lymphocytes incubated with interleukin 2 (IL-2) were shown selectively to lyse fresh tumour cells in vitro. The basic principles of IL-2–LAK therapy are illustrated in Figure 1. The patient is initially treated with either bolus or continuous infusion of recombinant IL-2 for 3–5 days. During the latter stages of IL-2 infusion and immediately after stopping there is a rebound lymphocytosis. The patients are then leukopheresed to collect peripheral white blood cells (i.e. patients connected to a blood cell separator which separates out the buffy coat and

IL–2–LAK therapy   TIL cells

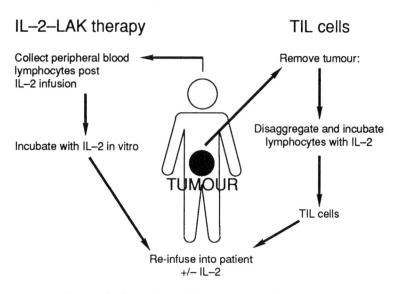

Collect peripheral blood
lymphocytes post
IL–2 infusion

Remove tumour:

Incubate with IL–2 in vitro

Disaggregate and incubate
lymphocytes with IL–2

TUMOUR

TIL cells

Re-infuse into patient
+/– IL–2

Figure 1. Basic principles of IL-2–LAK and TIL cell therapy.

returns other blood components back to the patient). The collected white blood cells are incubated in vitro with recombinant IL-2 for a period of up to 7 days and then reinfused into the patient with concomitant IL-2 administration. Rosenberg et al (1985) demonstrated the antitumour activity of IL-2– LAK therapy in a cohort of patients with advanced refractory cancers, particularly in renal cell cancer and in melanoma. However, the original IL-2–LAK therapy protocol was associated with considerable toxicity and there is continuing controversy on the most effective regimen of IL-2 therapy in cancer. Rosenberg's group also demonstrated that lymphoid cells from tumours could be expanded in culture in vitro with IL-2 and develop tumour-specific cytotoxicity (Figure 1). These so-called 'TIL' cells (tumour infiltrating lymphocytes) have been shown to localize specifically to tumour sites on reinfusion into patients, and induce tumour regression in selected series of patients with melanoma (Rosenberg et al, 1988). Trials of intra- peritoneal IL-2–LAK and TIL therapy have been reported in patients with ovarian cancer. The feasibility of IL-2–LAK therapy in ovarian cancer is indicated by data showing the efficacy of intraperitoneal IL-2–LAK therapy in experimental animal models (Ortaldo et al, 1986), pharmacokinetic data showing prolonged retention of IL-2 in the peritoneal cavity (Chapman et al, 1988), and the demonstration that lymphocytes from the peritoneal cavity can be induced selectively to lyse autologous tumour cells in vitro (Ioannides et al, 1991).

Stewart et al (1990) reported a phase I trial in which patients refractory to standard therapy were treated with intraperitoneal IL-2 and LAK cells. The basic protocol consisted of intravenous administration of recombinant IL-2, followed by harvesting peripheral blood lymphocytes by blood cell separation (leukopheresis). The peripheral blood lymphocytes were incubated in vitro with IL-2 (i.e. activated to antitumour state), and administered with recombinant IL-2 back into the peritoneal cavity. The dose-limiting toxicity was abdominal distension and pain due to accumulation of ascites. Other toxic manifestations included fever, nausea and vomiting, diarrhoea and anaemia. No significant clinical responses were noted, and in at least one patient undergoing laparotomy, increased peritoneal fibrosis was seen as noted in a previous study (Lotze et al, 1986). A phase II study reported the combined use of intraperitoneal IL-2 and LAK cells in a total of 24 patients, 10 of whom had ovarian cancer and one endometrial cancer (Steis et al, 1990). Two of the 10 ovarian cancer patients were partial responders at laparoscopy. Peritoneal fibrosis was noted in 14 of the 24 patients and was a limiting factor in continued therapy. The toxicity of the regimen was severe to moderate, but the toxic manifestations improved following discontinuation of IL-2. From these studies it is evident that IL-2–LAK therapy in its present form is complex and toxic. Some of this toxicity may be avoided if LAK cells can be specifically targeted to the tumour cells, possibly using TIL cells and antibody-guided therapy.

Aoki et al (1991) have injected patients with advanced ovarian cancer with TIL cells (lymphocytes obtained from solid tumours or effusions and activated in vitro in the presence of IL-2), with and without cisplatin-based chemotherapy. In the patients treated with TIL cells only following a single injection of cyclophosphamide, one complete response and four partial responses were seen, although these were of short duration. The toxicity of therapy was minimal. TIL cells were successfully administered with cisplatin, and seven complete and two partial responses were noted. Although the concomitant use of chemotherapy in both patient groups made it difficult to assess the precise contribution of TIL cells to these responses, this study has demonstrated that it is technologically feasible to carry out TIL therapy in intraperitoneal cancers with considerably less toxicity than intraperitoneal IL-2–LAK therapy.

There have been no large trials of IL-2–LAK therapy in breast cancer. Phase I trials of IL-2 alone have not shown major responses in heavily pretreated patients (D. Miles, personal communication). Adler et al (1984) have conducted a pilot trial of intralesional injection of IL-2 activated autologous LAK cells in four patients with breast cancer, and noted regression in 25% of injected lesions.

Cytokines in the pathophysiology of gynaecological cancers

There is increasing evidence of dysregulated cytokine biology in cancers. Several actions of cytokines may contribute to tumour progression, including growth stimulation of tumour cells, and enhancement of metastasis. Cytokines may also mediate paraneoplastic phenomena, e.g. cancer associated hypercalcaemia, fever, weight loss and hypergammaglobulinaemia (Sato et al, 1987; Kishimoto, 1989; Malik, 1992).

Ovarian cancers have been shown to elaborate a number of cytokines, including TNF, M-CSF, IL-6, TGF-β, IL-1, and TGF-α (Malik and

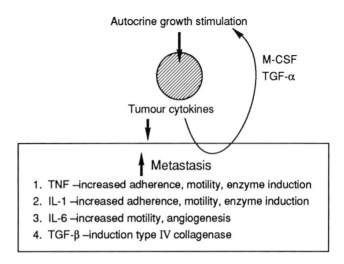

Figure 2. Cytokines and ovarian cancer pathophysiology.

Balkwill, 1991), that potentially contribute to tumour progression (Figure 2). Experimental data indicate that TNF production by ovarian cancers (Naylor et al, 1990; De Jaco et al, 1991; Takeyama et al, 1991) may be involved in a number of cancer-associated phenomena, such as metastasis (Malik et al, 1989, 1990), cancer-associated cachexia and anaemia (Oliff et al, 1987; Johnson et al, 1989), and hypercalcaemia (Yoneda et al, 1991). The expression of the M-CSF receptor and production of M-CSF by ovarian tumours suggests a potential autocrine growth promoting mechanism (Kacinski et al, 1990) in both ovarian cancers and uterine cancers (Kacinski et al, 1989a,b), and serum measurement of M-CSF levels may be of value in assessing disease status. Recent data also implicate TGF-α as an autocrine growth factor in ovarian cancer (Morishige et al, 1991). Erroi et al (1989) showed that tumour-associated macrophages from ovarian cancer patients spontaneously produce IL-6 and further investigations have shown production of IL-6 by ovarian tumour cells (Watson et al, 1990). Berek et al (1991) have shown that serum levels of IL-6 correlated with disease status in patients with ovarian cancer, suggesting that IL-6 is another potential serum marker in ovarian cancer. IL-6 may also theoretically enhance tumour progression by promoting angiogenesis and tumour cell motility (Tamm et al, 1989).

The major cytokine that may be involved in the pathogenesis of breast cancer is TGF-α (Saloman et al, 1991). Transgenic mice, i.e. genetically engineered mice, that overexpress the TGF-α gene developed mammary tumours and hyperplasia (Matsui et al, 1990). TGF-α expression in breast cancers has been shown by several investigators (Ciardiello et al, 1989; Lundy et al, 1991). TGF-α interacts specifically with the receptor for epidermal growth factor, the expression of which has been noted to correlate with the prognosis of breast cancer patients (Sainsbury et al, 1987). Recent data have shown that the overexpression of the c-*erb*-β2 oncogene product, which is a receptor similar to, but distinct from the epidermal growth factor receptor, may also indicate a worse prognosis for patients with breast cancer (Slamon et al, 1987; Berger et al, 1988; Tandon et al, 1989). The ligand for the c-*erb*-β2 encoded receptor is presumably an epidermal growth factor-like molecule that has yet to be identified. In contrast to TGF-α, TGF-β has been postulated to be a negative growth regulator in breast cancer. The expression of TGF-β can be regulated by oestrogens in breast cancer cell lines (Arrick et al, 1990), and experimental data suggest that tamoxifen may inhibit breast cancer cell growth by inducing TGF-β (Knabbe et al, 1987). TNF and M-CSF production by breast cancer cell lines has been noted (Spriggs et al, 1987), although there are no definitive data on the expression of these cytokines by breast tumours taken from patients.

SUMMARY

There have been major advances in our understanding of the cellular and humoral immune mechanisms involved in antitumour activities. The characterization of soluble mediators of the immune response and their synthesis as recombinant proteins has led to an explosion of research activity concerning their role as antitumour agents and also as contributors to the pathogenesis of cancer. It is evident that cytokine production is not restricted to cells of the immune system, and that cytokines are involved in a variety of cell regulatory processes ranging from embryonic development to tissue differentiation. Their production by immune cells may enable inter-actions between the immune system and other homeostatic systems of the body. The therapeutic role of some cytokines such as the interferons and IL-2 in the routine management of gynaecological cancers needs to be investigated further because of their promise as antitumour agents. The study of cytokine production and cytokine receptor expression by cancers is potentially of great therapeutic value. Identification of cytokines that contribute to tumour progression may paradoxically lead to the treatment of cancers by agents that antagonize their biological effects and to rational-ization of future trials of cytokine therapy.

REFERENCES

Adler A, Stein JA, Kedar E et al (1984) Intralesional injection of interleukin-2 expanded autologous lymphocytes in melanoma and breast cancer patients. A pilot study. *Journal of Biological Response Modifiers* 3: 491–500.
Alberts DS, Moon TE, Stephens RA et al (1979) Randomized study of chemoimmunotherapy for advanced ovarian carcinoma: a preliminary report of a Southwest Oncology Group study. *Cancer Treatment Reports* 63: 325–331.
Alberts DS, Mason-Liddil N, O'Toole RV et al (1989a) Randomized phase III trial of chemoimmunotherapy in patients with previously untreated stage III and IV suboptimal disease ovarian cancer: a Southwest Oncology Group study. *Gynecologic Oncology* 32: 8–15.

Alberts DS, Mason-Liddil N, O'Toole RV et al (1989b) Randomized phase III trial of chemoimmunotherapy in patients with previously untreated stage III, optimal disease ovarian cancer: a Southwest Oncology Group study. *Gynecologic Oncology* **32:** 16–29.

Allevana P, Peccatori D, Maggioni D et al (1990) Intraperitoneal recombinant γ-interferon in patients with recurrent ascitic ovarian carcinoma: modulation of cytotoxicity and cytokine production in tumor associated effectors and of major histocompatibility antigen expression on tumor cells. *Cancer Research* **50:** 7318–7323.

Aoki Y, Takakuwa K, Kodama S et al (1991) Use of adoptive transfer of tumor-infiltrating lymphocytes alone or in combination with cisplatin-containing chemotherapy in patients with epithelial ovarian cancer. *Cancer Research* **51:** 1934–1939.

Arrick BA, Korc M & Derynck R (1990) Differential regulation of expression of three transforming growth factor β species in human breast cancer cell lines by estradiol. *Cancer Research* **50:** 299–303.

Balkwill FR (1989) *Cytokines in Cancer Therapy*. Oxford: Oxford University Press.

Balkwill F & Burke F (1989) The cytokine network. *Immunology Today* **10:** 299–303.

Balkwill FR, Griffin DB & Lee A (1989) Interferons alpha and gamma differ in their ability to cause tumour stasis and regression in vivo. *European Journal of Cancer and Clinical Oncology* **25:** 1481–1486.

Balkwill FR, Lee A, Adlam G et al (1986) Human tumour xenografts treated with recombinant human tumour necrosis factor alone or in combination with interferons. *Cancer Research* **46:** 3990–3993.

Bast R, Berek JS, Obrist R et al (1983) Intraperitoneal immunotherapy of human ovarian carcinoma with intraperitoneal *Corynebacterium parvum*. *Cancer Research* **43:** 1395–1401.

Berek JS, Hacker NF, Lichtenstein A et al (1985) Intraperitoneal recombinant α-interferon for 'salvage' therapy in stage III epithelial ovarian cancer: a gynecological oncology group study. *Cancer Research* **45:** 4447–4453.

Berek JS, Chung C, Kaldi K et al (1991) Serum interleukin-6 levels correlate with disease status in patients with epithelial ovarian cancer. *American Journal of Obstetrics and Gynecology* **164:** 1039–1043.

Berger MS, Locher GW, Saurer S et al (1988) Correlation of c-*erb*β-2 gene amplification and protein expression in human breast carcinomas with nodal status and nuclear grading. *Cancer Research* **48:** 1238–1243.

Bookman MA & Bast Jr RC (1991) The immunobiology and immunotherapy of ovarian cancer. *Seminars in Oncology* **18:** 270–291.

Buzdar AU, Blumenschein G, Gutterman JU et al (1979) Postoperative adjuvant chemotherapy with fluorouracil, doxorubicin, cyclophosphamide and BCG vaccine: a follow-up report. *Journal of the American Medical Association* **242:** 1509–1513.

Carswell EA, Old LJ, Kassel RJ et al (1975) An endotoxin-induced serum factor that causes necrosis of tumors. *Proceedings of the National Academy of Sciences (USA)* **72:** 3666–3670.

Chapman PB, Kolitz JE, Hakes T et al (1988) A phase I trial of recombinant interleukin-2 in patients with advanced ovarian cancer. *Investigational New Drugs* **6:** 179–188.

Ciardiello F, Kim N, Liscia DS et al (1989) mRNA expression of transforming growth factor alpha in human breast carcinomas and its activity in effusions of breast cancer patients. *Journal of the National Cancer Institute* **81:** 1165–1171.

Coley WB (1896) The therapeutic value of mixed toxins of the streptococcus of erysipelas and *Bacillus prodiogosus* in the treatment of inoperable malignant tumors with a report of one hundred and sixty cases. *American Journal of Medical Science* **112:** 251–260.

D'Aquisto R, Markman M, Hakes T et al (1988) Phase I trial of intraperitoneal gamma-interferon in advanced ovarian carcinoma. *Journal of Clinical Oncology* **6:** 689–695.

Davidovich CR, Guglielmineti A, Zorzoupulos J, Criscuolo M & Diaz A (1989) Disappearance of dysplastic cervical lesions treated with leucocyte interferon with persistence of viral signs. *Journal of Interferon Research* **9(supplement 2):** S119.

DeCicco F, Sica G, Benedetto MT et al (1988) In vitro effects of beta-interferon on steroid receptors and prostaglandin output in human endometrial carcinoma. *Journal of Steroid Biochemistry* **30:** 359–362.

De Jaco P, Asselian B, Orlandi C, Fridman WH & Teillaud P (1991) Evaluation of circulating tumour necrosis factor-α in patients with gynaecological malignancies. *International Journal of Cancer* **48:** 375–376.

Diehl V, Pfreundschuh M, Steinmetz MT & Schaadt M (1987) Phase I studies of recombinant human tumour necrosis factor in patients with advanced cancer. In Bonavida B, Clifford G, Kirchner H & Old L (eds) *Tumour Necrosis Factor and Related Cytokines*, pp 183–188. Basel: Karger.

Durham AM, McCartney JC, McDance DJ & Taylor RW (1990) Effect of perilesional alpha-interferon on cervical intraepithelial neoplasia and associated human papillomavirus infection. *Journal of the Royal Society of Medicine* 83: 490–492.

Einhorn N, Cantell K, Einhorn S et al (1982) Human leukocyte interferon therapy for advanced ovarian carcinoma. *American Journal of Clinical Oncology* 5: 167–172.

Einhorn N, Ling P, Einhorn S et al (1988) A phase II study of escalating interferon therapy for advanced ovarian carcinoma. *American Journal of Clinical Oncology* 11: 3–6.

Erroi A, Sironi M, Chiaffarino F, Zhen-Guo C, Mengozie M & Mantovani A (1989) IL-1 and IL-6 release by tumour associated macrophages from human ovarian carcinoma. *International Journal of Cancer* 44: 795.

Freedman RS, Gutterman JU, Wharton JT et al (1983) Leucocyte interferon in patients with epithelial ovarian carcinoma. *Journal of Biological Response Modifiers* 2: 133–138.

Freedman RS, Edwards CL, Bowen JM et al (1988) Viral oncolysates in patients with advanced ovarian cancer. *Gynecologic Oncology* 29: 337–347.

Freedman RS, Patenia R, Rashed S, Platsoucas CD & Ioannides CG (1990) T cell functions in ovarian cancer patients treated with tumour cell vaccines. Increased helper cell activity to immunoglobulin production. *FASEB Journal* 4: A1718.

Frost L, Skajaa K, Hvidman LE, Fay SJ & Larsen PM (1990) No effect of intralesional injection of interferon on moderate intraepithelial neoplasia. *British Journal of Obstetrics and Gynaecology* 97: 626–630.

Gall SA, Blessing JA, DiSaia PJ & Creasman WT (1980) The effect of chemoimmunotherapy in the treatment of primary stage III epithelial ovarian cancer: a gynecology oncology group study. In *Immunotherapy of Cancer: Present Status of Trials in Man*, p 13. Bethesda, Maryland: Bethesda National Cancer Institute.

Graham JB & Graham RM (1962) Autogenous cancer vaccine in cancer patients. *Surgery, Gynecology and Obstetrics* 114: 1–4.

Granger GA & Williams TW (1968) Lymphocyte cytotoxicity in vitro: activation and release of a cytotoxic factor. *Nature* 312: 721–724.

Grimm EA, Mazumder A, Zhang HZ et al (1982) Lymphokine activated killer cell phenomenon: lysis of fresh solid tumor cells by interleukin-2 activated autologous peripheral blood lymphocytes. *Journal of Experimental Medicine* 155: 1823–1841.

Hird V, Snook D, Kosmas C et al (1990) Intraperitoneal radioimmunotherapy with yttrium-90-labelled immunoconjugates. In *Monoclonal Antibodies: Applications in Clinical Oncology*. New York: Chapman and Hall.

Hubay CA, Pearson OH, Manni A et al (1985) Adjuvant endocrine therapy, cytotoxic chemotherapy and immunotherapy in stage II breast cancer: 6-year result. III. Anti-estrogens in combination with chemotherapy in early breast cancer. *Journal of Steroid Biochemistry* 23: 1147–1150.

Ioannides CG, Platsoucas CD, Radshed S et al (1991) Tumor cytolysis by lymphocytes infiltrating ovarian malignant ascites. *Cancer Research* 51: 4257–4265.

Isaacs A & Lindemann J (1957) Virus interference. I. The interferon. *Proceedings of the Royal Society (Series B)* 157: 259–267.

Johnson RA, Boyce BF, Mundy GR & Roodman GD (1989) Chronic exposure to tumor necrosis factor in vivo preferentially inhibits erythropoiesis in nude mice. *Blood* 74: 130–138.

Jones AL & Selby P (1989) Tumour necrosis factor: clinical relevance. *Cancer Surveys* 8: 817–836.

Kacinski BM, Carter D, Mittal SK et al (1989a) High level expression of *fms* protooncogene mRNA is observed in clinically aggressive human endometrial carcinomas. *International Journal of Radiation: Oncology–Biology–Physics* 15: 823–829.

Kacinski BM, Stanley ER, Carter D et al (1989b) Circulating levels of CSF-1 (MCSF), a lymphopoietic cytokine, may be a useful marker of disease status in patients with malignant ovarian neoplasms. *International Journal of Radiation: Oncology–Biology–Physics* 17: 159–164.

Kacinski BM, Carter D, Mittal K et al (1990) Ovarian cancers express fms-complementary transcripts and fms antigen, often with co-expression of CSF-1. *American Journal of Pathology* **137**: 135–147.

Kelly S, Malik STA & Balkwill F (1990) Cytokines in cancer therapy. In Waring M & Ponder BJ (eds) *The Science of Cancer Treatment. Cancer and Biology Series B*, Chapter 8, pp 127–160.

Kirby TK, Keviat N, Beckman A et al (1988) Tolerance and efficacy of human recombinant interferon-γ in the treatment of refractory genital warts. *American Journal of Medicine* **85**: 183–188.

Kishimoto T (1989) The biology of interleukin-6. *Blood* **74**: 1.

Klein E, Holtermann O, Milgrom N et al (1976) Immunotherapy for accessible tumors utilizing delayed hypersensitivity reactions and separated components of the immune system. *Medical Clinics of North America* **60**: 389–418.

Knabbe C, Lippman ME, Wakefield LM et al (1987) Evidence that transforming growth factor-β is a hormonally regulated negative growth factor in human breast cancer cells. *Cell* **48**: 417–428.

Levin L, McHardy JE, Curling OM & Hudson CN (1975) Tumour antigenicity in ovarian cancer. *British Journal of Cancer* **32**: 152–159.

Lotze MT, Custer MC & Rosenberg SA (1986) Intraperitoneal administration of interleukin-2 in patients with cancer. *Archives of Surgery* **121**: 1373–1379.

Lundy J, Schuss A, Stanick E, McCormack ES, Kramer S & Sorvillo JM (1991) Expression of neu protein, epidermal growth factor receptor, and transforming growth factor alpha in breast cancer. *American Journal of Pathology* **138(6)**: 1527–1534.

Malik STA (1992) Tumour necrosis factor roles in cancer pathophysiology. *Seminars in Cancer Biology* **3**: 27–33.

Malik STA & Balkwill FR (1991) Epithelial ovarian cancer: a cytokine propelled disease? *British Journal of Cancer* **64**: 617–620.

Malik STA & Balkwill FR (1992) Antiproliferative and antitumour activity of TNF in vitro and in vivo. In Aggarwal BB & Vilcek J (eds) *Tumor Necrosis Factors: Structure, Function, and Mechanism of Action.* New York: Marcel Dekker Inc.

Malik STA, Griffin DB, Fiers W & Balkwill FR (1989) Paradoxical effects of tumour necrosis factor in experimental ovarian cancer. *International Journal of Cancer* **44**: 918–925.

Malik STA, Naylor MS, Oliff A & Balkwill FR (1990) Cells secreting tumour necrosis factor show enhanced metastasis in nude mice. *European Journal of Cancer* **26**: 1031–1034.

Malik STA, East N, Knowles R et al (1992) Antitumor activity of gamma interferon in ascitic and solid intraperitoneal models of human ovarian cancer. *Cancer Research* **51**: 6643–6649.

Manetta A, Podczacski E, Zaino RJ & Satyaswaroop PG (1989) Therapeutic effect of recombinant tumor necrosis factor in ovarian carcinoma xenograft in nude mice. *Gynecologic Oncology* **34**: 360–364.

Marth C, Muller-Holzner E, Greiter E et al (1990) Gamma interferon reduces the expression of the protooncogene c-*erb*-B2 in human ovarian carcinoma cells. *Cancer Research* **50**: 7037–7041.

Matsui Y, Halter SA, Holt JT, Hogan BLM & Coffey RJ (1990) Development of mammary hyperplasia and neoplasia in MMTV-TGFα transgenic mice. *Cell* **61**: 1147–1155.

Morishige K, Kurachi H, Amemiya K et al (1991) Evidence for the involvement of transforming growth factor α and epidermal growth factor receptor autocrine growth mechanism in primary human ovarian cancers in vitro. *Cancer Research* **51**: 5322–5328.

Nardi M, Cognetti F, Pollera CF et al (1990) Intraperitoneal recombinant interferon alpha-2-interferon alternating with cisplatin as salvage therapy for minimal residual disease ovarian cancer: a phase II study. *Journal of Clinical Oncology* **8**: 1036–1041.

Nauts HC (1987) Beneficial effects of acute concurrent infection, fever, or immunotherapy (bacterial toxins) on ovarian and uterine cancer. *Cancer Research Institute Monographs* **17**: 1–122.

Nawa A, Nishiyama Y, Yamamoto N et al (1990) Selective suppression of HPV type 18 mRNA level in HeLa cells by interferon. *Biochemical and Biophysical Research Communications* **170**: 793–796.

Naylor MS, Malik STA, Stamp G & Balkwill FR (1990) Demonstration of mRNA for tumour necrosis factor in human ovarian cancer by in situ hybridisation. *European Journal of Cancer* **26**: 1027–1030.

Niloff JM, Knapp RC, Jones G et al (1985) Recombinant leucocyte alpha interferon in advanced ovarian carcinoma. *Cancer Treatment Reports* **69:** 895–896.

Okamura K, Hamazaki Y, Yajima A & Noda K (1989) Two randomised controlled studies of patients with cervical cancer. *Biomedicine and Pharmacotherapy* **43:** 177–181.

Oliff A, Defeo-Jones D, Boyer M et al (1987) Tumours secreting human TNF/cachectin induce cachexia in mice. *Cell* **50:** 555–563.

Ortaldo JR, Porter HR, Miller P et al (1986) Adoptive cellular immunotherapy of human ovarian cancer xenografts in nude mice. *Cancer Research* **46:** 4414–4419.

Papermaster BW, Holtermann OA, Klein E et al (1976) Preliminary observations on tumor regressions induced by local administration of a lymphoid cell culture supernatant in patients with cutaneous metastatic lesions. *Clinical Immunopathology* **5:** 31–47.

Pardridge DH, Sparks FC, Goodnight JE et al (1979) Intratumor bacillus Calmette-Guerin therapy for chest wall recurrence of carcinoma of the breast. *Surgery, Gynecology and Obstetrics* **148:** 867–871.

Peters WP (1991) The myeloid colony stimulating factors. *Seminars in Haematology* **28:** 1–5.

Pujade-Lauraine E, Guastella JP, Colombo N et al (1991) Intraperitoneal human r-IFN gamma as treatment of residual ovarian carcinoma at second look laparotomy. *Proceedings of the American Society for Clinical Oncology* **10:** 195.

Pulley MS, Nagendrian V, Edwards JM et al (1986) Intravenous, intralesional and endo-lymphatic administration of lymphokines in human cancer. *Lymphokine Research* **5:** 5157–5163.

Rambaldi A, Introna M, Colotta F et al (1985) Intraperitoneal administration of interferon-beta in ovarian cancer patients. *Cancer* **56:** 294–301.

Rath U, Kaufmann M, Schmid H et al (1991) Effect of recombinant human tumour necrosis factor alpha in malignant ascites. *European Journal of Cancer* **27:** 121–125.

Rosenberg SA, Lotze MT, Muul LM et al (1985) Observations on the systemic administration of autologous lymphokine activated killer cells and recombinant interleukin-2 to patients with metastatic cancer. *New England Journal of Medicine* **313:** 1485–1492.

Rosenberg SA, Packard BS, Aebersold PM et al (1988) Use of tumor infiltrating lymphocytes and interleukin-2 in the immunotherapy of patients with metastatic melanoma. *New England Journal of Medicine* **319:** 1676–1680.

Sainsbury JR, Farndon JR, Needham GK et al (1987) Epidermal growth factor receptor status as a predictor of early recurrence of and death from breast cancer. *Lancet* **i:** 1398–1402.

Salomon DS, Kim N, Saeki T & Ciardiello F (1990) Transforming growth factor-α: an oncodevelopmental growth factor. *Cancer Cells* **2:** 389–397.

Sato K, Fuji Y, Ono M, Nomura H & Shizume K (1987) Production of interleukin 1 alpha-like factor and colony-stimulating factor by a squamous cell carcinoma of the thyroid (T3M-5) derived from a patient with hypercalcemia and leukocytosis. *Cancer Research* **47:** 6474.

Scambia G, Panici PB, Battaglia F et al (1991) Effect of recombinant human interferon alpha(2b) on receptors for steroid hormones and epidermal growth factor in patients with endometrial cancer. *European Journal of Cancer* **27:** 51–53.

Slamon DJ, Clark GM, Wong SG et al (1987) Human breast cancer: correlation of relapse and survival with amplification of the HER-2/neu oncogene. *Science* **235:** 177–182.

Smyth MJ, Pieteresz A & McKenzie IFC (1988) Increased antitumor effect of immuno-conjugates and tumor necrosis factor in vivo. *Cancer Research* **48:** 3607–3712.

Spriggs D, Imamura K, Rodriquez M, Horiguchi J & Kufe DW (1987) Induction of tumor necrosis factor expression and resistance in a human breast tumor cell line. *Proceedings of the National Academy of Sciences (USA)* **84:** 6563–6566.

Steis RG, Urba WJ & Vandermolen LA (1990) Intraperitoneal lymphokine-activated killer cell and interleukin-2 therapy for malignancies limited to the peritoneal cavity. *Journal of Clinical Oncology* **8:** 1618–1629.

Stewart JA, Nelinson JL, Moore AL et al (1990) Phase I trial of intraperitoneal recombinant interleukin-2/lymphokine activated killer cells in patients with ovarian cancer. *Cancer Research* **50:** 6302–6310.

Takeyama H, Wakamiya N, O'Hara C et al (1991) Tumor necrosis factor expression by human ovarian carcinoma in vivo. *Cancer Research* **50:** 2538–2542.

Tamm I, Cardinale I, Drueger J, Murphy JS, May L & Seghal PB (1989) Interleukin 6 decreases cell–cell association and increases motility of breast carcinoma cells. *Journal of Experimental Medicine* **170:** 1649.

Tandon AK, Clark GM, Chamness GC, Ullrich A & McGuire WL (1989) HER-2/neu oncogene protein and prognosis in breast cancer. *Journal of Clinical Oncology* **7:** 1120–1128.

Wanebo HJ, Ochoa M, Gunther U et al (1979) Randomized chemoimmunotherapy trial of CAF and intravenous *C. parvum* for resistant ovarian carcinoma. Preliminary results. *Proceedings of the American Association for Cancer Research* **18:** 225.

Watson JM, Sensintaffar JL, Berek JS & Martinez-Maza O (1990) Constitutive production of interleukin-6 by ovarian cancer cell lines and by primary ovarian tumor cultures. *Cancer Research* **50:** 6959.

Welander CE, Homesley HD, Reich SD et al (1988) A phase II study of the efficacy of recombinant interferon gamma in relapsing ovarian carcinoma. *American Journal of Clinical Oncology* **11:** 167–172.

Willemse PHB, DeVries EGE, Mulder NH et al (1990) Intraperitoneal human recombinant interferon alpha-2b in minimal residual disease ovarian cancer. *European Journal of Cancer* **26:** 353–358.

Yliskoski M, Cantell K & Syrjanen S (1990) Topical treatment with human leukocyte interferon of HPV16 infections associated with cervical and vaginal intraepithelial neoplasms. *Gynecologic Oncology* **36:** 353–357.

Yoneda T, Alsina MA, Chavez JB et al (1991) Evidence that tumor necrosis factor plays a pathogenetic role in the paraneoplastic syndromes of cachexia, hypercalcemia, and leukocytosis in a human tumor in nude mice. *Journal of Clinical Investigation* **87:** 977–985.

14

Overview and future perspectives

GORDON M. STIRRAT
JAMES R. SCOTT

INTRODUCTION

Our understanding of the immune system has increased dramatically over the last two decades predominantly as a result of the introduction of monoclonal antibody technology and protein sequencing. An explosion of knowledge is beginning, brought about by molecular cloning and sequencing of genes coding for surface molecules. By the time of the 4th International Workshop on Human Leucocyte Differentiation Antigens in 1989 almost 90 distinct human leukocyte surface molecules had been identified by monoclonal antibodies (Knapp et al, 1989). They have been given the prefix CD for 'cluster determinant' (sometimes CDw denoting provisional designation by the workshop). It is clear that many of them are broadly distributed over a variety of types of leukocyte and some are present on seemingly totally unrelated cell types, e.g. platelets, epithelial cells and brain cells. Thus 'immunology now finds itself within the mainstream of classical molecular biology, its central phenomena providing a fertile hunting ground for clues to the basis of cell signalling, differentiation and growth control' (Nossal, 1988).

CELL ADHESION MOLECULES—FAMILIES AND SUPERFAMILIES

Other strands of evidence point ineluctably in the same direction as suggested by Nossal (1988). For example, at least four families of cell-surface molecules regulate the migration of lymphocytes and their interaction during immune responses (Springer, 1990; Mallett and Barclay, 1991). Several members of these families also subserve non-immunological functions within other systems in the body. The first of these families to be described was the immunoglobulin superfamily (IgSF). Some of its members are described in Table 1. The most significant feature of this family is that its members share 90–100 amino acids ('the immunoglobulin domain') suggesting that, despite their varied functions, they originally sprang from a common primeval gene. It is, therefore, likely that the IgSF are related in evolution and share the functional property of involvement in recognition

Baillière's Clinical Obstetrics and Gynaecology—
Vol. 6, No. 3, September 1992
ISBN 0–7020–1634–9

Table 1. Some members of the immunoglobulin supergene family (IgSF).

Immunoglobulins	IgG, IgM, IgA, IgD, IgE
Major histocompatibility antigens	MHC class I & class II
β_2-microglobulin	B2m
Several T cell antigens	CD1, 2, 4 & 8
T cell receptor	Tcr (CD3)
Macrophage Fc receptor	FcR
Carcinoembryonal antigens	CLA
Colony stimulating factor I receptor	CSF-IR
Platelet derived growth factor receptor	PDGFR
Neural cell adhesion molecule	N-CAM
Myelin-associated glycoprotein	MAG
Major glycoprotein of peripheral myelin	Po
Lymphocyte-related function antigen 2	LFA-2
Lymphocyte-related function antigen 3	LFA-3
Intercellular cell adhesive molecule 1	ICAM-1
Intercellular cell adhesive molecule 2	ICAM-2

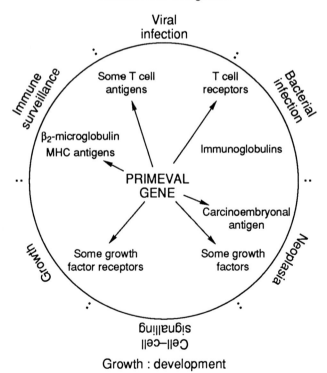

Figure 1. Immunoglobulin supergene family.

events at the cell surface (Williams, 1984). Williams suggested that molecules corresponding to a single immunoglobulin domain were first expressed at cell surfaces at an early stage in the evolution of multicellular organisms and that these molecules interacted with receptors on other cells as an integral part of cellular interactions. Increasing diversity and sophistication of both arms of this recognition system allowed specificity of cell interactions in development and tissue formation. It is suggested that it was from these primitive recognition systems that self/non-self recognition evolved into the immune system. Figure 1 provides a paradigm for this process.

The second major cell-adhesion family and among the most versatile, is that of the integrin adhesion receptors (Springer, 1990). Like many receptors, integrins transduce information from the outside to the inside of the cell. Growth and differentiation of a variety of connective tissues and nervous system cells are dependent on the integrins. They contain α- and β-subunits of between 750 and 1100 amino acids. The α-subunits are up to 65% identical and the β-subunits up to 45% identical in amino acid sequence. These subfamilies of integrins are distinguished by their β-subunits known as β_1-, β_2- and β_3-integrins. The β_1-subfamily includes receptors which bind to the extracellular matrix components fibronectin, laminin and collagen found within the tissues and basement membranes of, for example, muscle, the nervous system and epithelium including endothelium. Among the integrins with immune regulatory functions are lymphocyte-related function antigen 1 (LFA-1) and very late activation molecules VLA-4, 5 and 6.

LFA-1, restricted to leukocytes, is involved in T helper and β-lymphocyte responses, natural killer (NK) cell function, antibody-dependent mediated cytotoxicity, and adherence of leukocytes to endothelial cells, fibroblasts and epithelial cells (Springer, 1990). The counter-receptors or ligands for LFA-1 on the target cell are ICAM-1 or 2 (for intercellular cell adhesive molecules), both of which are members of the IgSF. In contrast to the restricted expression of LFA-1, ICAM-1 is found on a wide variety of cells particularly during inflammatory responses in which it is intimately involved. LFA-2 and 3 are also members of the IgSF, the latter being the counter-receptor on the target cell for the former on the lymphocyte (the idiosyncrasy and inconsistency of the nomenclature must soon be sorted out!).

Figure 2 illustrates how the IgSF and LFA-1 function as recognition molecules during antigen-specific T cell interaction. This is discussed in greater detail in Chapter 1. Less is known about a third family known as 'selectins' which are involved in cell interactions in the vascular tree and are expressed on leukocytes and endothelial cells (Springer, 1990). The selectins have sequences of amino acids in common with several lectins (proteins which activate lymphocytes), epidermal growth factor (EGF) and many complement regulatory proteins (see Chapter 3).

So far, three selectins have been identified and found to regulate leukocyte binding to endothelium at inflammatory sites (Springer, 1990). Mel-14 and endothelial leukocytes adhesion molecule (ELAM-1) bind neutrophils

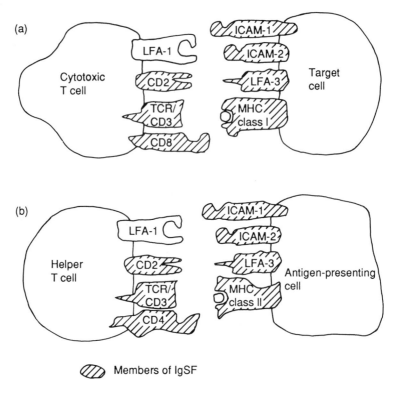

Members of IgSF

Figure 2. Antigen-specific T cell interaction (adapted from Springer, 1990). This shows the important role of members of the IgSF and the integrin LFA-1 as receptors on T cells and counter-receptors on target or antigen-presenting cells. The main purpose of these adhesion receptors is cell–cell signalling.

to the endothelium, but the former is quickly released from the cell surface and the latter rapidly inactivated. Integrins, which remain permanently upregulated on the activated neutrophil, then take over to achieve trans-endothelial migration.

A fourth superfamily of cell surface proteins has recently been described (Mallett and Barclay, 1991). Its members are related to the nerve growth factor receptor (NGFR) found on neural cells and within it are the B cell antigen designated CD40, the activated T cell antigen OX-40, and two receptors for tumour necrosis factor (TNF) called TNFR-I and TNFR-II and found on a variety of cell types. Most of the current functional information exists about NGFR and TNFR-I and II which are cytokine growth factor receptors.

THE IMMUNE SYSTEM AS PART OF A GREATER CELL–CELL SIGNALLING SYSTEM

It is, therefore, clear that the 'immune system' is not as discrete an entity either functionally or in terms of its effectors and receptors as had been originally believed. On one hand, polypeptides produced by activated cells initially named interleukins then lymphokines (because they were thought to be produced solely by leukocytes), are now called cytokines because the same polypeptides are produced by a variety of cell types. In addition the same cytokine can function within several cells and tissues. For example, cytokines are crucial mediators between vascular cells and leukocytes (Mantovani and Dijana, 1989). Endothelial cells which function like mononuclear phagocytes in their production and response to various cytokines are active participants in the induction and regulation of coagulation, inflammation and immunity. In addition there is such a strong link between immunology, growth and differentiation, and oncology that categorization becomes meaningless. Several proto-oncogenes code either for cytokine growth factors or their receptors (see Table 2) (Adamson, 1987). Similarly, some cytokines cause transcription of cellular proto-oncogenes.

Table 2. Some proto-oncogenes (c-*onc*) and their products.

c-*onc*	Product	Putative function
c-*sis*	Platelet derived growth factor (PDGF) β-chain	Growth factor in embryogenesis (?) Mitogenesis
c-*myc*		Proliferation Regulation of DNA synthesis
c-*erb*-A	Thyroid hormone receptor	Regulator of growth and metabolism
c-*erb*-B	Epidermal growth factor receptor (EGFR)	Signal transduction in mitogenesis and differentiation
c-*fms*	Colony stimulating factor 1 receptor (ISF-IR)	Signal transduction in mitogenesis and differentiation

Exactly the same diversity of expression and function applies to the families of cell adhesion receptor molecules such that the conceptual boundaries between, for example, the immune system, the vascular system, and the nervous system are now at least blurred if not non-existent. Janeway (1988) has pointed out that the immune and nervous systems are often compared. Both react in a very specific manner to signals, both have memory, and the cellular organization of both is highly complex in which cells with similar outward appearance have widely different functions. The main feature which distinguishes them is their very different anatomical organization. The immune system is highly mobile whereas the nervous system is relatively static. However, even this difference is lessening because it has now been demonstrated that one particular subset of lymphocytes has a very precisely defined anatomy. Lymphocytes have classically been described as having receptors with variable chains designated α and β. A small subset has now been discovered with different variable chains now called γ and δ. These lymphocytes are only found in epithelia and two of the most important are the dendritic epithelial cells (DEC) in skin and the intestinal epithelial lymphocytes (IEL). The α/β T cells are the dominant immunological effector cells characterized by their recirculation capacity and specialization for MHC recognition. The γ/δ T cells seem to be less sophisticated in their antigen specificity and memory. This has led to the speculation (Mantovani and Dijana, 1988) that epithelial surfaces were the site at which cell-mediated immunity originally developed in evolutionary terms. The γ/δ T cell system may, therefore, be the progenitor of the α/β antigen-specific T cell.

SOME OTHER EXAMPLES OF SEQUENCE HOMOLOGY AND THEIR CONSEQUENCES

Structural homology is not only a feature of the families and superfamilies of cell adhesion molecules. Many major antigens recognized during a wide variety of bacterial and parasitic diseases belong to conserved protein families which share extensive amino acid sequences identical with the surface molecules on the host's cells (Cohen and Young, 1991). For example, the induction of heat shock proteins (hsp) is brought about by cellular 'stress' in any type of cell, from prokaryotic to human. Infection of the body by bacteria and many protozoan and helminthic parasites results in antibody responses to hsps. The protein structure of members of the hsp family is remarkably similar: more than 50% of the amino acid sequences are shared by, for example, bacterial and mammalian hsps. This produces a problem for 'classical' immunology because bacterial hsps are strongly immunogenic to the mammalian immune system despite containing a series of epitopes which are also 'self' to that animal. One might predict that immune reactions to hsps might be associated with autoimmune disease. This is in fact the case (reviewed in Cohen and Young, 1991): immunity to mycobacterial hsp 65 is associated with autoimmune arthritis and diabetes. Immunity to hsps 70 and 90 is linked with systemic lupus erythematosus (SLE). The puzzle is not that this happens but why it occurs so infrequently. Cohen and Young (1991) pose the questions—what is the point of the immune system focusing on the very molecules that the infective agent shares with the host: how is this focus of attention encoded within the system: and how is the chance of auto-immune disease reduced or eliminated? In trying to answer these questions about 'self' and 'non-self' they draw an analogy with the nervous system 'homunculus' to be found in all physiology textbooks. The neurological homunculus draws a functional picture of the body in terms of the domi-nance of the neural networks within different organs or structures. Thus the tongue and fingers are much more prominent in the homunculus than the trunk. The 'self' seen by the nervous system is different from that described anatomically. They invoke the presence of immune networks centred around a selected few 'self-antigens' which encode the dominance of these antigens as a result of preformed lymphocyte networks. This produces an alternative 'homunculus' in which the immune system 'sees' some parts of self as being dominant. This is illustrated in Figure 3. Each dominant

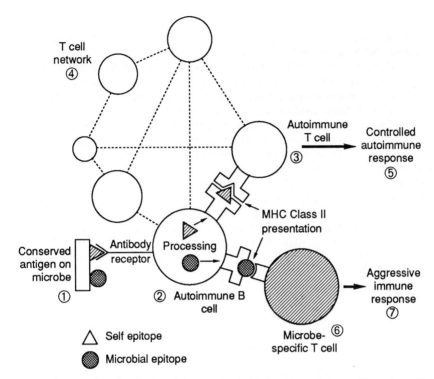

Figure 3. Immune homunculus lymphocyte network (derived from Cohen and Young, 1991). 1, The conserved antigen on the microbe is recognized by a natural autoimmune B cell (or macrophage); 2, the self and microbial epitopes are processed by the B cell which presents them on its cell surface; 3/4, the response to the self epitope is regulated by the lymphocyte network; 5, this results in a controlled autoimmune response; 6/7, T cells recognize the microbial antigen and are free to respond aggressively.

self-antigen is, they suggest, served by an interacting set of T and B cells some of which suppress and others stimulate. As a result of connections between various interacting lymphocytes in the network, some lymphocytes can become activated even without being driven by contact with a specific immunogen. They argue that this immunological homunculus hypothesis would allow the immune system to deal with self molecules efficiently and predictably. The dominance of a few selected self-antigens 'blinds' the system to other competing 'recessive' self-antigens to which it is, therefore, tolerant. It also links immunological dominance with control. Autoimmune responses are channelled and controlled so that autoimmunity is graded, guarded and usually transient.

Hsp molecules have been conserved because they are essential to both the host and parasite. In immune terms the body has made a virtue out of necessity. If, of course, the immune homunculus errs by omission or commission frank autoimmune disease can result. The ideal therapy for auto-immune disease is not, therefore, general suppression of the immune system or inflammatory responses but restoration of the connections between the natural T and B cell networks and the autoimmune effector cells, e.g. by vaccination using attenuated autoimmune cytotoxic T cells (reviewed in Cohen and Young, 1991).

Biochemical similarities between the mechanisms within the human body and lower orders is not confined to hsps. There is clear peptide sequence homology between the MHC system of vertebrate and invertebrate chordates (Reinisil and Litman, 1989). This has been a neglected area of study but from it has arisen the observation that cell surface adhesion molecules involved in MHC recognition (Figure 2) may share characteristics with those involved in sperm recognition of the envelope of the ovum. In addition, it is now becoming clear that MHC associated immune functions in all classes of vertebrates derive from genes and gene products similar to those in mammals. Chicken MHC class II B genes are related to mouse and human class II two genes to the same extent. Gene duplications probably occurred independently in the avian and mammalian lineages and subsequently in different groups of placental mammals.

OVERVIEW

As a result of these developments in our understanding of the immune system, the genes controlling it, its products and their receptors, it is apparent that:

1. The immune system is an integral part of a generalized cell–cell signalling system which, among its functions, has developed the ability to recognize self and non-self.
2. The genes coding for the immune system developed from a primitive progenitor, developing antigen specificity in the process. In doing so the humoral immune system became linked opportunistically with the classical pathway of complement activation (Atkinson and Farries, 1987). The so-called 'alternative' pathway is probably phylogenetically older than the 'classical' pathway (see Chapter 3).

   The immune system has also turned potentially serious phylogenetic problems, such as the sharing of heat shock proteins with pathogens, into advantageous mechanisms for controlling autoimmunity while still retaining the ability to eliminate the infective agents.
3. The fundamental purpose of cell adhesion molecules, originally described in relation to immune regulation, is to do with the regulation of development and differentiation (Cunningham, 1991). One of the outstanding features is the dynamic pattern of their expression during development (for references see Cunningham, 1991). Their expression and that of their receptors is often coded for by proto-oncogenes (c-*onc*) which are also crucially involved in growth regulation and differentiation (Adamson, 1987) (see Table 2). The roles of the c-*onc*s may vary with the stage of development. Eades et al (1988) found tumour necrosis factor receptor (TNFR) in a purified plasma membrane preparation of human villous trophoblast. Among the proto-oncogenes expressed on

extravillous trophoblast are c-*sis* and c-*erb* (see Table 2), which code for PDGF β-chain and EGFR respectively (Gousti et al, 1985; Venter et al, 1987). Tavare and Holmes (1989) observed receptors for epidermal growth factor (EGFR) and insulin throughout gestation on syncytiotrophoblast. On first-trimester cytotrophoblast, however, the expression of EGFR decreased as the cytotrophoblast columns invade the maternal decidua whereas the expression of insulin receptors remained constant. This differential expression is probably relevant to placental development.

CONSEQUENCES FOR IMMUNE DISEASES IN OBSTETRICS AND GYNAECOLOGY

1. The clear placement of the immune system within a generalized system regulating cell–cell signalling and fundamentally involved in development gives obstetricians and gynaecologists and scientists involved in research on reproductive biology and immunology a highly privileged position for advancing understanding of these crucial areas.

   The messages which pass between mother and fetus as a result of cell–cell signalling from the earliest point in implantation throughout the whole of pregnancy are highly relevant to the normal fetomaternal immune relationship (Chapter 2) and pregnancy disorders consequent on pathology within the placental bed (Chapter 4). This could also play a role in pregnancy loss (Chapter 5). Now that the lack of classical MHC antigens on syncytiotrophoblast and the non-classical nature of the MHC antigens on other populations of trophoblast has been established beyond peradventure (see Chapter 2), more attention can be focused on developmental questions posed by the possible functions of the non-classical HLA-G found there, and of the profusion of cell adhesion molecules and their receptors on trophoblast. Holmes and Simpson (Chapter 3) have already given new evidence for the importance of complement regulatory protein expression at the fetomaternal interface and this story will be developed over the next few years.

   The model of sperm–egg interactions as an illustration of the involvement of cell surface adhesion molecules in MHC recognition (Reinisil and Litman, 1989) (and vice versa) may be initially useful as reproductive biologists try to understand the former and immunologists the latter.

2. The immunological homunculus hypothesis of Cohen and Young (1991) is of considerable relevance to further developments in our understanding of autoimmune conditions in pregnancy (Chapter 9), and the anti-cardiolipin antibody (ACA) syndrome discussed in Chapter 6. Because of the 'partial self' nature of the fetus in respect of the mother (and vice versa) it may also shed light on Rhesus disease and such 'alloimmune' conditions as thrombocytopenia (Chapter 8). In addition, the attempts to develop contraceptive vaccines (Chapter 12) may be facilitated by some of the concepts outlined by Cohen and Young (1991).

3. The cytokine link between leukocytes and endothelial cells raises interesting questions about the pathogenesis of pre-eclampsia addressed in Chapter 10.
4. Regrettably, several cell adhesion receptors are subverted as virus receptors (White and Littman, 1989). Of more than 100 distinct rhinovirus variants, 90% bind to the IgSF member, ICAM-1. Rhinoviruses use the immune response to induce sneezing and the secretion of mucus which facilitates spread to other individuals. CD4, a member of the IgSF, acts as a receptor for HIV which then infects and kills or renders functionless CD4+ T helper cells and downregulates CD4 expression. It also spreads by fusion of infected with uninfected cells to form syncytia by involving the integrin LFA-1. This is of relevance to the discussion of HIV infection in pregnancy in Chapter 11.
5. The increasingly obvious overlap between immunology and oncology in the context of recognition systems which are fundamentally to do with cell differentiation and development (Nossal, 1988) are highly relevant to the discussions on gestational trophoblastic tumours (Chapter 7) and gynaecological cancer (Chapter 13). Malik and Epenetos (Chapter 13), for example, have elegantly presented the role of cytokines in pathophysiology and potential for treatment of gynaecological cancers.

CONCLUSION

The 'state of the art' consideration of the immune system in health and disease in obstetrics and gynaecology contained in this volume illustrates well the value of an interdisciplinary approach to a subject. This will become increasingly important now that the artificial barriers between physiological systems is being broken down. Our understanding of what is scientifically and clinically relevant to obstetricians, gynaecologists, reproductive biologists or immunologists can only increase if unhelpful barriers with other clinicians and scientists are also removed. Cassius says in Shakespeare's *Julius Caesar*: 'There is a tide in the affairs of men which, taken at the flood leads on to fortune.' The biochemical and molecular biological technology now (and increasingly) at our disposal means that, by interdisciplinary and, sometimes, lateral thinking, we are at a watershed in the scientific understanding of the pathophysiological processes involved in development and differentiation. Who knows what scientific fortunes could result if these opportunities are taken; or to what intellectual or clinical 'shallows and miseries' we will be bound if we do not.

REFERENCES

Accolla RS, Auffray C, Singer DS & Guardiola J (1991) The molecular biology of MHC genes. *Immunology Today* **12**: 97–99.
Adamson ED (1987) Oncogenes in development. *Development* **99**: 449–471.
Atkinson JP & Farries T (1987) Separation of self from non-self in the complement system. *Immunology Today* **8**: 212–215.

Cohen IR & Young DB (1991) Auto-immunity, microbial immunity and the immunological homunculus. *Immunology Today* **12:** 105–110.

Cunningham BA (1991) Cell adhesion molecules and the regulation of development. *American Journal of Obstetrics and Gynecology* **164:** 939–948.

Eades DK, Cornelius P & Fekala PH (1988) Characterisation of the tumour necrosis factor receptor in human placenta. *Placenta* **9:** 247–251.

Gousti AS, Betsholtz C & Pfeifer-Chisson S (1985) Co-expression of the *sis* and *myc* proto-oncogenes in developing human placenta suggests autocrine control of trophoblast growth. *Cell* **41:** 301–312.

Janeway CA (1988) Frontiers of the immune system. *Nature* **333:** 804–806.

Knapp W, Rieber P, Dorken B et al (1989) Towards a better definition of human leucocyte surface molecules. *Immunology Today* **10:** 253–261.

Mallett S & Barclay AN (1991) A new superfamily of cell-surface proteins related to the nerve growth-factor receptor. *Immunology Today* **12:** 220–223.

Mantovani A & Dijana E (1989) Cytokines as communication signals between leucocytes and endothelial cells. *Immunology Today* **10:** 370–375.

Nossal GJ (1988) Triumphs and trials of immunology in the 1980's. *Immunology Today* **9:** 286–291.

Reinisil CL & Litman GW (1989) Evolutionary immunobiology. *Immunology Today* **10:** 278–281.

Springer TA (1990) Adhesion receptors of the immune system. *Nature* **346:** 425–434.

Tavare JM & Holmes CH (1989) Differential expression of the receptors for epidermal growth factor and insulin in the developing human placenta. *Cell Signalling* **1:** 55–64.

Venter DJ, Tusi NK, Kumar S & Gullick WJ (1987) Over expression of the c-*erb*B-2 onco-protein in human breast carcinomas: immunohistological assessment correlates with gene amplification. *Lancet* **ii:** 69–72.

White JM & Littman DR (1989) Viral receptors of the immunoglobulin superfamily. *Cell* **56:** 725–728.

Williams AF (1984) The immunoglobulin superfamily takes shape. *Nature* **308:** 12–13.

Index

Note: Page numbers of article titles are in **bold** type.

Abortion, 472–473
  antinuclear antibodies and, 494–495
  antipaternal cytotoxic antibodies, 495
  MLC and, 496
  parental HLA and, 495–496
  SLE and, 570–571
  see also under Recurrent pregnancy loss
Accreta, *see* Placenta accreta
Acetylcholine receptors, 581–588
Adaptive immunity, 393–394
AIDS, *see* HIV
Alloimmune thrombocytopenia, 555–557
Alloimmunity, in pregnancy, **541–563**
Amniocentesis, 546
Amniotic fluid bilirubin, 543–544
Antibody deficiency block, 491–492
Anticardiolipin antibodies, *see under* Anti-
  phospholipid antibodies
Anti-D titre, 543
Antifetal antibody, 423–424
Antigen-presenting cells, 393–397
  and MHC, 394–397
Antigen recognition, 400–403
  B-cell activation, 403
  MHC restriction, 400–401
  T-cell activation, 401–402
Antigens, 394–398
  hCG, 636
  MHC deficiency, 491
  oocyte, and, 633–634
  placental, 634–635
  spermatozoal, 631–633
  trophoblast, 421–422
Antigen sensitization, 553–555
  red blood cells and, 541–542
Anti-HLA antibody, 424–426
Anti-Kell antibody, 554–555
Antimalarials, 576
Antinuclear antibodies, 494–495
Antipaternal cytotoxic antibodies, 495
Antiphospholipid antibodies, **507–518**, 571
  diagnostics and, 511–514
  history of, 507–508
  implications of, 509–510

  and pregnancy loss, 510–511, 514
Arterial subinvolution, 478
Aspirin, 571, 577
Autoantibodies, 428–429
  in pre-eclampsia, 609
Autoimmune disease, **565–600**
Autoimmune thrombocytopenia, 577–581
  pregnancy and, 577–581
Autoimmune thyroid disease, *see* Thyroid
  disease
Azathioprine, 576

Bacterial infections, in AIDS, *see* HIV
Bacterial sepsis, 412
B-cell activation, 403
  see also Lymphocytes
BCG, 641–642
β-core fragment, of hCG, 526–528
Bilirubin, 543–544
Blood coagulation, and antiphospholipid
  antibodies, **507–518**
Breast cancer, and TGF-α, 650–651
Breast milk, 583
  and HIV, 622
  IgA antibodies, 431–432

Cancer, **519–539, 641–656**
  active immunotherapy of, 641–643
  cytokines and, 643–651
  and HIV, 625
  trophoblast, 480–482
Candidiasis, 624
C3 convertase, 445–446
CD46, 464
CD59, 448
Cell adhesion molecules, 657–660
Cell–cell signalling, and the immune system,
  661–662
Cell-mediated maternal immunity, in pre-
  eclampsia, 607
Cervical intraepithelial neoplasia, 625, 646
Chemotherapy, in gestational trophoblastic
  tumours, 530–538
  in cancer, 530–538

Chemotherapy, in gestational trophoblastic tumours—(*cont.*)
   side effects of, 535–536
Chlorambucil, 576
Choriocarcinoma, 480, 482, 521–522
Chronic villitis, 475–476
Ciprofloxacin, 626
Complement, and pregnancy, **439–460**, 474, 480
   membrane regulators, 442–448
   overview of, 439–442
   pre-eclampsia and, 609–610
   pregnancy and, 455–456
   trophoblast and, 448–455
Complete hydatiform mole, 521
Computed tomography, 623
Congenital heart block, 573
Congestive heart failure, 585
Contraception, 626
   HIV and, 626
   see also Immunological contraception
Cord blood sampling, 429–430, 544–546
Cordocentesis, 580–581
Corticosteroids, 583
Corynebacterium parvum, 641–642
Cromer antigen genes, 456
Cyclophosphamide, 576, 619
Cyclosporin, 499
Cytokine therapy, in cancer, 643–651
Cytokines, 397–398, 468, 492–494
   and lymphokines, 410
Cytotoxicity, 403–407

Decay accelerating factor (DAF), 446–456
Decidua, 464–465, 474, 490
   stromal cells and, 470
Dehydroepiandrosterone, 408–409
Dexamethasone, 581, 587
Doppler flow-velocity analysis, 547–548

Embryo development, 418–419
Embryonic antigenic contraception, 634–635
Endometrial granulated lymphocytes, *see* Granulated lymphocytes
Endometrial stromal cells, 470
Enzymes, trophoblastic, 462–464
Epidermal growth factor, 659, 665
Escherichia coli, 412
Extravillous trophoblast, 461–464

Fetal anaemia, 542
Fetal growth retardation, 475–476
Fetal immunocompetence, 432–433
Fetomaternal immune relationship, **417–438**, **439–460**
Fetomaternal interface, 419–420
Fragmented hCG, 526–528

Genital ulcers, 626

Gestational trophoblastic tumours, **519–539**
   chemotherapy of, 530–536
   clinical presentation, 528–529
   epidemiology of, 522–524
   follow-up, 529–530, 535–536
   genetics of, 525–527
   prognosis, 530–531
   risk status, 531–535
   staging of, 530–531
   treatment of, 531–535
   see also specific disorders and also Cancer
Glanzmann's thrombasthenia, 581
Glucocorticosteroids, 408–409, 591
Glucose metabolism, 476
GM-CSF, 405
Gold salts, 591
Graft-versus-host disease, 429, 557–559
Granulated lymphocytes, 465–468
Granulated metrial gland cells, 467–468
Graves' disease, *see* Thyroid disease
Growth factors, 403–405, 493–494
Growth retardation, intrauterine, 475–476

Haemolytic anaemia, 456
Hashimoto's thyroiditis, *see* Thyroid disease
Health, and immune system, **393–416**
Heart block, *see* Congenital heart block
High endothelial venules, 398–399
HIV, **617–628**
   immunology, 617–619
   management, 620–621, 625–626
   perinatal infections, 619–620
   pregnancy, treatment in, 622–624
   prevention of, 624–625
HLA, 464
   anti-, antibody, 424–426
   antibodies, and pre-eclampsia, 608
   antigen-deficient trophoblast, 422
   parental profiles, abortion and, 495–496
   and pre-eclampsia, 604–605
Homing, of lymphocytes, 398
Human chorionic gonadotrophin (hCG), 526–528
   as an immunological contraceptive, 635–638
      hCG antigens, 636
      vaccine development, 636–638
Human papillomavirus, 625, 641, 645–646
   see also HIV
Hydatiform mole, 480, 521
   chemotherapy of, 530
   complete, 521
   genetics of, 524–525
   invasive, 521
   partial, 521
Hydrocortisone, 576
Hydrops, 547
Hypertension, in pregnancy, *see* Pre-eclampsia
Hyperthyroidism, *see* Thyroid disease

Hypothyroidism, 586–587
    see also Thyroid disease

IgA, 608
    antibodies, in breast milk, 431–432
IgD, 608
IgE, 608
IgG, 426–428, 608
Immune system—
    origins of, 433–434
    response regulation, 407–411
    see also specific aspects of
Immunity ontogeny, 431–434
    innate vs. adaptive, 393–394
Immunodystrophism, 492–494
Immunoglobulins, 426–428, 608
    and pre-eclampsia, 608
Immunoglobulin superfamilies, 657–660
Immunological contraception, **629–640**
    advantages, 629
    hCG, 635–638
    oocyte antigens, 633–634
    placental antigens, 634–635
    spermatozoal antigens, 631–633
    vaccines, development of, 630–631
Immunotherapy—
    of cancer, 641–643
    spontaneous abortion, 496–499
Implantation, 419
Inab phenotype, 456
Increta, see under Placenta accreta
Infections, 412
    maternal, 478–480
    parasitic, 411–412, 479–480
Infertility, unexplained, 471–477
Innate immunity, 393–394
Insemination, 417–418
Interferons, 644–647
    α, 645–646
    γ, 645–646
Interleukin-2, 647–649
Interleukins, 397–398
Intrauterine growth retardation, 475–476
Intrauterine intraperitoneal transfusion, 549–
    550
    and intravascular, 550–552
Intrauterine intravascular transfusion, 550–
    551
    and intraperitoneal, 555
Invasive hydatiform mole, 521
Isoantibodies, 428

Joints, see Rheumatoid arthritis

Kell antigen, 554–555
Ketoconazole, 624

Laminin, 470
Lectins, 462

Leishmaniasis, 411–412
Leukocytes, 606–607
Leukotrienes, 409–410
Listeria, 478
Lymphocyte-activated killer cells, 647–649
Lymphocyte networks, 662–664
Lymphocyte-related function antigens, 659–
    660
Lymphocytes, 398–399, 465–468, 491–492
    TIL, 648–649
    see also B cells and also T cells
Lymphokines, 403–407
    cytokine regulation, 410
    prostaglandins and, 409–410
    steroid hormones, 408–409

Macrophages, 468–469
Magnesium sulphate, 583
Malaria, 478–480
    antimalarials and, 576
Maternal decidua, 464–465
Maternal infections, 411–412, 478–480
M-CSF, 649–651
Membrane attack complex (MAC), 447–448
Membrane-bound trophoblastic complement
    proteins, 448–455
Membrane co-factor protein, 445–447
Membrane regulators, of complement
    system, 442–448
    DAF and, 446
    MAC, 447–448
    MCP, 446–447
    tissue distribution, 448
Mestinon, 582
MHC, 394–397, 464, 491, 664
    restriction, 400–401
Migration, of lymphocytes, 398–399
Milk, breast, see Breast milk
Milk, IgA antibodies, 431–432
Mixed lymphocyte cultures, 491–492, 496
Molar pregnancy, 480
Myasthenia gravis, 581–588
Mycobacterium tuberculosis, 624

Natural killer cells, 405–407, 422, 467, 607
Neonatal growth, 573
Neonatal lupus, 573–575
Neonatal myasthenia, see Myasthenia gravis
Nicked hCG, 526–528
Nifedipine, 499
Nippostrongylus brasiliensis, 411

Oestrogen, 409
OK-432, 462
Oncogenes, 493–494
Oncolysates, 643
Oocyte antigenic contraception, 633–634
Ovarian cancer, and cytokines, 649–651
Oxpentifylline, 499

Paracetamol, 591
Parasitic infections, 411–412, 478–480
Parental HLA, and spontaneous abortion, 495–496
Paroxysmal nocturnal haemoglobinuria, 455–456
Partial hydatiform mole, 521
Passive immunity, 426–429
  autoantibodies, 428–429
  IgG, 426–428
  isoantibodies, 428
Pelvic inflammatory disease, 626
Pentamidine, 623
Pentoxyfylline, 499
Percreta, *see under* Placenta accreta
Placenta, 420–422
  accreta, 477
  decidua, 464–465
  decidualized endometrial stromal cells, 470
  extravillous trophoblast, 461–464
  granulated lymphocytes, 465–468
  IgG transfer, 426–428
  macrophages, 468–469
  pre-eclampsia and, 605–606
  T cells and, 469–470
  uterine spiral arterials, 470–471
  see also Trophoblast
Placental antigenic contraception, 634–635
Placental site trophoblastic tumour, 482, 522
  genetics, 525–526
Plasmodium, 478–480
Pneumocystis carinii, 622–623
  see also HIV
Polyhydramnios, 547
Polymorphic epithelial mucin, 643
Polymorphonuclear cell function, 607
Prednisone, 571, 576, 581
Pre-eclampsia, 473–475, **601–615**
  complement and, 609–610
  genetic factors, 603–604
  HLA and, 604–605, 608
  immune mechanisms, 601–603, 609
  immunoglobulins, 608
  leukocytes, 606–607
  maternal cell-mediated immunity, 607
  placenta and, 605–606
  PMN function, 607–608
  SLE and, 571–573
Pregnancy—
  and spontaneous abortion, *see* Abortion
  alloimmunity and, **541–563**
  antifetal antibody, 423–424
  anti-HLA antibody, 424–426
  antiphospholipid antibodies, 510–511, 514
  autoimmune thrombocytopenia, 577–581;
    see also Autoimmune disease
  complement, **439–460**
  cord blood sampling, 429–430
  diabetes mellitus, 476

GVHD, 429
  infertility, unexplained, 471–472
  intrauterine growth retardation, 475–476
  loss, recurrent, **489–505**
  myasthenia gravis, 581–588
  placenta accreta, 477
  placental bed pathology, **461–488**
  rheumatoid arthritis, 589–591
  SLE, 476, 567–577
  thyroid disease, 583–589
  trophoblastic tumours, **519–539**
  uteroplacental artery subinvolution, 478
Progesterone, 409, 499
Propranolol, 588
Propylthiouracil, 586–587
Prostacyclin, 410
Prostaglandins, 398–399, 409–410, 468–469
Protein C, 510
Proto-oncogenes, 661–662
Pyridostigmine, 582

RCA cluster, 445–447
Recurrent pregnancy loss, **489–505**
  antiphospholipid antibodies and, 510–511, 514
  blocking antibody deficiency, 491–492
  factor deficiency, 490
  immunodystrophism, 492–494
  immunotherapy, 496–499
  MHC and, 491
  suppressor cells, 490
  see also Abortion
Red blood cell antigen sensitization, 541–542
Rheumatoid arthritis, 589–591
Rh-immunized pregnancy, 542–543
  anti-D titres, 543
  antigen sensitization, 553–555
  bilirubin, 543–544
  cord blood, 544–546
  Doppler flow-velocity analysis, 547–548
  intrauterine transfusions, 549–552
    intraperitoneal, 549–550, 552
    intravascular, 550–552
Rh isoimmunization, 541–542

Sex steroids, 408–409
Sizofuran, 642
SLE, 476
  classification of, 566
  pre-eclampsia, 572
  pregnancy and, 567–577
    loss, 570–571
    management, 575–577
    neonatal, 573–575
    pre-eclampsia, 571–573
    SGA infants, 573
Small for gestational age, 475, 476, 573
Spermatozoa, 417–418

Spermatozoal antigenic contraception, 631–633
Spiral arteries, 470–471
Spontaneous abortion, 472–473
Steroids, and lymphokines, 408–409
Stromal cells, 470
Suppressor cells, 490
Systemic lupus erythematosus, *see* SLE

T cell activation, 401–402
T cells, 405–407, 409–410
    CD4+, 400–408, 410–411
    trophoblastic cancer and, 480–482
    see also Lymphocytes
Th1 CD4+ T cells, 407–408
Th2 CD4+ T cells, 407–408
Thrombocytopenia, 555–557, 577–581
Thymectomy, 583
Thyroid disease, 583–589
Thyrotoxicosis, *see* Thyroid disease
Thyroxine, 586; *see also* Thyroid disease
Toxoplasmosis, 623–624
Transforming growth factors, 650–651
Transfusions, intrauterine, 549–552
Trimethoprim/sulphamethoxazole, 622, 626
Trophoblast, 421–422
    antigenic status, 421–422
    deportation, 430–431
    enzymes, 462–464
    extravillous, 461–464

HLA antigen deficiency, 422
immune attack, 422
membrane-bound complement regulation proteins, 448–455
tumours and, 480–481
Trophoblast-lymphocyte cross-reactivity, 492
Trophoblastic tumours, *see* Gestational trophoblastic tumours
TSH, *see* Thyroid disease
'Tumour infiltrating lymphocytes', 648–649
Tumour markers, 526–528
Tumour necrosis factor, 397–398, 647
Tumours, *see* Cancer

Ultrasound, 547
Umbilical cord blood, 541–546
Unexplained infertility, 471–472
Uterine spiral arteries, 470–471
Uteroplacental artery subinvolution, 478

Vaccines—
    hCG, 636–638
    for immunological contraception, 630–631
Villitis, 475–476
Viral oncolysates, 643
Viruses, *see under* HIV

Zidovudine, 618, 624
Zona pellucida antigens, 633–634
ZP-3 peptide, 634